Best Practices in
Educational Interpreting

Related Titles

Deaf People: Evolving Perspectives from Psychology, Education, and Sociology
Jean F. Andrews, Irene W. Leigh, and Tammy Weiner
ISBN: 0-205-33813-5

Language Learning in Children Who Are Deaf and Hard of Hearing: Multiple Pathways
Susan R. Easterbrooks and Sharon Baker
ISBN: 0-205-33100-9

Counseling Children with Hearing Impairments and Their Families
Kristina M. English
ISBN: 0-205-32144-5

Learning American Sign Language, Second Edition
Tom L. Humphries and Carol A. Padden
ISBN: 0-205-27553-2

Learning American Sign Language Video: Levels I & II—Beginning & Intermediate, Second Edition
Tom L. Humphries and Carol A. Padden
ISBN: 0-205-27554-0

Psychosocial Aspects of Deafness
Nanci A. Scheetz
ISBN: 0-205-34347-3

Language and Literacy Development in Children Who Are Deaf, Second Edition
Barbara R. Schirmer
ISBN: 0-205-31493-7

Psychological, Social, and Educational Dimensions of Deafness
Barbara R. Schirmer
ISBN: 0-205-17513-9

Counseling the Communicatively Disabled and Their Families: A Manual for Clinicians
George H. Shames
ISBN: 0-205-30799-X

Sign Language Interpreting: Its Art and Science
David A. Stewart, Jerome D. Schein, Brenda E. Cartwright
ISBN: 0-205-27540-0

Teaching Deaf and Hard of Hearing Students: Content, Strategies, and Curriculum
David A. Stewart and Thomas N. Kluwin
ISBN: 0-205-30768-X

For further information on these and other related titles, contact:
College Division
ALLYN AND BACON, INC.
75 Arlington Street, Suite 300
Boston, MA 02116
www.ablongman.com

SECOND EDITION

Best Practices in Educational Interpreting

Brenda Chafin Seal

James Madison University

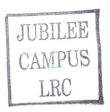

PEARSON

Boston • New York • San Francisco
Mexico City • Montreal • Toronto • London • Madrid • Munich • Paris
Hong Kong • Singapore • Tokyo • Cape Town • Sydney

Executive Editor and Publisher: *Stephen D. Dragin*
Senior Editorial Assistant: *Barbara Strickland*
Manufacturing Buyer: *Andrew Turso*
Marketing Manager: *Tara Whorf*
Cover Designer: *Joel Gendron*
Editorial-production Service: *Stratford Publishing Services*
Electronic Composition: *Stratford Publishing Services*

Library of Congress Cataloging-in-Publication Data

Seal, Brenda Chafin.
    Best practices in educational interpreting / Brenda Chafin Seal.—2nd ed.
      p. cm.
    Includes bibliographical references and index.
    ISBN 0-205-38602-4
    1. Interpreters for the deaf—United States.   2. Deaf—Education—United States.
I. Title.
    HV2402.S42 2003
    419'.071—dc21

1006265751

                                                                    2003045308

Printed in the United States of America

10   9   8   7   6   5   4   3   2   1   05   04   03

To Mom,
your loss was my gain.

CONTENTS

PREFACE

The field of educational interpreting is rapidly growing. Since the first edition of this book, several changes have occurred that suggest continued development and maturation in this new profession. One of these changes involves our student consumers. Never before have our students been so diverse in their hearing loss, their language and cultural backgrounds, their learning abilities and disabilities, and their communication skills and needs. Our current practices in educational interpreting are heavily influenced by the diversity of communication skills found within the population of today's students who use sign language and spoken language. Research in childhood acquisition of languages is also accelerating, particularly at two polar ends—language learning in infants, and language learning in older children and adolescents. Furthermore, our knowledge of American Sign Language continues to proliferate as research in ASL phonology, semantics, syntax, and pragmatics advances beyond the pioneer work of the late William Stokoe. The literature in childhood language acquisition and in ASL are particularly relevant to educational interpreters who use ASL or any of its features in their interpreting and transliterating with students, both young and old.

Another change influencing educational interpreting and its future involves the widespread acknowledgment that continued education and training are critical to effective practices. Web-based offerings of videotapes, computer disks, and distance learning opportunities rival weekly bulk-mail offerings of training workshops, materials, and courses that focus on improving interpreting skills. Nationally, the Registry of Interpreters for the Deaf (RID) has expanded efforts to support and recognize educational interpreters as a critical part of the organization. At its national and regional conferences, RID and its special interest group, the Educational Interpreters and Transliterators of RID (EdITOR), offer an attractive agenda of presentations that are both research- and practice-based. State conferences in deaf education, speech-language-hearing, special education, and interpreting frequently feature speakers who address issues and topics in educational interpreting.

Visibility of educational interpreting as a profession has been achieved nationally with support from the U.S. Department of Education (ED), the Office of Special Education and Rehabilitative Services (OSERS), and the National Association of State Directors of Special Education (NASDSE) (Linehan, 2000). The National Clearinghouse for Professions in Special Education (1997) offers information on educational interpreting at its web site. Both state education agencies (SEAs) (for example, Florida Department of Education, 1998) and local education agencies (LEAs) recognize the importance of educational interpreting in the menu of services that ensure least restrictive environments for students who are deaf and hard-of-hearing. Interpreter training programs continue to flourish, with at least 112 ITPs offered in 41 different states and 14 undergraduate and three graduate degree programs in 13 different states (Linehan, 2000). It was not unusual in the 1990s for a school administrator to use the phrase "educational interpreting" with rising intonation. Today, administrators in rural, suburban, and urban schools, colleges, and universities are more likely to talk about their efforts to recruit and retain educational interpreters who meet licensing and certification regulations.

Another change that impacts our current and future practices is technology, not just cochlear implant technology that affects the services we provide this growing student population, not just web-based technology that affects our access to resources, and not just multimedia technology that affects our classroom experiences, but also communication technology that affects our daily interactions (Hallett, 2002). Pagers, faxes, e-mail, instant messaging, wireless messaging, text messaging, Internet Protocol (IP) relay, voice-activated software, and high-speed video streaming are accelerating changes in our communication patterns in ways unprecedented in the history of the world (Bowe, 2002; Nelson, 2002). We are using briefer utterances, key-word topicalization, acronyms, and turn-taking strategies in our technology-based communication exchanges that will eventually infiltrate our interpreting. Consumer expectations for quick access and reduced ambiguity are sure to raise the expectations for increased efficiency in our educational interpreting.

We are changing because of the influences just mentioned, and also as a result of the natural momentum that empowers us to change. Like a toddler whose biological clock and environmental experiences work in tandem to enable greater strides, more efficient moves, and improved security in going forward, educational interpreting's *biological clock* is set to take greater strides, and to move forward with efficiency and improved security. Embracing these changes is critical in introducing the changes in this book. Clearly, the responsiveness of school systems, training programs, and educational interpreters to the first edition of *Best Practices in Educational Interpreting* has been gratifying and deserves a promise to retain its desirable features in this revision. The call for a second edition occurred rather quickly, and once again, the analogy to a young child's rapid growth seems appropriate in introducing this 2004 publication—where did the time go?

So what will you find in this second edition? The format of the first edition has been preserved. Each chapter follows much like the previous edition's chapters with questions that introduce topics, cases that expose real-world issues surrounding the profession and those who practice it. The new information is largely directed to the opening topics mentioned here: changing consumers, changing knowledge of language acquisition, changing technology, and changing visibility of the profession. Research and scholarship that has both influenced and resulted from these changes is infused within the respective chapters and in the final chapter on research. New cases are offered to reflect the dynamics of our encounters and interpretation of ethical codes. The Appendix has been revised to include RID's Standard Practice Paper on Interpreting in Educational Settings (K–12) (2000). Hopefully, these changes improve the timeliness of the book and encourage positive direction for future growth and development. To the end that *Best Practices in Educational Interpreting, Second Edition* encourages any of you as readers to contemplate new or replicated research, new or revised resources, and new or reconsidered practices, then this book is a success.

With best wishes,

Brenda Chafin Seal, Ph.D., CSC

REFERENCES

Bowe, F. G. (2002). Relay Online. *NADmag, 2,* 19.

Florida Department of Education. (1998). *Competencies of educational interpreters.* [Online]. Available: *http://www.fsdb.k12.fl.us/eit/98competencies.html*

Hallett, T. L. (2002). The impact of technology on teaching, clinical practice, and research. *The ASHA Leader, 7,* 4–7, 13.

Linehan, P. (2000). Educational interpreters for students who are deaf and hard of hearing. *Project Forum at NASDSE.* U.S. Office of Special Education Programs.

National Clearinghouse for Professions in Special Education (1997). Careers in special education and related services: Interpreter for students who are deaf or hard of hearing. Reston, VA: Council for Exceptional Children.

Nelson, J. (2002). The state of the wireless industry. *NADmag, 2,* 20–21.

Professional Standards Committee. (2000). Interpreting in Educational Settings (K–12). RID Standard Practice Paper. Alexandria, VA: RID Publications.

ACKNOWLEDGMENTS

My sincerest appreciation is extended to all those, both named and unnamed in the following pages, who molded my opinions and challenged my thoughts to the end that a book was written.

Appreciation goes to the following reviewers for their comments on the manuscript: Brenda Cartwright, Lansing Community College, Lansing, Michigan; Brian Edward Cerney, Community College of Allegheny, Pittsburgh; and Peter V. Paul, Ohio State University, Columbus; Nanci A. Scheetz, Valdosta State University; and Jean S. Moeller, Georgia Perimeter College.

CHAPTER 1

Educational Interpreting:

An Introduction

Interpreting and Inclusion

Educational interpreting is the most rapidly growing deafness-related profession in our American schools, colleges, and universities. Even though Thomas Hopkins Gallaudet served as an educational interpreter for Laurent Clerc in the early 1800s (Frishberg, 1990; Lane, 1984) and interpreters have been common in schools for the deaf for decades, today's widespread use of educational interpreters is unprecedented. This growth is largely a product of social and legislative acts of the 1970s, 1980s, and 1990s that enabled deaf and hard-of-hearing students to move from residential programs, day schools, and college programs for the deaf to their local schools and college programs (e.g., Dahl & Wilcox, 1990; Gustason, 1985; Zawolkow & DeFiore, 1986). Today, the trend toward integrating students with hearing loss into classrooms with hearing students is referred to as *inclusion*. Philosophically, inclusion implies more than mainstreaming. Inclusion refers to full membership in a regular classroom, full ownership of the student's education by both special and general educators, and collaborative efforts among teachers and special service providers to make curricular content accessible (Brinton, Fujiki, Montague, & Hanton, 2000; Sailor, Gee, & Karasoff, 1993).

The inclusion philosophy has been controversial among educators, parents, and those who have a vested interest in deaf and hard-of-hearing students (Johnson & Cohen, 1994). Some advocate a philosophy that supports different types of instruction for different student needs, such that *all* instructional programs, including schools for the deaf, are *included* in the options made available to parents and students (Seal, 1997). These advocates contend that different students have different learning, social, and communication needs, and that no one program or type of class, nor any one learning environment, can satisfy the multitude of different needs that students who are deaf and hard-of-hearing bring to their educational years. Those who oppose inclusion often voice concerns about the elimination of special schools that serve students who are deaf and hard-of-hearing. They are likely to resent the reduced enrollments observed in schools for the deaf as a cultural threat. Opponents of inclusion may also advocate specially trained teachers who provide special instruction in special environments where deaf students are the social majority (Lane, 1995). They may warn against programs that lack deaf adult role models and deaf peers, whose communication enhances social and academic learning. Opponents of inclusion are likely to recommend an educational placement that emphasizes inclusion in, not exclusion from, the Deaf[1] culture (Lane, Hoffmeister, & Bahan, 1996). Most professionals involved in deaf education, even those who support inclusion, are similarly opposed to inclusion when it satisfies an educational trend without full commitment to the academic, social, and communication needs of the students (Ramsey, 1997; Winston, 2001).

Recent demographics indicate about 83% of students with hearing loss are taught in mainstreamed, integrated, and/or inclusive settings. The U.S. Department of Education's Twenty-third Annual Report to Congress on the Implementation of the Individuals with Disabilities Education Act (2001) listed close to 72,000 students from ages 6 through 21 who have hearing impairments. This number represents more than a 21% increase from the previous decade. The large increase is due to both legislative and technological changes that occurred during the 1990s. The Individuals with Disabilities Education Act (IDEA) (1997) requires states to identify preschoolers with disabilities. Earlier identification in the preschool years leads to more accurate identification of students once they enter first grade. At the same time, technological advances in testing hearing has made a tremendous difference in identifying infants with hearing loss. Universal Newborn Hearing Screenings now permit diagnoses as early as the first few months of life. Infants who are identified early are more likely to receive early intervention, and early intervention is more likely to transfer to improved census and educational intervention during the formal school years (Yoshinago-Itano, 2000). The National Association of State Directors of Special Education (NASDSE) reported in 2000 that about 8,000 school-aged students were receiving educational interpreting services in the 17 states that had census data (Linehan, 2000). Applying this figure to all 50 states would indicate that as many as 24,000, or approximately one-third of all deaf and hard-of-hearing students in our kindergarten through 12th grades (K–12), are consumers of educational interpreting services. That number is considerably larger when we include deaf students from residential programs and those in higher education programs where educational interpreting services are also provided. Gary Sanderson, Linda Siple, and Bea Lyons (1999) reported that another 10,000, or about half of the more than 20,000 deaf and

[1]Many terms are used to refer to individuals who are deaf and hard-of-hearing. Terms such as "Deaf," "hearing impaired," "hard of hearing," and "individuals with hearing loss" are common to the books and articles used as references for this book. When a particular author or resource used a particular term (as in "hearing impaired"), that term is also used in this book. Where the language is my own, however, the terms "deaf" and "hard-of-hearing" are used to refer to persons who are distinguished by their hearing loss.

hard-of-hearing students attending post-secondary programs in the United States use an interpreter. These data point to two fundamental facts that are critical to the contents of this book: Thousands of students who are deaf and hard-of-hearing are being educated in their local school systems, and the primary tool for educating many of these students in inclusion programs is to provide them with an interpreter.

Because educational interpreting represents one of the most dramatic changes in educating deaf and hard-of-hearing students since the 1970s, a brief look at the events that led to its rise is appropriate. Several laws have led to the increasing use of interpreters in schools: (1) Section 504 of the Rehabilitation Act of 1973 and its 1998 Amendments; (2) Public Law 94-142, the Education of All Handicapped Children Act of 1975; (3) the 1997 reauthorization of the 1990 amendment, the Individuals with Disabilities Education Act (IDEA); (4) the Education of the Deaf Act of 1986; and (5) the Americans with Disabilities Act of 1990 (ADA). Another law, the Federal Bilingual Education Act, 1968–2002, has probably also influenced the widespread acceptance of interpreters, although its influence has been indirect, not direct.

Passage of the 1973 Rehabilitation Act had its most immediate impact on adult students, both those who were entering college programs as first-year students and those who were returning to the college scene to continue their education. Many of these students who were deaf and hard-of-hearing preferred to take courses that met their educational goals in their local colleges and universities. Their enrollment in these local programs was formally sanctioned by the Rehabilitation Act and resulted in the hiring of educational interpreters (usually part-time) by colleges and universities (Paul & Quigley, 1990). Originally, the educational interpreters in these higher-education settings took their knowledge of and skills in interpreting from other settings (medical, religious, and/or legal) into the college classroom. Some of these interpreters were successful in generalizing their knowledge and skills to the higher-education setting, but some were failures. Those who succeeded recognized that the educational setting is a unique setting. They honed their skills and expanded their knowledge to meet the needs of the setting and of the adult deaf and hearing consumers for whom they interpreted.

At the other end of the student continuum, in the mid-1970s and early 1980s, were deaf and hard-of-hearing students whose parents opted to enroll them in local elementary and secondary schools. Although Public Law 94-142 is most often discussed relevant to its impact on the enrollments of residential schools for the deaf, its impact on local school systems likewise has been dramatic. For the first time ever, many school administrators found themselves in the position of being unable to refer a child to a school for the deaf. These administrators could no longer deny a student enrollment because of a lack of services or unqualified teachers. Parents exercised their legal rights to demand of these local schools a free and appropriate education. Many parents assumed that their local schools represented the least restrictive environment for their deaf or hard-of-hearing children. Local school administrators, especially those faced with the enrollment of just one or two deaf or hard-of-hearing students, scrambled to meet the standards of the law. They hired teachers of the deaf and set up self-contained classrooms, resource classrooms, and mainstream opportunities for deaf and hard-of-hearing students.

In the early years of mainstreaming, and for those students who used sign language,[2] it was not uncommon for teachers of the deaf to arrange their schedules to go into mainstream classes with their students. There the teachers would interpret, facilitate, and monitor as the students' needs in these classes dictated. In recent years, however, the trend toward hiring professional interpreters has replaced the trend toward using (and maybe abusing) teachers of the deaf as interpreters. We recognize today that professional interpreters for deaf students have unique roles and responsibilities that stand apart from the roles and responsibilites of teachers, both teachers in regular education and teachers of the deaf.

The Individuals with Disabilities Education Act further supported the regulations set forth by Public Law 94-142 and extended a free and appropriate education in the least restrictive environment to children from birth to 36 months of age. The 1997 reauthorization of IDEA further amended the statute to require that individual states establish entry-level standards for all personnel providing special education or related services, including sign language interpreters. Congress has appropriated millions of dollars in recent years for interpreter training. A growing number of SEAs are using these training dollars to improve the knowledge and skills of educational interpreters who have not met their newly developed regulations.

The Education of the Deaf Act of 1986 is most often recognized for renaming Gallaudet College as Gallaudet University and its establishment of the Commission on Education of the Deaf. The Commission's findings that "the present status of education for persons who are deaf in the United States, is unsatisfactory. Unacceptably so . . . " (Commission on Education of the Deaf, 1988, p. viii) led to 52 recommendations for improving the quality of education for students with hearing loss. Among the recommendations is one devoted to educational interpreters, Recommendation 36:

> The Department of Education, in consultation with consumers, professionals, and organizations, should provide guidelines for states to include in their state plans such policies and procedures for the establishment and maintenance of standards

[2]Many terms are used to refer to sign language. Terms, such as "sign language," "Sign Language," "signed languages," "Pidgin Sign English," "Pidgin Sign Language," "Manually Coded English sign systems," "English-based sign systems," "Contact Signing," and "Signed English" are common to the books and articles used as references for this book. When a particular author or resource used a particular term (as in "Pidgin Sign English"), that term is also used in this book. Where the language is my own, however, the term "sign language" is used to refer to any language or system that uses signs and fingerspelling to communicate. (*See also* D. Moores's discussion of ASL as an "inclusive" term, 1996.)

to ensure that interpreters in educational settings are adequately prepared, trained, and evaluated (p. xxi).

The Americans with Disabilities Act of 1990 further upheld standards established by the Rehabilitation Act of 1973. ADA prohibits discrimination for individuals who have disabilities and extends their rights to include "access" to institutions of higher education. ADA further defined a "qualified interpreter as one who is able to interpret effectively, accurately and impartially, both receptively and expressively, using any necessary specialized vocabulary" (Kincaid, 1995, p. 1). The Association on Higher Education and Disability (AHEAD) and the American Council on Education (ACE) have joined together to assist colleges and universities in interpreting the law and its regulations. Members of AHEAD may also join a special-interest group that focuses on issues, including educational interpreting, in the education of deaf and hard-of-hearing students in higher-education settings. Numerous agencies within deafness professions (like the Post-secondary Education Programs Network or PEPNet) and outside deafness professions (like the American Chemical Society) also promote educational interpreting in their workshops and publications.

Finally, the Bilingual Education Act, 1968–2002 (see Grosjean, 1982, for a more thorough discussion), provided that children of "limited English proficiency" (LEP) be taught in their native language by teachers who are sensitive to their cultural heritage. The direct impact of this law on public schools has been the development of classes and programs for hearing students who must learn English as a second language (or ESL). The impact of this law on the education of deaf and hard-of-hearing students, however, also has been substantial. The Commission on Education of the Deaf, for example, recommended that the Department of Education extend "practices under the Bilingual Education Act that seek to enhance the quality of education received by limited English-proficiency children whose native (primary) language is American Sign Language" (p. xvii). Bob Johnson, Scott Liddell, and Carol Erting (1989), in their paper *Unlocking the Curriculum*, further recommended that deaf children be provided American Sign Language (ASL) as their first or native language and that ASL be the formal language for teaching ESL. School administrators who have attempted to honor parents' request for this sequence have opened their school doors to increasing numbers of educational interpreters.

The Rehabilitation Act, IDEA, the Education of the Deaf Act, and ADA have been important catalysts, but these laws did not contribute solely to the current movement that has created the educational interpreting boom. Educational reform is widely supported today by politicians, parents, educators, and consumers alike. Political movements that call for excellence in education promise to raise literacy levels, improve graduation rates, and make higher education more affordable and available in the twenty-first century. More and more parents are demanding excellence in the educational programs we offer their deaf and hard-of-hearing children. More and more deaf and hard-of-hearing adults are demanding excellence in what was previously known as a demand for equal access. The President's Commission on Excellence in Special Education (2002) called for excellence in all special education programs for students with disabilities. Standards for excellence in educational interpreting have never been higher, nor will they likely ever return to previously accepted levels.

The Scope of Practice for Educational Interpreters

The scope of practice for educational interpreting is both broad and deep. Any teaching-learning situation can be an educational interpreting situation. Consider a 40-year-old taking scuba diving lessons, a 25-year-old in a Lamaze class, a 62-year-old taking "Alternatives to Smoking" classes, or an 8-year-old in a summer soccer camp. Educational interpreting can and does occur in each of these settings; but only one setting, the school setting, provides a scope of practice that can include units on scuba diving, natural childbirth, the dangers of smoking, and the basics of soccer in the same 6-hour day that also includes units in mathematics, reading, writing, and on and on. Educational interpreting itself is *all-inclusive*.

Educational interpreters are those individuals who provide interpreting services in an educational setting. Although they may carry a generic title and perform conventional interpreting tasks, educational interpreters also must demonstrate special skills necessary for the demands of the educational setting (Stuckless, Avery, & Hurwitz, 1989). Educational interpreters most often provide sign language interpreting and transliterating; some provide cued speech transliterating; and a few provide oral interpreting or transliterating services within the educational environment. As Cokely (1992) explained, educational interpreters, like all language interpreters, serve to equalize the target language (tL) and the source language (sL). In most classrooms around the country today, the sL is a spoken language, usually English. For most students whose hearing loss is severe or profound, the tL is a sign language or sign system. Pidgin Sign English or an English-like signing system is most common to the educational setting (Paul & Quigley, 1990; Woodward & Allen, 1988), although ASL, the language that is indigenous to the Deaf culture of the United States, is being increasingly prescribed in Individualized Education Programs (IEPs), and Individual Family Service Plans (IFSPs).

In equalizing the tL and sL, the educational interpreter may need to demonstrate proficiency in multiple languages (e.g., ASL, English) and multiple modes (e.g., manual, oral, written) of communication. The educational interpreter may need to be versed in multiple topics and subject areas. The educational interpreter may need to work with students of different age ranges, different hearing levels, different cognitive levels, different cultural levels, and varying levels of language competency. The educational interpreter may need to work with teachers of multiple disciplines whose previous experiences with students who have a hearing loss may prove to be a bonus or a hindrance, or may be altogether nonexistent.

The educational interpreter may play various roles in various settings for various individuals. The educational interpreter's work, like the breadth and depth of the scope of his or her practice, can be *all-inclusive*.

Current Practices

Current educational reform movements and consumer demands combine with the all-inclusive scope-of-practice demands for educational interpreters to surface issues that never before have surfaced. At the same time, deaf and hard-of-hearing students have never been so diverse (Schildroth & Hotto, 1995). The growing number of infants identified through newborn hearing screenings, the growing number of cochlear implant students, of students from homes where English is not the native language, of students who use American Sign Language and other sign systems, and the growing number of students with multiple disabilities characterize the most heterogenous population of "hearing-impaired" students ever in the history of our country (see Easterbrooks & Baker, 2002, for a detailed discussion of the "Heterogeneity of the Population"). Colleges and universities offer rigorous curriculums that include courses for educational interpreters in their interpreter training programs (Shroyer & Compton, 1994). Parents of deaf students expect school systems to provide qualified and competent educational interpreters for their children. School systems expect college programs to train qualified and competent educational interpreters. SEAs expect LEAs to hire and retain educational interpreters who meet the regulations and guidelines provided by their departments and boards of education.

All this has happened quickly (Frishberg, 1990; Gustason, 1985) and without precedence. Consequently, many "seat-of-the-pants" decisions have been made. Some of these decisions reflect positively on the collective efforts of those whose responsibility it is to systematize the interpreting curriculum and standards for advancing within that curriculum. Some decisions reflect positively on the educational interpreter who takes his or her general training and customizes it to the educational setting with a high standard of performance. In time, some practices will be reexamined and abandoned for better practices. At the moment, however, it is important to document those practices that are judged to be *best practices* in educational interpreting. Documentation is critical in assessing where the profession is today so that both those involved in and those impacted by the profession can make changes for a better future.

The term *best practices* implies tried practices that have brought success, not necessarily success for all deaf and hard-of-hearing students, or success for all interpreters, or in all educational settings, but practices that are considered successful enough to warrant sharing. That is what this book is about, documenting—in order to share and examine—practices that occur in educational interpreting settings today and are being promoted as *best practices in educational interpreting*. Many of the practices discussed in this book have been field-tested (i.e., many of the procedures and cases used to illustrate the variety of issues that surface in educational interpreting have been presented to audiences of educational interpreters and to student consumers for their feedback and recommendations). Other practices and cases are presented merely in the name of good common sense; often these *common sense* practices are common to all interpreting settings, not just educational settings. Those practices supported by professional literature are discussed with appropriate citations and references. Those practices for which no previous research has been established are discussed from my personal perspective, a perspective heavily influenced by personal experiences and experiences shared by colleagues and consumers.

The Audience and Contents of This Book

This book is written for several audiences. Primarily, it is directed to the 8,000 educational interpreters who are currently serving the 24,000 or more deaf and hard-of-hearing students in primary and secondary schools, and the thousands more who are providing services to students in post-secondary educational programs. It is for and about these interpreters that this book was conceived. This book is also intended for students in the 120-plus interpreter training programs (ITPs) across the United States (Linehan, 2000), especially to those who take an educational interpreting position. Faculty in ITPs are encouraged to guide these students in their readings and discussion of these chapters, to provide them with a supportive environment where reactions that trigger meaningful dialogue and debate are nurtured. This book is also written for educators, both special educators and their administrators, who hold expert knowledge in the fields of deafness, and for regular educators and their administrators who have limited knowledge of and limited experiences with students who are deaf and hard-of-hearing. The joint responsibilities that teachers and administrators share in their work with and support of students who have interpreters can be overwhelming. Finally, this book is written for deaf and hard-of-hearing students, across all ages, whose access to their education is partially or totally through interpreters. Student reactions to the practices presented here, especially reactions that are grounded in firsthand experiences, should serve to validate or to challenge current practices in the name of an improved future for educational interpreting.

A brief look at what each of these different audiences will encounter is appropriate. This first chapter, of course, is intended as an overview, to offer introductory information on the historical background and current trends in education. This information should assist readers in developing a point of reference for the future chapters.

Chapter 2, "Best Practices in the Administration of Educational Interpreting Services," deals with the role and characteristics of the administrator, with the educational interpreter position description, contract, the policy procedures manual, and procedures for evaluating the interpreter and interpreter mentor program. Cases[3]

---

[3]Many individual names are used in the cases presented in Chapters 2 through 6; all are fictional. The situations that depict the individual cases, however, are based on true stories—often embellished, with details changed to protect the confidentiality of the persons involved.

representing difficult situations and suggested best practices for handling them are presented at the end of the chapter.

Chapter 3, "Best Practices in Educational Interpreting in the Primary Grades Setting," deals with the cognitive, linguistic, and social needs of students in preschool and primary settings, and the different roles the interpreter must assume to meet diverse student needs. In this chapter language learning is discussed with emphasis on the role of the interpreter as a language facilitator, language teacher, and as a language reporter. Issues surrounding interpreting for young children with cochlear implants and children with multiple disabilities are discussed in this chapter. Practices that involve fingerspelling, spatial propositions and perspective, and inventing signs are discussed, as well as the challenges of interpreting booksharing. In conclusion, and common to each chapter, difficult situations and suggested practices for handling them are offered.

Chapter 4, "Best Practices in Interpreting in the Elementary- and Middle-School Setting," deals with social and curriculum issues that impact on educational interpreting for students in this changing developmental period. Unique to this chapter are concerns about interpreting textbook material, interpreting curriculum that is not text dependent, and curriculum that is technology-dependent. Issues surrounding interpreting tests and interpreting for students who have a "mixed" communication profile, including students with cochlear implants and the diversity of their interpreting needs, are included. Difficult situations and recommended best practices also are presented in this chapter.

Chapter 5, "Best Practices in Interpreting in High School and Vocational Settings," focuses primarily on the process of interpreting, particularly from a metacognitive perspective. The concept of tracking, common to the secondary curriculum, is discussed with a focus on the general curriculum, the college-preparatory curriculum, and the vocational-preparatory curriculum, and the impact that the different curricula have on the interpreter. Issues of teacher pace, compatibility and incompatibility of delivery style and simultaneous and consecutive interpreting, and issues of scheduling are discussed for their importance to optimum interpreter services. Issues surrounding interpreting multimedia presentations, technology classes, and interpreting with supportive technology are raised. Consumerism is discussed with emphasis on the interpreter's role in nurturing consumerism. Then, in keeping with the previous chapters, difficult situations are presented as cases with suggestions for best practices.

Chapter 6, "Best Practices in Interpreting in Higher Education Settings," focuses on college settings. The themes of this chapter, diversity and individuality, are represented in issues involving curriculum and instruction. Communication breakdowns and repairs—or the process of miscue analysis—are discussed with guidelines for reducing and correcting interpreter errors. Unique to this chapter, yet in keeping with its themes, are portions of three interviews: (1) an interview with Steve Nover, who used sign language interpreters in his doctoral coursework at the University of Arizona; (2) an interview with Bonnie Poitras Tucker, a professor at Arizona State University, who used oral interpreters in her teaching; and (3) an interview with Donna Panko, a sign language interpreter who interpreted in a doctoral program at the University of Virginia. Discussion of *educated* educational interpreters focuses on the need for continuing education, lifelong learning, and mentoring relationships. Finally, difficult situations and suggested best practices conclude the chapter.

Chapter 7, "Educational Interpreting Research," begins with a brief explanation as to the need for research in educational interpreting and concerns about the difficulties involved in conducting research in this behavioral and social science. A literature review that spans the years from 1986 to 2002 organizes the existing research into four areas. An annotated bibliography of this research is provided in table form. Concerns raised from the literature review over the lack of attention to the consumer or the student who is expected to learn through an interpreter are met with suggestions about how to approach data collection that focuses on the student. Recent research on the psychological profiles of educational interpreters is added. Chapter 7 concludes with a list of questions that are offered for practicing interpreters, interpreter trainers, school administrators, and students (both consumers and those in training programs) to pursue research in this newly developing discipline.

Finally, the Appendix provides resources that should be helpful to any of the intended readers. These include RID's Standard Practice Paper on Educational Interpreting, Code of Ethics, and Certification Maintenance Program. Information from the Training, Evaluation, & Certification Unit (the TECUnit) on the Cued Speech Transliterator Levels of Certification and Credentials are provided as supplementary readings.

Time for a Change

Chapters 3, 4, 5, and 6 are presented with a chronology that moves our focus from the young child as a student to the adult student. Table 1.1 provides a look at this sequence. This developmental approach is used for several reasons.

One important reason takes us back to the history of professional interpreting and the earlier discussion of the impact of the Rehabilitation Act on higher education. The first efforts at promoting professional interpreting came about in 1964 at Ball State Teacher's College in Indiana where a group of interpreters established themselves as an official organization—the National Registry of Professional Interpreters and Translators for the Deaf (Frishberg, 1990; Witter-Merithew & Dirst, 1982). Financial support for this organization was soon to follow when the Rehabilitation Services Administration (RSA) officially recognized and sanctioned the group (in 1965, its name was changed to the Registry of Interpreters for the Deaf) and promoted testing and certification for its members. This support soon interfaced with Section 504 of the Rehabilitation Act, and by the mid-1970s, colleges and universities were hiring interpreters for their adult deaf students. We owe much to those early interpreters who met in Indiana and to the RSA that fostered the development of interpreting as a profession, but we need to recognize that their pioneer work focused on interpreting for adults.

TABLE 1.1   Developmental Stages and the Educational Years

School Classification	Chronological Age	Corresponding Grades
Early Childhood	3–5 years old	Preschool
Primary	5–8 years old	Kindergarten, 1st, 2nd, and 3rd
Elementary: Middle- to Upper-Middle School	8–11 years old 11–14 years old	3rd, 4th, 5th, 6th 6th, 7th, and 8th
Secondary: Junior High and High School	14–21 years old	8th and 9th 10th, 11th, and 12th
Higher Education (College)	18–22 years old and beyond	Freshman, sophomore, junior, senior, graduate student
Continuing Education	Adult years	Graduate school, workshops, conferences, special classes, conventions, etc.

The knowledge and skills that have been gained from interpreters and consumers in higher education and in other noneducational settings, unfortunately, have served as the foundation for the knowledge and skills applied to interpreting for children (see Figure 1.1). We have assumed a "top-down" model; that is, we have proliferated downward what is known about interpreting for adults to apply to what we do when we interpret for children. As logical as it may seem for interpreters in elementary and secondary settings to borrow knowledge from interpreters and consumers at higher levels, reliance on the "top-down" model has probably been detrimental to our practices.

The current shift in our thinking about educational interpreting takes a "bottom-up" approach. We need to establish a foundation of practices that work for primary students because primary students are different from adult students. In addition, we need to change our practices as young students mature, as their cognitive, communication, and social needs change. I am not suggesting that we abandon all we have learned about interpreting for adults; rather, I support a developmental approach to practices of educational interpreting that values all interpreters at all levels. This approach does not place interpreters with better skills in higher grades where the curriculum is assumed to be more demanding and put interpreters who have underdeveloped skills at lower grades because the demands are assumed to be less. A developmental approach recognizes that the demands at each chronological and cognitive stage, and at each academic level, warrant the *best* interpreter who provides the *best* possible practices. Those early

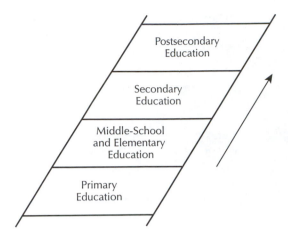

**FIGURE 1.1   A Developmental (Bottom-Up) Approach to
Educational Interpreting**

pioneers who paved our way 40 years ago would surely agree that anything less
than this today is wrong for our children.

The need for a change in our attention to educational interpreting is also
supported by the changing demographics that are found in today's schools. During the early days of mainstreaming, students who were deaf (or Deaf) were more
likely to be referred to schools for the deaf, while students who were hard-of-
hearing (or more hearing-like) in their communication, social, and learning profiles were more likely to be mainstreamed. Educational interpreters who worked
in these earlier mainstream settings were more likely to prescribe to a Manually
Coded English system and rely on the student's hearing and speechreading to pick
up the "incidentals." Today's student profiles are mixed or heterogenous. Any
local school system may have enrolled any one or any combination of these students, such that a variety of communication skills, communication modes, and
communication needs becomes the rule, not the exception to the rule. As a consequence of this heterogeneity, the notion of being or having a "total communication" program, or an "auditory–oral" program, or a "bilingual–bicultural" program
is not as common in local schools as is the notion of having a variety of multiple
program options—three students could have ASL interpreters, two students could
have cued speech transliterators, and seven students could have Signed English
transliterators, with one student scheduled in five classes without an interpreter
and in one class with an oral interpreter. This diversity is also common to postsecondary settings where an interpreter might provide ASL interpretation for a deaf
undergrad in her five weekly classes. The same interpreter might work with a
recorder who provides real-time captioning in one of these classes, a team interpreter in another, and notetakers in all five classes.

This heterogeneity of communication needs is similarly met with a heterogeneity of cultural needs. The changing cultural demographics of American school children in general is represented in the changing cultural demographics of deaf and hard-of-hearing children. The U.S. Census Bureau identified 8.8 million children who speak a language other than English (Spanish, Vietnamese, Hmong, Cantonese, Russian, French, Korean, Cambodian, Arabic, and Tagalog) in their homes (cited by the American Speech-Language-Hearing Association, 2002). The 200 different languages spoken in a city the size of Chicago (Langdon, 2002) are similarly represented in smaller towns like Harrisonburg, Virginia where 24 different languages are used by its 40,000 residents (Mellott, 2002). The U.S. Department of Education (2001) reported that 41% of the students ages 6 through 21 who have hearing loss represent minority and ethnic distributions. Educational interpreters who ascribe to a bilingual-bicultural model for their interpreting are now expected to expand their cultural learning and sensitivity. This expansion goes beyond learning whether a deaf or hard-of-hearing student is from a Deaf home where ASL is the first language, or a hearing home where spoken English is the first language, to learning whether the hearing parents speak Spanish or the deaf parents use Chinese Sign Language. Students with multiple language and cultural backgrounds bring challenges to all educators, but especially to educational interpreters who work to make the language of the classroom accessible for their learning. Multilingual–multicultural environments are fast becoming the rule, not the exception, in educational settings.

A final area of change in the student profile that requires a change in our attention to educational interpreting involves the heterogenous learning needs of deaf and hard-of-hearing students. At least one-third of all students diagnosed with hearing loss present with disabling conditions or special learning needs (Karchmer, 1985; Paul & Quigley, 1990). Students with cerebral palsy, mental retardation, learning disabilities, autistic disorder, attention deficits, and special medical needs have the same broad range of communication and cultural differences that students who are "just deaf" have. Interpreters who expect all deaf and hard-of-hearing students to learn equally well or to attend to them with the same level of maturity are prone to be disillusioned. Interpreters who approach each student with the attitude that "I will work to provide my *best* interpreting skills to match this student's learning needs" become integral members of each child's educational team and make a positive difference in the student's learning.

How to Read the Chapters for Maximum Learning

Because the material each chapter presents builds on material presented in previous chapters, readers who select a chapter according to their area of practice or interest may find the isolated chapter to be more meaningful if they read the previous chapter(s) first. Likewise, I encourage readers who start at this beginning chapter to complete the later chapters. Some of the practices and cases presented in later chapters have applications in earlier chapters; these practices were placed in later chapters because of their apparent relevance to the general age group, grade levels, or topics of interest. The topic of cochlear implants is discussed in Chapter 3, the chapter on interpreting in primary grades, and in Chapter 4, interpreting in elementary- and middle-school grades. Cochlear implants are also mentioned in Chapter 2, the administration chapter, Chapter 5, the secondary school chapter, and in Chapter 6, the postsecondary chapter. The topic of continuing education is also mentioned in Chapter 2, but discussed at length in Chapter 6. This discussion could easily have been placed in this first chapter or mentioned in some detail in each chapter. Indeed, interpreters who are considering continuing education units (CEUs) for their work with this book might begin by formulating their goals for independent study according to the questions listed in this book's Contents (*see also* the Certification Maintenance Program [CMP] in the Appendix). A review of the questions in the Contents, in light of the CMP procedures found in the Appendix, and reading from the beginning to the end of this book should provide a holistic view of the material. A holistic view of the material should lead to improved comprehension of particular topics when particular chapters or sections are revisited to determine if independent study goals were met.

Each of the topics found in the chapters is introduced with a question. The question–answer format seems appropriate to a book on educational interpreting for at least two reasons: (1) The question–answer style of discourse is more commonly found in the classroom than in any other communication setting; and (2) we have an abundance of questions about this phenomenon called educational interpreting. The questions posed in this book and their attempted answers are relevant for today's interpreting practices; but over time, they should lead to more questions that will lead to improved practices. In each chapter that concludes with difficult cases, for example, I have added "departure" questions which are intended to generate additional thinking and problem solving. In fact, when I teach educational interpreting at workshops and in courses, I try to encourage participants and students to ask questions about the material presented. I strongly believe that the standards set for our interpreting practices are improved when we become active learners, and I believe that active learners are those who think and question.

Finally, may I offer a bit of personal introduction and humility. No single individual has all the answers or even all the questions where human communication is concerned. My questions and answers are merely the product of my experiences, my work, my life—as the daughter of a hard-of-hearing parent (my mother has a severe conductive loss as a result of scarlet fever when she was a little girl); as a former speech-language pathologist and teacher of deaf children in a residential school for the deaf; as a university professor of students who aspire to work with and interpret for deaf and hard-of-hearing children and adults; as a supervisor in a university clinic that serves deaf and hard-of-hearing clients; as a freelance interpreter; as a part-time educational interpreter; as a researcher who studies educational interpreting; as a consultant to school systems that employ educational interpreters; as a friend and colleague of other interpreters and other consumers of interpreting; and, finally, as a lifelong learner. My experiences and thoughts are likely to resemble those of others who wear any of these hats; they are also likely to differ. In either regard, I offer them with best wishes for challenging and enjoyable reading.

REFERENCES

Brinton, B., Fujiki, M., Montague, E. C., & Hanton, J. C. (2000). Children with language impairment in cooperative work groups: A pilot study. *Language, Speech, and Hearing Services in Schools, 31,* 252–264.

Cokely, D. C. (1992). *Interpretation: A sociolinguistic model.* Silver Spring, MD: Linstok Press.

Commission on Education of the Deaf. (1988). *Toward equality: Education of the deaf—A report to the President and the Congress of the United States, February.* Washington, DC: U.S. Government Printing Office.

Dahl, C., & Wilcox, S. (1990). Preparing the educational interpreter: A survey of sign language interpreter training programs. *American Annals of the Deaf, 135,* 275–279.

Easterbrooks, S. R., & Baker, S. (2002). *Language learning in children who are deaf and hard of hearing: Multiple pathways.* Boston: Allyn & Bacon.

Frishberg, N. (1990). *Interpreting: An introduction.* Silver Spring, MD: RID Publications.

Grosjean, F. (1982). *Life with two languages: An introduction to bilingualism.* Boston: Harvard University Press.

Gustason, G. (1985). Interpreters entering public school employment. *American Annals of the Deaf, 130,* 265–266.

Johnson, R. C., & Cohen, O. P. (Eds.) (1994). *Implications and complications for deaf students of the full inclusion movement.* Gallaudet Research Institute Occasional Paper 94-2. Washington, DC: Gallaudet University.

Johnson, R. C., Liddell, S. K., & Erting, C. J. (1989). *Unlocking the curriculum: Principles for achieving access in deaf education.* Gallaudet Research Institute Working Paper 89-3. Washington, DC: Gallaudet University.

Karchmer, M. A. (1985). A demographic perspective. In E. Cherow, N. D. Matkin & R. J. Trybus (Eds.), *Hearing-impaired children and youth with developmental disabilities: An interdisciplinary foundation for service* (pp. 36–56). Washington, DC: Gallaudet College Press.

Kincaid, J. M. (1995). *Legal issues specific to serving students who are deaf or hard of hearing in institutions of higher education.* Columbus, OH: AHEAD Publications.

Lane, H. (1984). *When the mind hears: A history of the deaf.* New York: Random House.

———. (1995). The education of deaf children: Drowning in the mainstream and the sidestream. In D. P. Hallahan & J. M. Kauffman (Eds.), *The illusion of full inclusion* (pp. 275–287). Austin, TX: Pro-Ed.

Lane, H., Hoffmeister, R., & Bahan, B. (1996). *A Journey into the Deaf-World.* San Diego, CA: Dawn Sign Press.

Langdon, H. W. (2002). Language interpreters and translators: Bridging communication with clients and families. *The ASHA Leader, 7,* 14–15.

Linehan, P. (2000). Educational interpreters for students who are deaf and hard of hearing. *Project Forum at NASDSE.* U.S. Office of Special Education Programs.

Mellott, J. (2002, July 18). Retreat touches on ESL: School board setting up panel to research options. *Daily News Record,* p. 9.

Moores, D. F. (1996). *Education the deaf: Psychology, principles and practices* (4th ed.). Boston: Houghton Mifflin.

Paul, P. V., & Quigley, S. P. (1990). *Education and deafness.* White Plains, NY: Longman.

President's Commission on Excellence in Special Education (2002) *A new era: Revitalizing special education for children and their families.* [online]. Available: http://www.ed.gov/inits/commissionsboards/whspecialeducation/index.html.

Ramsey, C. (1997). *Deaf children in public schools: Placement, context, and consequences.* Washington, DC: Gallaudet University Press.

Sailor, W., Gee, K., & Karasoff, P. (1993). Full inclusion and school restructuring. In M. Snell (Ed.), *Instruction of students with severe disabilities* (4th ed.) (pp. 1–30). New York: Merrill.

Salend, S. J., & Longo, M. (1994). The roles of the educational interpreter in mainstreaming. *Teaching Exceptional Children, 26,* 22–28.

Sanderson, G., Siple, L., & Lyons, B. (1999). *Interpreting for postsecondary deaf students.* A report of the national task force on quality of services in the postsecondary education of deaf and hard of hearing students. Rochester, NY: Northeast Technical Assistance Center, Rochester Institute of Technology.

Schildroth, A. N., & Hotto, S. A. (1995). Changes in student and program characteristics, 1984–1985 and 1994–1995. *American Annals of the Deaf, 141,* 68–71.

Seal, B. C. (1997). Educating students who are deaf and hard-of-hearing. In L. Power-deFur & F. Orelove (Eds.), *Inclusive education for students with disabilities: A practical guide to meeting the least restrictive environment requirements* (pp. 259–272). Gaithersburg, MD: Aspen Publishers.

Shroyer, E. H., & Compton, M. V. (1994). Educational interpreting and teacher preparation: An interdisciplinary model. *American Annals of the Deaf, 139,* 472–479.

Stuckless, E. R., Avery, J. C., & Hurwitz, T. A. (Eds.) (1989). *Educational interpreting for deaf students: A report on the national task force on educational interpreting.* Rochester, NY: NTID/RIT.

U.S. Congress (1973). The Rehabilitation Act. [online]. Available: www.ed.gov/offices/OSERS/RSA/Policy/Legislation/rehabact.doc.

U.S. Congress (1986). Education of the Deaf Act of 1986. [online]. Available: http://www4.law.cornell.edu/uscode/20/index.html.

U.S. Congress (1990). The Americans with Disabilities Act. [online]. Available: http://nationalrehab.org/website/history/ada.html.

U.S. Congress (1997). Individuals with Disabilities Education Act, Amendments of 1997 Regulations, Number 48, Volume 64. *Federal Register,* § 300.23, 300.135, 300.136.

U.S. Congress (1998). Rehabilitation Act Amendments. [online]. Available: www.ed.gov/offices/OSERS/RSA/Policy/Legislation/rehabact.doc.

U.S. Department of Education (2001). Twenty-third annual report to Congress on the implementation of the Individuals with Disabilities Education Act. Washington, DC: Author.

What languages do we speak? (2002, April 2). *The ASHA Leader, 7,* 10.

Winston, E. (1994). An interpreted education: Inclusion or exclusion? In R. C. Johnson & O. P. Cohen (Eds.), *Implications and complications for deaf students of the full inclusion movement.* Gallaudet Research Institute Occasional Paper 94-2. Washington, DC: Gallaudet University.

Winston, E. (2001, Winter/Spring). Visual inaccessibility: The elephant (blocking the view) in interpreted education. *Odyssey, 2,* 5–7.

Witter-Merithew, A., & Dirst, R. (1982). Preparation and use of educational interpreters. In D. G. Sims, G. G. Walter, & R. L. Whitehead (Eds.), *Deafness and communication: Assessment and training* (pp. 395–406). Baltimore: Williams & Wilkins.

Woodward, J., & Allen, T. (1988). Classroom use of artificial sign systems by teachers. *Sign Language Studies, 61,* 405–418.

Yoshinago-Itano, C. (2000). Successful outcomes for deaf and hard-of-hearing. *Seminars in Hearing, 21,* 309–326.

Zawolkow, E., & DeFiore, S. (1986). Educational interpreting for elementary- and secondary-level hearing-impaired students. *American Annals of the Deaf, 131,* 26–28.

2 Best Practices in the Administration of Educational Interpreting Services

Much of our knowledge on the administration of educational interpreting services comes from the comprehensive work of members of a National Task Force on Educational Interpreting. In 1985, Ross Stuckless, Joseph Avery, and Alan Hurwitz (from the National Technical Institute of the Deaf) convened a group of leaders from the American Society for Deaf Children, the Alexander Graham Bell Association of the Deaf, the Convention of American Instructors of the Deaf, the Conference of Interpreter Trainers, the National Association of the Deaf, and the Registry of Interpreters for the Deaf (RID) to embark on a longitudinal study of educational interpreting services for deaf students. In the four years that followed, and with financial support from the U.S. Department of Education, the Task Force collected hundreds of documents from hundreds of school systems across the United States and Canada. The Task Force's 1989 report, *Educational Interpreting for Deaf Students: Report of the National Task Force on Educational Interpreting*, provided the first comprehensive body of information on issues related to the administration and provision of educational interpreting services for students in kindergarten through twelfth grades (K-12).

The National Technical Institute for the Deaf (NTID) also stepped forth as a leader in educational interpreting services in higher education in the 1970s and early 1980s. The Educational Support Service Program (ESSP) at NTID served as a model to many college programs in its provision of interpreting, tutoring, notetaking, counseling services, and technological instructional aids to deaf students (Hurwitz & Witter, 1979; Hurwitz, 1980). One of the critical outcomes of this pioneer program involved its internal evaluation of services and the questions it generated for other programs to ask when designing their own support services program for deaf students.

The questions raised and guidelines provided during these early years were fundamental to today's educational interpreting programs. Many state education agencies (SEAs), local education agencies (LEAs), and higher education programs have established their own interpreter guidelines and disability service protocols that reflect these previous efforts, and, at the same time, reflect current trends and responses to legislation. Information provided by several SEAs (Ohio, as an example), LEAs (San Diego City Schools, as an example), the Association on Higher Education and Disability (AHEAD), the Gallaudet University Regional Centers (GURC), and the Postsecondary Education Consortium and its network of programs (PEPNet) served as resources for much of the information provided in this chapter.

Question 1: Who is responsible for administering educational interpreting services?

The administration of educational interpreting services is likely to be the responsibility of a central administrator, usually a special education director or disability services coordinator. This person may work with a building principal, director of personnel or human resources, dean of student affairs, or other administrators to set up a position description for educational interpreters; draw up contracts or agreement documents; write policy statements; and hire, supervise, and evaluate interpreters. This person may also work with a representative from the SEA in implementing statewide guidelines for educational interpreting or a representative from the Department of Rehabilitation Services in implementing federal guidelines for transitioning students to postsecondary programs.

In school systems where the incidence of hearing loss is relatively high, the administrator of educational interpreting services is likely to be a person whose knowledge of deafness and support services is already established. In smaller school systems or schools where the incidence of deaf and hard-of-hearing students is low, the administration for educational interpreting services is frequently an add-on responsibility of someone who may already wear a number of hats. Adding the hiring, programming, and supervising of educational interpreters to the job of a person who works to establish eligibility criteria for students with special needs, satisfy placement issues, determine and manage special education funding, supervise the special education personnel, and serve as the school's representative to parents, students, faculty, other administrators, and other agencies must be done carefully, so that existing programs do not suffer.

Regardless of the size of the school program, these characteristics are expected in the administrator of an educational interpreting services program:

- The administrator is knowledgeable about hearing loss and deafness, the impact of hearing loss on learning, and issues surrounding the communication needs of deaf and hard-of-hearing students. The administrator prioritizes the student's learning needs in all decisions that involve interpreting.
- The administrator is knowledgeable about the legal basis for the provision of educational interpreting services, particularly Section 504 of the Rehabilita-

tion Act of 1973, the Individuals with Disabilities Education Act (IDEA), and the Americans with Disabilities Act (ADA). The administrator values the legal rights of students who are deaf or hard-of-hearing.

- The administrator recognizes the need for assistance and is able to tap the knowledge of other individuals and other resources when issues surrounding the provision and administration of educational interpreting services require such. The administrator values a network of supportive colleagues, including members of the deaf community (Seal, 1997).

- The administrator is able to administer the educational interpreting services program efficiently and successfully, documenting policies, issues, and program data that support the successful and efficient administration of the program to higher-level administrators, school boards, or personnel committees. The administrator values meaningful documentation.

- The administrator is able to evaluate the effectiveness of the program and adjust it to meet changing needs as they occur. The administrator values ongoing evaluation.

- The administrator provides support to the educational interpreters and to the educator and student consumers of interpreting services with orientations, inservices, workshops, conferences, and other opportunities for professional development.

Question 2: What is involved in the position description for an educational interpreter?

Position descriptions for educational interpreters are most likely to be found in progressive school systems in which the administration meets the profile just specified. The importance of a position or job description is clear to these administrators in that it not only benefits the educational interpreter and the administration, but also benefits parents, teachers, and student consumers. The position description specifies job title, job responsibilities relevant to the title, and conditions under which the job is to be performed. Salary information may not be appropriate to the position description, although salary conditions (full-time, part-time, hourly wage, annual contract, and so on) may be mentioned in the position description. Similarly, interpreter credentials may not be specified in the position description but may be alluded to in the qualifications for the position.

The educational interpreter position description is sometimes part of a larger document, such as a handbook or manual on the educational interpreting services program. When this occurs, the position description is generally referenced as a sample job description for educational interpreters. In some school systems, this sample position description is replaced with several job descriptions, sometimes differentiated by name; "Interpreter I," "Interpreter II," and "Lead Interpreter," as examples, may indicate a hierarchy of skill level, experiences, credentials, or qualifications. They may also indicate a hierarchy of placement through the school system from the primary setting to the middle-school setting to the secondary setting. Various names or titles may also be used to refer to different types of interpreters (Stuckless, Avery, & Hurwitz, 1989). "Cued Speech Transliterator," "ASL Interpreter," "Signed English Transliterator," "Interpreter Aide," again as examples, may indicate a division of responsibility that is not found in the generic title of "Educational Interpreter." The importance of the position description to the administrator, then, is to clarify the position to the greatest extent possible for hiring and evaluating purposes. The importance of the position description for the interpreter and the student and teacher consumer is to clarify the responsibilities of the position.

Sample job descriptions can be obtained from various resources. SEAs, personnel departments, interpreter training programs, and advocacy agencies representing interpreters, deaf, and hard-of-hearing people frequently have sample position descriptions. The sample job description offered in Table 2.1 has been adapted from the National Task Force on Educational Interpreting (Stuckless, Avery & Hurwitz, 1989). It can be further tailored to fit a particular program's needs.

Question 3: What is involved in the contract for an educational interpreter?

Programs that have sufficient numbers of deaf and hard-of-hearing students at various grades, levels, and/or ages are likely to hire several interpreters on a contractual basis. A staff of interpreters is a desirable feature of educational interpreting programs in larger schools and is often used in promotions to attract additional staff. School systems that have only one or two deaf or hard-of-hearing students and at disparate grades or levels may have difficulty in justifying a staff of interpreters. These smaller school systems are more likely to contract with individual interpreters on an hourly or part-time basis.

Procedures for determining the size of the interpreting staff and for determining the nature of the individual contract should always be driven or dictated by the needs of the student(s). In higher education programs, student needs are generally determined by student requests or written work plans (IPEs). In schools serving students in K–12, student needs are determined by an educational team that is likely to designate whether the interpreting services should be provided during parts or all of the student's day. The IEP may indicate interpreting as an accommodation or related service, and a student's successful use of interpreting services may be written as an annual goal. Although an interpreter may not be part of the first IEP, subsequent reviews, particularly annual reviews of the IEP, should involve the interpreter's participation. Interpreters who are participating in the IEP conference cannot interpret the proceedings for other participants whose full access and full participation in the meeting requires an interpreter. In some cases, the participation of the interpreter in an annual review of the IEP may indicate an automatic renewal of the interpreter's contract. A continuation of the

TABLE 2.1   Educational Interpreter Position Description

Overview of Position

The Educational Interpreter is an integral member of the educational team serving students who are deaf or hard-of-hearing. The educational interpreter provides interpreting and/or transliterating skills in the educational environment. This environment includes classroom, laboratory, field trip, assembly, and other educational sites that are deemed appropriate for student learning. The educational interpreter works to equalize the target language with the source language in maximizing the learning situation for all involved.

Qualifications

A qualified interpreter is defined in the Americans with Disabilities Act as one who can interpret effectively, accurately and impartially, both receptively and expressively, using any necessary specialized vocabulary. In addition, the educational interpreter must show evidence of at least two of the following:

a. Certificate of Interpretation (CI), Certificate of Transliteration (CT), Comprehensive Skills Certificate (CSC), Oral Transliteration Certificate (OTC), or Certified Deaf Interpreter (CDI) from the Registry of Interpreters for the Deaf (RID); Level 4 (Advanced) and Level 5 (Master) certification from the National Association of the Deaf[1]; and/or Cued Speech Transliteration Certifications, TSC:3 (Competent) or TSC: 4 (Expert), through the TECUnit;

b. Certificate or documentation of state-level screening from the appropriate state agency;

c. Transcript or documentation of completion of an interpreter training program from an appropriate college or university;

d. Transcript or documentation of enrollment in an interpreter training program from an appropriate college or university;

e. Documentation of successful experience as an educational interpreter (e.g., letters of recommendation from school personnel, parents, and/or hearing-impaired students);

f. Successful interviewing with the search committee.

Responsibilities

The Educational Interpreter is responsible for each of the following:

a. to interpret and/or transliterate according to the specifications of the student's Individual Educational Program (IEP), Individual Plan for Employment (IPE), or request for such accommodations to meet access needs;

b. to utilize planning time to meet with teachers and staff as deemed appropriate by the educational team and/or supervisor;

c. to prepare for demanding course material (teacher lectures, videotapes, tests) as necessary for successful interpreting and/or transliterating;

---

[1]The National Association of the Deaf (NAD) and the Registry of Interpreters for the Deaf, Inc. (RID) have joined forces to develop a new joint certification test for interpreters. The joint task force is referred to as the National Council on Interpreting. The new certification test and levels of certification are forthcoming (Bublitz, 2002).

(continued)

TABLE 2.1   continued

Responsibilities
  d. to demonstrate professionalism in all interactions with administrators, teachers, and staff, with parents and students, and with visitors or individuals unfamiliar with the educational setting;
  e. to demonstrate professionalism in all ethical areas, especially in applying the Code of Ethics to the educational setting;
  f. to participate in educational team meetings, particularly those that address communication issues;
  g. to participate in self-evaluations as determined appropriate by the supervisor.

same interpreter for the same student may be desirable. Likewise, in school systems where interpreters are assigned to particular grades or subject areas, the interpreter's continued contract may be contingent on having sufficient numbers of younger deaf students matriculating from lower to higher grades. It is certainly not unusual for school systems to vary in their contract procedures from year to year and from interpreter to interpreter. Whenever variation becomes the norm, procedures for securing and maintaining qualified interpreters probably begin with an attractive contract package.

Contracts that provide competitive salaries, secure benefits, and promise of continued and progressive employment are far more likely to attract successful interpreters than contracts that are vaguely written with only immediate needs acknowledged. Determining competitive salaries is frequently a matter of comparing market value with agencies that provide or contract freelance interpreters. State registers of interpreters, state departments of education, and other agencies that provide interpreter registers are most likely to have information about current market value in specific localities. Logically, interpreters in metropolitan areas are accustomed to salaries that are higher than those in rural areas. Matching or even raising salaries of educational interpreters to those of freelance interpreters, however, may place unreasonable demands on the school. Failing to meet the salary needs of an interpreter who can secure a better hourly wage as a community interpreter could also diminish the value placed on providing a successful interpreter in the school setting.

Many school systems are forced to seek out compromise, frequently a compromise that a part-time contractual interpreter can provide. The part-time interpreter may be willing to work for a higher hourly salary and at fewer hours per week than the full-time interpreter who is offered a lower hourly wage. At the same time, some interpreters enjoy the hours and security of the teaching day and perfer to work on a full-time contractual basis where the demands are known and the salary is constant, rather than interpreting in freelance situations where the demands change and the assignments and salaries are more sporadic. One of the common guidelines school programs use in moving from hourly contracts to salaried contracts is that when the dollar amount for vendor services approaches or surpasses the salary of a full-time staff person, a staff position for educational interpreting services is easy to justify.

Negotiating different types of contracts with different interpreters is more likely to occur when the interpreting pool is sufficiently large. When the interpreting pool is limited, the school system becomes more limited in its ability to negotiate. Unfortunately, many rural school administrators find themselves faced with a single deaf student whose IEP calls for an interpreter in mathematics, science, and social studies. Even creative scheduling may not attract a qualified interpreter for what appears to some to be a competitive salary. (See Chapter 5 for more on scheduling.) In these cases, when an interpreter is simply not available, school administrators are wise to work with neighboring school systems, pooling resources to provide more attractive contract packages. Nurturing a team of interpreters across school systems may prove to be a proactive approach for short-term needs. Working with interpreter training programs to set up practicum sites may also provide the necessary catalyst for building a successful interpreting staff with commensurately attractive contracts.

Having a staff of interpreters is also beneficial when team interpreting is needed. Team interpreting involves the simultaneous use of two or more interpreters working supportively with each other to ensure the highest level of accuracy and the lowest risk of repetitive motion injury. Team interpreting is recommended in several situations: in classes in which the lecture or discussion is fast-paced; in classes that extend beyond the usual 50 or 60 minutes; in classes in which the content is particularly complicated or cognitively demanding; in classes where different deaf consumers have different language levels (e.g., students with minimal language skills educated alongside students with age-expected communication skills); and in classes where dialects require intense discrimination skills. Determining the pace of a lecture or the challenge of a dialect is not as easy as determining the length of a class. We generally expect spoken language to be about 120 words per minute. Reading rates and emotionally charged language are both faster, so a class that lasts only 50 minutes might be too difficult for one interpreter if the teacher uses lots of read-alongs or engages in volatile discussion. Nonmainstream dialects are also difficult to interpret, particularly until the interpreter acclimates to the dialect. Team interpreters work together intellectually as well as physically, correcting errors, confirming sign and word choices, and generally supporting each other with turn-taking (Stewart, Schein, & Cartwright, 1998). Teams may include hearing interpreters paired with Deaf interpreters, newly hired interpreters paired with seasoned mentors, and male interpreters paired with female interpreters. Teaming is a growing practice in educational interpreting, quite possibly because the stakes for excellence and the ramifications of liability are higher than ever.

Finally, hiring educational interpreters who themselves are educated generally makes good sense to knowledgeable administrators. Educated interpreters, those with at least an associate's degree, but preferably those with bachelor's degrees or higher, present a profile that may not be observed in interpreters without postsecondary degrees. This profile includes evidence of sufficient intelligence to

have met competitive entrance requirements and evidence of sufficient commitment to have met competitive graduation requirements. Educated interpreters are
also more likely to be viewed by other members of the educational staff as colleagues, rather than as assistants.

Question 4: What is involved in the policy manual or guidelines for educational interpreting services?

All school systems have policy manuals, handbooks, or guidelines that serve to set
the pace of the working day. These manuals are generally reviewed annually and
changes are made to accommodate the changing needs of the school system.
Although the educational interpreter should be given the general policy manual
for the school program in which he or she is employed, this manual is probably
insufficient in detailing procedures that are specifically relevant to educational
interpreting services. As such, an additional manual or policy statement that
details guidelines is appropriate.

The contents of the policy manual vary from general dos-and-don'ts to
detailed case scenarios. Although the responsibilities of the educational interpreter typically are itemized in the position description, the details of those
responsibilities and further role delineations are likely to be itemized in the policy
manual. Policy manuals that are written in a proactive style, rather than in a
punitive or negative style, set a more positive and professional tone and are likely
to be better received by the reader.

The policy manual, like the position description, may have an introductory
philosophy page or statement. This statement may reflect the philosophy of the
entire school system or it may be particular to the educational interpreting services
or disability services program. Philosophy statements generally underscore the
importance of educational interpreting services and the role of interpreting services
in the overall program for students who are deaf and hard-of-hearing. The policy
manual also may include any number of responsibilities delegated to the interpreter.
Table 2.2 lists sample responsibilities that are commonly found in a policy manual.

Policy manuals frequently match the interpreter responsibilities with a delin-
eation of teacher and student responsibilities. A critical need for clear policies and
procedures exists, particularly in light of the reported conflicts in perception of the
interpreter's role (Antia & Kreimeyer, 2001; Ramsey, 1997; Turner, 2001; Warren-
Norman, 2002). Shared knowledge of these procedures is just as critical for the
teacher and student consumers as it is for interpreters (refer to the RID Standard
Practice Paper on Interpreting in Educational Settings in the Appendix). Teachers
who have participated in orientation or inservice meetings on the responsibilities of
and how to work with educational interpreters have reported them to be beneficial
in increasing their understanding and expectations (Beaver, Hayes, & Luetke-
Stahlman, 1995). Even then, conflicts in role perceptions (Ramsey, 1997) can occur

TABLE 2.2   Responsibilities of the Educational Interpreter

- To facilitate communication within the educational setting (e.g., interpreting student dialogues not intended for the entire classroom to hear; interpreting procedures during tests, field trips, assemblies)
- To set up the physical setting for the most successful interpretation (e.g., determining the best physical arrangement for the interpreter in relation to the teacher's presentation style and movement within the classroom; working with the teacher to accommodate lighting needs during movies, filmstrips, use of overhead projector)
- To follow extracurricular policies when extracurricular activities occur (e.g., procedures for interpreting or not interpreting PTA meetings, school club, sorority, fraternity, advising, and other organizational meetings)
- To follow absentee policies when student is absent (e.g., procedures for notifying interpreter; adjusting interpreter schedule for teaming or observing)
- To prepare for the interpreting assignment (e.g., determining availability of resources during planning period, scheduling teacher and team meetings)
- To follow disciplinary policies when disciplinary matters occur (e.g., procedures for reporting or not reporting the student who does not attend to the interpreter, incidences of cheating, offensive or vulgar language, missed information)
- To follow policies for interpreting in difficult situations (e.g., procedures for reporting concerns about the student's role in using the interpreter, interpreting behind-the-wheel instruction in driver education class, interpreting for teachers who read lecture notes at a rapid rate, interpreting in foreign language classes)
- To work with other faculty, staff, and students as expected (e.g., procedures for conducting orientation sessions at the onset of the school year, working with other support personnel such as occupational therapists, speech-language pathologists)
- To comply with responsibilities in hyphenated roles—interpreter–notetaker, interpreter–aide, interpreter–tutor, interpreter–teacher (e.g., procedures for moving from one role to another within the hyphenated position)
- To comply with noninterpreting assignments (e.g., procedures for bus duty, bulletin-board duty, lunchroom duty, teaching sign language classes)
- To pursue professional growth and development (e.g., expectations for continuing education activities, attending conferences, teacher workdays, workshops, procedures for self-evaluation)
- To educate consumers as needed (e.g., training students to use interpreters, mentoring new interpreters, inservicing teachers)
- To follow absentee policies when unable to interpret (e.g., procedures for securing substitute interpreters, for reporting or taking sick-leave, emergency leave)

in the most enlightened. Imagine, for example, a teacher's anticipation of the interpreter's help when individual seatwork occurs. The interpreter who approaches the deaf student's desk as the teacher starts to roam around the desks of hearing students may give the impression that she is responsible for helping the deaf student with his seatwork when, more appropriately, the interpreter is merely positioning herself to interpret when the teacher approaches the deaf student's desk. This subtle yet critical error in perceptions can create ethical issues for the interpreter, the teacher, and the student. The administrator may also find it uncomfortable explaining to disgruntled parents why an otherwise qualified teacher is deferring instruction to an interpreter who, although qualified to interpret, is probably not qualified to teach.

Orientations, or inservice training, was identified as the number-one technical assistance need by SEAs responding to a U.S. Department of Education survey on educational interpreting services (Linehan, 2000). Guidelines on providing supportive inservices for teachers who work with interpreters can be found in *RID's Educational interpreting: A collection of articles from Views: 1996–2000.* "A well-planned, conscientiously conducted inservice can set the stage for meaningful partnerships that mature over the months of the school year" (Seal, 2000, p. 15). Follow-up meetings or focus group discussions are also valuable throughout the semester or year, especially when they address provocative questions such as these: What should the interpreter do when the teacher is talking to an individual student at his or her desk? What should the teacher do if the interpreter appears to be chatting with the deaf student? What should the teacher do when the deaf student doesn't pay attention? (Seal, 2000, p. 14) What should the interpreter do when a deaf student has to go to the emergency room? What should the interpreter do if a deaf student verbally assaults a teacher? What should the interpreter do if a student cheats during a test? (Warren-Norman, 2002). Answers to these questions are likely to vary, depending on the parties involved. Discussions that air different perspectives without imposing absolute rights and wrongs are more desirable than discussions in which the "musts" are dictated.

Question 5: How should the interpreter be evaluated?

The process of evaluating an educational interpreter raises questions and concerns for both the interpreters and those responsible for evaluating the interpreters. *Evaluation*[2] is an integral part of all that we *value*. All teaching–learning experiences and all teaching–learning relationships involve some kind of evaluation. Evaluation may be ongoing, incidental, or scheduled at predetermined dates. Evaluation may involve formal observation or casual observation. Evaluation may be extrinsic, involving feedback provided by others, or intrinsic, involving feedback to self. There is no single evaluation method that works for all teaching–learning experiences or relationships.

The evaluation of educational interpreters can be viewed from several perspectives. An interpreter who holds a certificate of performance from RID or a

---

[2]Material in this section was originally printed in Seal, B. C. (1995). Evaluating the educational interpreter. *RID Views, 12,* 17, 38. Reprinted with permission from The Registry of Interpreters for the Deaf, Inc., Silver Spring, MD.

comparable state agency may be seen as having already been evaluated by authorities who are more capable of conducting an evaluation that those in the typical school system. Schick and Williams (1994) suggested that traditional evaluation methods, which rated an interpreter's use of one sign language system or another, are *not* appropriate for evaluating the educational interpreter. They recommended an alternative process for appraising the educational interpreter. Their Educational Interpreter Performance Assessment (EIPA) is described as an approach that utilizes a team of evaluators (including deaf individuals) and videotaped samples from the interpreter's actual day, to provide feedback to the interpreter and to the school program in improving the skill and placement of interpreters. The EIPA has gained widespread use by many administrators across different states. Positive features include the use of evaluators from outside the school, authenticity of a system that evaluates interpreters in their actual work, and the usefulness of the diagnostic feedback that is returned to interpreters with their videotape (Budding, 2001). Negative features of the EIPA include the potential for administrators to remove themselves or to feel dismissed from the evaluation process once they contract with the EIPA developers. (See the Appendix for the EIPA in its entirety.)

Under no circumstances should a single appraisal instrument serve as the *only* assessment instrument for the educational interpreter. A multiple-person, multiple-instrument assessment process is recommended for a comprehensive and valid evaluation. This multiple-instrument process, which is described here as a formal approach, also has merit for informal and ongoing evaluation.

The building administrator's assessment instrument

The evaluation instrument used by the building administrator typically focuses on issues that are within his or her purview. These issues include observations or assessments of the interpreter's promptness, ability to get along with others, acceptance of responsibility, and so on. The instrument used to assist evaluation in these areas may be the same one that is used with other school personnel. The procedures for its use may differ, however, especially if the interpreter is itinerant and moves from one building to another. The National Task Force on Educational Interpreting (Stuckless, Avery, & Hurwitz, 1989) proposed certain "overall job performance" tasks that are appropriate for the administrator's assessment instrument. According to these tasks, the educational interpreter should:

1. demonstrate the ability to understand and follow instructions;
2. be reliable in meeting responsibilites;
3. be supportive toward the program in which he or she is employed;
4. be constructive in his or her advocacy for quality;
5. have good interpersonal relationships with staff, particularly with the teachers and others providing services to the deaf students;
6. be effective with the deaf students and their hearing peers;
7. be flexible in adapting to change;

8. observe school policies and procedures;
9. use good judgment and decision making in work-related situations;
10. have an acceptable personal appearance for the work setting.

The supervisor's assessment instrument

The evaluation process for the educational interpreter should include an assessment by the immediate supervisor or, if the supervisor is not knowledgeable in the communication modes used in interpreting, the supervisor's appointed designee(s). This particular assessment should focus on the educational interpreter's actual interpreting skills. An instrument that can be used during "directed observation in selected aspects of the interpreting service provision process" (Conference of Interpreter Trainers, 1994, p. 13) is recommended. This instrument should focus on competencies demonstrated by the educational interpreter. These competencies, as detailed by the CED/RID Ad Hoc Educational Interpreter Committee (1993) include: (1) the ability to provide interpreting services in a wide variety of content areas within the school's overall curriculum, (2) the ability to work with a variety of deaf and hard-of-hearing students of different ages and grade levels, (3) basic knowledge of the process of interpreting, and (4) the ability to work cooperatively with numerous other persons and to contribute specialized knowledge.

Detailed "Competencies of Educational Interpreters" are also available from the Florida Department of Education (1998). A statewide task force developed a comprehensive list of more than 150 competencies across eight areas for the Florida Department of Education. These competencies are behaviorally written and have transfer value to evaluation instruments. The sample evaluation instrument in Figure 2.1 includes ten of these competencies.

FIGURE 2.1 Assessing the Educational Interpreter

Name of Interpreter: _____

Interpreting Situation/Class: _____

Time of Observation: _____

Rating Scale: 1–2 Unsatisfactory 3–4 Needs Work 5–6 Average 7–8 Good
9–10 Very Good

1. Produces clear and readable signs: _____
2. Uses appropriate nonmanual markers to convey moods: _____
3. Produces accurate, readable fingerspelling at an
   appropriate rate: _____
4. Uses specific technical sign vocabulary appropriate to the
   subject area and the grade level of the student: _____
5. Selects conceptually accurate sign vocabulary: _____
6. Uses facial expressions appropriate to the mood, spirit,
   and intent of the speaker: _____

FIGURE 2.1   (continued)

7. Utilizes signing space appropriately: _____
8. Provides a smooth flow while signing: _____
9. Interprets idioms with conceptual accuracy: _____
10. Formulates grammatically correct sentences: _____

Comments: _____

_____

_____

_____
Observer's Signature

_____
Date

The teacher's assessment instrument

Although the teacher's assessment may be part of the supervisor's evaluation process, it is probably more appropriate for the teacher to participate in the evaluation procedures with an instrument that focuses exclusively on the instructional situation. This instrument could be viewed as a questionnaire that is used as a portion of the total evaluation process. Sample items for this questionnaire-type instrument could include:

1. When I give directions to the class and the deaf student appears not to understand, I:
   a. ask the interpreter if everything's all right;
   b. approach the student and repeat the directions for the interpreter to repeat;
   c. assume that the interpreter will take care of it;
   d. depend on the interpreter to let me know if indeed the student is not understanding;
   e. other _____.
2. When I call on the deaf student to answer a question and the answer is only partially intelligibile, I:
   a. ask the interpreter to ask the student to repeat her or his answer to the interpreter, so that the interpreter might answer for all to understand;
   b. thank the student for answering but indicate that we had trouble understanding the answer and ask him or her to repeat the answer, leaving the sign-to-voice interpreting decision up to the student and the interpreter;

   c. thank the student for answering but indicate that we had trouble understanding the answer and prefer the interpreter to voice the answer;

   d. provide the class with what I think is the answer given;

   e. other _____ .

Customizing this type of questionnaire should be relatively easy, given that the teacher and interpreter can specify the details that should be included. Examples of customized items include these: performance during oral reading time for a third-grade reading class, performance during small-group problem-solving time for a ninth-grade civics class, performance during lecture-with-Power Point for a twelfth-grade English literature class, performance during lecture-with-map for a fifth-grade geography class, and so on. With these individual situations in mind, then, the questionnaire becomes directly applicable to the evaluation process.

More general evaluations are also available that encourage teacher input on interpreter evaluations. Figure 2.2 provides an example of a general assessment instrument used at New River Community College and at James Madison University, both in Virginia.

FIGURE 2.2   Faculty Evaluation of Interpreter

Directions

Please rate this interpreter on the characteristics below. Place the appropriate number of your rating on the line preceding the characteristics.

Feel free to add any comments that you desire to each characteristic in the appropriate space provided.

Note that the *evaluation is for the interpreter* and not the office that he or she may represent. The following rating scale is to be used for all items. Use **only whole numbers** in your rating.

Rating Scale:	1 = Needs Improvement (Requires Note of Explanation)
	2 = Fair
	3 = Average
	4 = Good
	5 = Excellent (Requires Note of Explanation)

INTERPRETER'S NAME: _____

_____ Meets classes/appointments promptly

_____ Demonstrates concern for the student as a person

_____ Sensitive to the needs of the class as a whole

_____ Effectively facilitates communication during classroom lectures, classroom
discussions, and meetings

_____ Creates a comfortable setting for faculty, student, and interpreter

FIGURE 2.2 (continued)

_____ Enthusiastic team member

_____ Exhibits a positive attitude

_____ Flexible and willing to work as a team member

_____ Shares knowledge and skills in the areas of deafness and interpreting

_____ Exhibits professional integrity

Comments:

Signature:_____

The student's evaluation instrument

The older deaf or hard-of-hearing student should participate in the evaluation process in much the same way that the teacher is expected to participate. That is, the evaluation format should focus explicitly on communication in specific situations. The following are examples of questions that belong in a student questionnaire:

1. When I don't understand my interpreter, I:
    a. let her know at the end of class what I didn't understand;
    b. raise my hand and ask the teacher to explain again;
    c. pretend I do understand;
    d. become frustrated and/or angry;
    e. other _____.
2. When my teacher calls on me to answer, I:
    a. respond with spoken English and then ask the teacher if everyone understood me;
    b. look to my interpreter to alert him that I need a sign-to-voice interpretation;
    c. ask my interpreter what I should do;
    d. tell my teacher that I don't know the answer;
    e. other _____.

Like the teacher questionnaire, this student instrument can be customized to reflect a particular communication situation or a particular classroom's interaction style. If a single questionnaire is used, multiple applications of the questionnaire may need to be administered. That is, the use of a questionnaire to assess the interpreter and interpreting situation in first-period math should not preclude its repeated use in fourth-period computer class and in sixth-period physical education class. Chapter 5 includes an assessment instrument for middle-school and secondary students, and Figure 2.3 is recommended for postsecondary students.

FIGURE 2.3   Student Evaluation of Interpreter

Interpreter's Name _____   Semester/Program _____

Please check the answers that best describe this interpreter. All information will be kept private and will be used to provide you with better interpreting services. Please be as honest as possible; we are interested in your feedback.

1. The interpreter's signs are:
   _____ Very Good   _____ Good   _____ Average   _____ Poor

2. The interpreter's sign vocabulary for this class is:
   _____ Very Good   _____ Good   _____ Average   _____ Poor

3. The interpreter's fingerspelling is:
   _____ Very Good   _____ Good   _____ Average   _____ Poor

4. The interpreter's speed of signing is (keeps up with the instructor):
   _____ Very Good   _____ Good   _____ Average
   _____ Too Fast   _____ Too Slow

5. The interpreter's lip movements are:
   _____ Very Good   _____ Good   _____ Average   _____ Poor

6. The interpreter's facial expressions are:
   _____ Very Good   _____ Good   _____ Average   _____ Poor

7. I understand what the interpreter is signing:
   _____ All of the time _____ Most of the time _____ Some of the time
   _____ I do not understand the interpreter most of the time.

8. When I ask a question in class, the interpreter:
   _____ Understands ALL of what I say and is able to tell the instructor.
   _____ Understands MOST of what I say and is able to tell the instructor.
   _____ DOES NOT understand what I say.
   _____ I DO NOT use the interpreter to ask a question.

9. The interpreter makes me feel comfortable communicating with hearing students:
   _____ All of the time _____ Most of the time
   _____ Sometimes   _____ Never

10. The interpreter follows the "mood" of the instructor (if the instructor is interesting/boring, the interpreter is interesting/boring):
    _____ All of the time _____ Most of the time
    _____ Sometimes   _____ Never

FIGURE 2.3   (continued)

11. The interpreter shows up for class:
    _____ All of the time _____ Most of the time _____ Often misses class

12. The interpreter arrives at class on time:
    _____ All of the time _____ Most of the time _____ Is often late

13. The interpreter wears appropriate clothing (not distracting):
    _____ All of the time _____ Most of the time _____ Sometimes _____ Never

14. The interpreter is enthusiastic and shows a positive attitude:
    _____ All of the time _____ Most of the time _____ Sometimes _____ Never

15. I am comfortable discussing an interpreting problem with the interpreter when a problem occurs:
    _____ All of the time _____ Most of the time _____ Sometimes _____ Never

16. In general, the interpreter behaves professionally:
    _____ All of the time _____ Most of the time _____ Sometimes _____ Never

17. Please indicate how you feel about having this interpreter again:
    _____ I wish I had this interpreter more often.
    _____ I would not mind having this interpreter again.
    _____ I would rather have another interpreter.
    _____ If possible, I do not want this interpreter again.

18. In what ways could this interpreter change or improve to make your interpreting services more beneficial?

The interpreter's self-evaluation instrument

Self-evaluation instruments have been reviewed extensively in supervision literature in communication sciences and disorders (Anderson, 1988). Indeed, one of the critical purposes of evaluation is to enhance the professional development of the person being evaluated. A continuum is described in supervision literature that operates on the assumption that professionals move from a stage in which they need and benefit from directed observation, feedback, and evaluation to a stage in which they can self-analyze and alter behavior appropriately as a result of the analysis. This independent stage does not imply that observation and feedback are not important; but at the independent stage, the professional seeks collegial consultation from peers rather than detailed how-did-I-do feedback. The self-evaluation instrument could be general in its design, or it could be task-specific. A sample self-evaluation instrument is shown in Figure 2.4.

FIGURE 2.4   An Educational Interpreter's Self-Evaluation

Name of Interpreter: _____

Interpreting Situation/Class: _____

Rating Scale: 1–2 Unsatisfactory   3–4 Needs Work   5–6 Average   7–8 Good
                 9–10 Very Good

   1. I was comfortable with the vocabulary: _____
   2. I used fingerspelling effectively: _____
   3. I succeeded in making the target language cohesive: _____
   4. I used phrasing appropriately: _____
   5. I used spatial markers appropriately: _____
   6. I used transition markers appropriately: _____
   7. I used nonmanual communication well: _____
   8. I was aware of communicaton breakdowns when they
         occurred and was able to repair appropriately: _____
   9. I used classifiers appropriately: _____
  10. I comprehended what I interpreted: _____

Comments: _____

_____

_____

                                    _____
                                                Signature

                                    _____
                                                Date

The Evaluation Process

Distributing and collecting the multiple assessment instruments should be the responsibility of a single administrator. Likewise, determining the frequency of use and the relative weight of each of the assessment instruments in the overall process should be the responsibility of a knowledgeable administrator. Procedures for evaluating the educational interpreter should be detailed in the hiring or orientation of the interpreter. A first-year interpreter may benefit from an evaluation early in the fall term, with a subsequent evaluation at midyear, and a final evaluation at the end of the year. Experienced interpreters may benefit more from an annual evaluation that weighs ongoing self-analysis as more important than the building administrator's annual assessment. Routine videotapes of the educational interpreter should serve many important purposes: (1) documentation of the interpreter's performance, (2) a resource for the evaluation conference, and (3) a comparison document that becomes a resource in future conferences.

Finally, it is critical that the process of evaluating the educational interpreter be *valued*. Administrators who approach evaluation with an attitude that the process is important to all involved is likely to instill that same attitude in others.

The evaluation process and product should provide the administrator with insight into the educational interpreting program. Spencer Salend and Maureen Longo (1994), in their article, "The Roles of the Educational Interpreter in Mainstreaming," recommended that the administrator examine the effectiveness of and satisfaction with the services the interpreter provides from several perspectives, including the perspective of the interpreter himself or herself. Salend and Longo indicated that a comprehensive evaluation enables administrators to answer questions that go beyond the details of the interpreter's performance in order to evaluate the program. Questions, such as the following, should come from the evaluation process even if they are not addressed as particulars within the evaluation:

1. Are teachers and the interpreter working cooperatively to deliver instruction to students?
2. What are the impacts of the interpreter on the student's peers and the social interactions between students with hearing impairments and their peers?
3. Has the interpreter aided professionals in communicating with parents who have hearing impairments?
4. Are administrative policies regarding the use of the interpreter appropriate? (Salend & Longo, 1994, p. 27)

Another question may be appropriate to add to this list: Would mentor relationships strengthen the educational interpreting services program? Mentoring has received popular support in many professional circles in recent years, including the interpreting profession. Mentors have also played an important role in the history of interpreting, particularly interpreters who were themselves nurtured by deaf consumers. The literature on mentoring tends to be descriptive with steps for establishing a mentorship program, strategies for giving effective feedback to the protégés (or mentorees), characteristics of effective mentors, phases or cycles in the mentorship process, and so on (Clark, 1995; Zachary, 2000). The NYC Metro RID's Mentoring Committee reported after the first ten-week cycle of its mentoring program that "selecting mentors and protégés was very challenging" and that "more hands-on [training] opportunities through role play and video work" were needed (Schwenke, Hoffman, & Nessanbaum, 2002, p. 6). Administrators who sponsor mentorship in their educational interpreting programs should add evaluation of the mentoring as part of the comprehensive evaluation protocol. Table 2.3 offers suggested questions for such an evaluation.

TABLE 2.3   Mentorship Program Evaluation

Please provide feedback on the effectiveness of the mentorship relationship you just experienced with answers to the following questions:

- Were the expectations of your mentor-protégé relationship clear?
- Were the goals well defined and clear?
- Were the responsibilities of each participant clear?
- Did you have a workable strategy for dealing with obstacles?
- Were you able to evaluate progress?
- What recommendations would you make for improving our mentorship program? (adapted from Zachary, 2000)

Question 6: What are the best practices for handling difficult administrative situations?

The following situations represent only a handful of potentially difficult situations administrators may experience within the educational interpreting services program. Because no specific right answers are available for these cases, the administrator may need to contemplate various practices that could be exercised in solving or resolving the dilemma. Consultations with other school administrators, particularly schools that have established interpreter service programs, should serve to validate decisions or provide alternative solutions when problems occur. The administrator's knowledge of a code of conduct or the Interpreter's Code of Ethics (RID, 1995) may be critical to the mediation and handling of some of these issues (see full text in the Appendix).

The Case of the Nonattending Student

James worked beautifully with his interpreter during the second and third grades. When she went on maternity leave in the spring, the school replaced her with an older woman from their substitute interpreter list. The substitute interpreter was hired later during the summer when the full-time interpreter decided not to return in the fall. James's attitude toward his new interpreter, Mrs. Ross, was unconscionable. He informed her on the first day of the school term that he didn't want her for an interpreter and would refuse to watch her. He stubbornly demanded that his favorite interpreter, Beth, be returned to her former role.

Mrs. Ross spoke to the administrator after the first week of school and called again during the second week to indicate that neither she nor the classroom teacher could secure James's attention. James's refusal to participate with the interpreter made the whole class uncomfortable. Both the teacher and the interpreter were at a loss as to the best approach to use with James. What's the best way to handle this situation?

Suggested Best Practice   The need for a conference is apparent. Whether a complete IEP or child study team needs to be convened, however, is unclear at this point. A first conference with the classroom teacher and with Mrs. Ross would likely be followed by a conference with James and his parents. A phone call to Beth to determine whether she had any similarly stubborn episodes and how she may have handled them might also be advantageous. In the meantime, a strategy that acknowledges James's ownership of responsibility is critical. The classroom teacher's treatment of James, in the same way as any other student in the class who fails to attend to instruction, directions, and assignments, should involve some natural consequences—most obviously, failure. In addition, James's behavior is potentially disruptive to the other students who are concerned about his unwillingness to attend.

Describing the consequences of disruptive behavior to James is also a natural strategy. Who should interpret this conference, this communication with James? In this case, another interpreter, one removed from the situation, should be called on. If James's behaviors continue to result in failure and disruption, the IEP or child study team would need to convene to determine an alternative placement or alternative approach to James's learning. Under no circumstances should Mrs. Ross be removed or replaced because James wants his former interpreter to return. Indeed, her input to the resolutions is critical. Sensitivity to the rapport between James and Mrs. Ross is also necessary on the part of the administrator in guiding the teacher, the interpreter, and the committee. Little attention has been given to personality types in interpreter–consumer relationships (Doerfert & Wilcox, 1986). It is highly unlikely, however, that administrators will ever have control over the many facets of personality in such a way that matching interpreter and child by personality types would be possible.

Departure Questions for Discussion

1. Why shouldn't the administration try to replace Mrs. Ross?
2. What's wrong with admitting that "it just isn't going to work"?
3. Isn't it reasonable to involve a counselor in this case?
4. What if James doesn't like his teacher and wants her replaced?
5. What affect does a negative interpreter–student relationship have on a student's learning? on the teacher's teaching? on the interpreter's interpreting?

The Case of the New Cochlear Implant

Mr. and Mrs. Ramsey had shared details about their six-year-old son's scheduled cochlear implant surgery weeks before the actual date of the surgery. The special education representatives voiced support and reconvened the IEP committee in February, five weeks after the first mapping. At that February meeting, the Ramseys requested an amendment to the IEP to halt the use of sign language with Jeremy and discontinue educational interpreting services. They requested instead a certified auditory verbal therapist (AVT) to work with Jeremy in individual sessions for 90 minutes daily. The speech-language pathologist and teacher of the deaf disagreed with the parents' claim that Jeremy would not have full benefit of his implant unless AVT were used exclusively. The general education teacher and educational interpreter both reported that although Jeremy was showing increased use of hearing, he also continued to rely on the interpreter. The administration suggested that the change to an oral-only approach with Jeremy be gradually implemented, so that documentation could guide the decision making. The Ramseys threatened due process if their requests were not honored. How should the adminstration handle their requests and threats?

Suggested Best Practice   Due process hearings are not only financially costly, but they can also drain a school system of its emotional reserves. Most administrators favor working with parents to avoid litigation.

Parents of older children who receive cochlear implants are often faced with new communication choices, sometimes out of hope that the previous choices will no longer be required, and sometimes out of misguided advice from medical professionals who promise cochlear implant technology as an immediate fix. Current research is not conclusive in support of any singular approach for all children with implants, although advocates of AVT commonly address improved speech intelligibility as a consequence of intense auditory training and in the absence of sign language or other visual support. Advocates of total communication programming are equally likely to address improved speech intelligibility and language development as a consequence of comprehensive services, including the presence of sign language and educational interpreting support.

Administrators facing conflicts such as this one are wise to seek input from unbiased experts and to communicate with parents from evidence-based reasoning. Holly Teagle and Jan Moore (2002), in their article on "School-Based Services for Children with Cochlear Implants," suggested that "children who use sign language as a primary communication mode at the time of implantation will likely continue to need sign support as they develop their listening and speaking skills" (p. 168). Documenting Jeremy's communication behaviors in these early weeks following the implant and over the weeks to come should provide critical evidence as to his changing needs. Encouraging the parents with offers of a combined approach seems reasonable, particularly in differentiating educational interpreting as a communication accommodation and auditory verbal therapy as an individual treatment approach. The customized use of both may be in Jeremy's best short-term and long-term interest.

Departure Questions for Discussion

1. Why not honor the parents' request, eliminate the sign language and educational interpreting services, and let Jeremy "sink or swim"?
2. Isn't auditory verbal therapy to be used *without* sign language or speechreading? How can it be customized if it's an exclusive approach?
3. What happens if the parents refuse this compromise? Isn't it possible that a due process hearing could be the quickest solution?

The Case of the Moving Family

Ms. Martin had voiced several complaints about the interpreters and teachers over the previous school year. In fact, her presence at the middle and elementary schools where her three deaf sons were enrolled was considerably stressful for the principals, teachers, and interpreters at the respective schools. Dr. Devereaux was not surprised when he received a call from one of the interpreters in early August indicating that she had heard Ms. Martin had moved across the state line to live with her sister. The interpreter also reported that Ms.

Martin and her boyfriend had been known to break up and get back together before, and, if this separation was like previous separations, the boys and their mom might well be back in a few months. The interpreter's question, in ending the conversation, was simply: Can I expect to have a job when we go back to school in three weeks? Dr. Deveraux's response that he would check into the matter raised several issues that he now has to address. First, verification of the move should eliminate any doubts about the rumor. Second, if the boys are not enrolled at the opening of the school year, Dr. Deveraux needs to determine whether to keep the three interpreters (only one of whom is certified) he had worked so hard to recruit over the previous two years. On the other hand, the family's absence from the school system could be a blessing, especially with the mom's frequent complaints, and, in these hard financial times, the money saved on the interpreting positions could really help the budget. Finally, if he did retain all three interpreters in anticipation of the family's return, what responsibilities should he assign them? They had all been outspoken about not doing aide work last year. What options does Dr. Deveraux have?

Suggested Best Practice   Re-entry students are not unusual in either small or large school communities. Today's multiple family types include those that are transient, sometimes in spite of their children's enrollment in good school programs and sometimes in search of school programs that better meet their children's needs. Ms. Martin's move, if verified, poses choices that have negative consequences, even in the best case.

Dr. Deveraux's first strategy should be to check the schools' respective offices for any notices or requests for student file transfers. Finding none, he still might need to prepare an alternative plan if the students don't show up on the first day of school. That plan would likely include alternate job assignments, particularly after discussing with the personnel director and building principals any possible reassignments and salaries that are attached to those reassignments. He should also be prepared to share with each of the interpreters the school system's position that their continued employment is desired, regretfully with reassignments and adjusted salaries, but also with hopes of returning them to their previous roles if the boys return. Presenting these options as offers and giving the interpreters time to contemplate them should reduce the negative consequences. Being prepared to lose the interpreters, even the certified interpreter, should also be part of the administrator's responsibilities when circumstances such as these occur.

Departure Questions for Discussion

1. What if the interpreters agree to stay but only at their current interpreting salaries?
2. What if one of the interpreters agrees to stay, and what if the boys move back when the other two interpreters, including the certified interpreter, have taken other jobs?
3. What if Ms. Martin returns her boys to the school system for a couple of months and then leaves again?

The Case of the Disgruntled Parents

Edward's parents call frequently to complain that he performed poorly on a test or missed a homework assignment or misunderstood the directions on a worksheet. The parents are adamant that the problem lies with the interpreters, not with Edward. They insist that Edward did fine in the middle school on his assignments and tests, but since he has been in high school and is working with three different interpreters, his schoolwork continues to go down. The parents request a meeting and expect a change in the interpreting situation. What should the administrator do?

Suggested Best Practice   The administrator who deals with disgruntled parents should approach the parents of a deaf child just as he or she would approach any parent of any child. Communication is critical! The administrator should be prepared to educate the parents about the school's interpreting policies and procedures. Written documents that serve to clarify the school's position in hiring and evaluating interpreters may be necessary during this communication. Such preliminary discussions may serve to alleviate or redirect the parents' concerns. If not, the administrator may need to include others as part of the communication link between the school and the parents. Guidance counselors or others trained in mediation may be important to the communication process. Under no circumstances should the administrator undermine or devalue the parents' concerns about their child's failure, but should always support the parents in their efforts to advocate for their child.

Presenting a "same-team" attitude that includes the interpreter as an important member of the team is critical to successful communication with unhappy parents and is also especially important in supporting the interpreters or any employees with whom parents find fault. Suggesting a series of steps to reach harmony may again prevent further insult, especially if the steps are mutually derived by parents and administrator. Some suggested strategies for that list of steps include: (1) discussion of the written documents after the parents have had opportunity to read and contemplate them, (2) providing classroom observations at scheduled intervals with follow-up discussions, and/or (3) hiring an outside consultant to mediate or negotiate other strategies. All school systems should be prepared, of course, to guide parents into a fourth step, due process proceedings, when no other recourse appears likely.

Departure Questions for Discussion

1. Who calls the shots when parents try to blame interpreters for a student's poor performance?
2. Where do the interpreters' rights begin and end?
3. Where do the teacher(s) come into play in cases like this?
4. Isn't this another case for a counselor?
5. What if due process is pursued?
6. Is the school responsible for the legal bills for the interpreters—if they're full-time? part-time?

The Case of Evaluating the Interpreter

Mrs. Smith worked with Bill, the sign language interpreter, all year. In May she requests a meeting with the administrator where she reports that Bill has become defiant in his acceptance of responsibilities and that she thinks his upcoming evaluation should reflect his arrogance. The administrator expressed that he had not been aware of a problem between the two earlier in the year, and Mrs. Smith responds that the change began after Bill went to a workshop on "The Role of the Classroom Interpreter" back in March. She says he flatout refuses to photocopy, to help her grade, to work with students one-on-one, and that Bill just acts "better than everybody else" now. What should be done?

Suggested Best Practice A preevaluation conference with Bill might be all that is required to support his need to "stretch" professionally. It is quite possible that teachers start to take their relationships with interpreters for granted, just as interpreters run the risk of taking their relationships with teachers for granted. Bill's newly demonstrated resistance is likely to be a symptom of his need for more respect. Acknowledging this need, while reminding Bill of his dual role and his upcoming end-of-the-year evaluation, should suffice in restoring Bill to his former cooperative self. If, however, his frustration with that dual role has truly interfered with his performance of that role, disciplinary steps may be in order. This is not to say that interpreters should be expected to photocopy or grade. It is to say, however, that Bill's role as it was established in the beginning of the year is the same role that he will be evaluated on at the end of the year. Conferencing with Bill regarding any limitations of his current role and negotiating ways to improve his job description for the future should show a good-faith effort to support him in his professional development.

Departure Questions for Discussion

1. How could problems like this be avoided?
2. What can be said of a school that supports its interpreters to attend workshops for professional development if the learning that occurs at that workshop is disregarded?
3. Does Bill get an opportunity to evaluate his teacher and her expectations of him?
4. Shouldn't the evaluation process involve reciprocity—the teacher provides input on the interpreter's evaluation and the interpreter provides input on the teacher's evaluation?

The Case of Equal Access to the Handouts

The Director of Disability Services at the Community College was excited to have its first deaf instructor in a class that did not involve sign language teaching. Thirty-eight students (2 deaf and 36 hearing) had registered for the "Human Growth and Development" course during the preregistration period. The instructor, Dr. Elliott, requested and was assigned two nationally certified interpreters for the weekly three-hour class.

The interpreters arrived early on the first night of class to meet Dr. Elliott, to discuss the course syllabus; her instructional plans; and her preferences for their seating, sign language usage, and so on. In their 20-minute conference, Dr. Elliott positioned them side-by-side about four feet in front of the podium, facing her with their backs to the students. Dr. Elliott also asked the two deaf students, when they arrived, to sit in front, flanking the interpreters for visual access to the interpreters and the rest of the students who sat behind the interpreters at desks in rows. After all students were seated, Dr. Elliott began by introducing herself and distributing the syllabus. She handed one copy of the syllabus to each of the deaf students, bypassed the interpreters, and proceeded to distribute a counted number of handouts to the first person in each of the rows. As Dr. Elliott walked back to the podium, one of the interpreters reached out to request a copy of the syllabus, but Dr. Elliot did not acknowledge the gestural request.

After the syllabus had been distributed and discussed, Dr. Elliott began lecturing. She used several transparencies during her lecture. The interpreters oriented to her delivery style and "smoothed out the wrinkles" in switching from sign-to-voice interpreting for the lecture information and deaf students' comments and questions to voice-to-sign interpreting for the hearing students' comments and questions. The class proceeded without incidence.

At the onset of the next class, a week later, the interpreters again arrived early to discuss the night's plans with Dr. Elliott. One of the interpreters asked if there were any handouts they could preview, but Dr. Elliott reported that she was going to use transparencies again. The class proceeded much like the first one, with this exception: Some of the transparencies were lengthy and required considerable time for the students to copy the information into their notes. Recognizing this as a potential problem, Dr. Elliott told the class that she would use handouts in future class meetings. As the two interpreters left that night, one commented to the other that she hoped Dr. Elliott was planning to give them a copy of the handouts. The other interpreter responded that she might continue to use the transparencies and that they could get the technical terminology and proper names from it if she did not distribute handouts to them.

During the third class meeting, Dr. Elliott did indeed distribute handouts to the students. As with the distribution of the syllabus, though, she did not offer the handouts to the interpreters. Very quickly into the lecture, the interpreters realized that she had removed the overhead projector. Their access to the information on the handouts was strictly through Dr. Elliott, who discussed language development in infants according to Furth, Piaget, Vygotsky, Chomsky, and others. The interpreters struggled with some of the individual names and technical words that Dr. Elliott fingerspelled. They "fed" to each other as much as possible, but both interpreters had to interrupt Dr. Elliott several times during the lecture to ask for repetitions. Dr. Elliott was visibly annoyed with their interruptions and asked them, after class, not to interrupt her again. In defense of their interruptions, one of the two interpreters explained that they needed to have a copy of the handouts, that they were unable to anticipate where her lecture was going without access to the handouts. Dr. Elliott countered their request with this comment: "I asked for qualified interpreters. Apparently, if you're unable to read me, you're not qualified for the job. I'll tell the Director of Disability Services tomorrow that she needs to get two interpreters who are qualified."

Dr. Elliott did indeed call the director the next morning with her complaint about the interpreters and a request to have them replaced by "qualified" interpreters. Her phone call, however, had been preceded by a visit from the two interpreters who shared the story as it is reported here. What should the Director do?

Suggested Best Practice   The Director of Disability Services may be able to reduce the tension that has been created in this case by calling a meeting of all those involved (with an additional interpreter to interpret during the meeting). *If* the Disability Services program has a policy manual or set of orientation guidelines that it uses with its hearing faculty, then the blame for the problem may well rest with the director for not providing the same manual or orientation guidelines to a faculty member who is deaf. Indeed, an apology for assuming that the deaf teacher did not need to be oriented could serve as an important lesson for all those involved.

An additional issue is clearly presented in this case, however, an issue of confidence. At this point in the course, the instructor's reported dissatisfaction with the interpreters represents a lack of confidence in their qualifications and skills. At the same time, the interpreters' reported concerns about the instructor's attitude toward them represents a lack of confidence in their ability to satisfy her. This mutual lack of confidence by the fourth week of the term could easily snowball by the semester's end and present a conflict that interferes with the students' learning. Administrators who are comfortable with conflict resolution recognize that mediation is a process. These administrators schedule meetings (both individual and joint conferences) and work to reach an agreement that is satisfactory to all parties. Administrators who are not comfortable with conflict resolution and the mediation process should involve counselors who are comfortable with conflict resolution where cases such as this one have potentially negative outcomes on student learning.

Departure Questions for Discussion

1. What if the Disability Services Program does NOT have a procedures manual or a set of orientation guidelines?
2. Can confidence in interpreters be restored after it's lost?
3. Can confidence in the instructor be restored after it's lost?
4. What if the instructor doesn't want to participate in mediation?
5. What if the interpreters refuse to participate in mediation?

The Case of Changing Technologies

The young deaf woman was entering her junior year at the university. She had presented several challenges to the Office of Disability Services during the two previous years, not necessarily because of her deafness, but mostly because of her unique communication needs. As a late-onset deafened individual, her spoken language was fully intelligible. Her speechreading skills were highly developed, but she had difficulty in large classes and with some teachers. So, accommodations during her freshman and sophomore years included oral interpreters in those classes in which she felt a need. The Office of Disability Services also provided her with a laptop computer so she could take her own notes; she didn't like the notetakers the office provided her during her first semester. The office provided her with a wireless pager; she insisted it was more practical than a TTY. The office had also provided her with a C-Print captionist; but she didn't like the intrusion of a second support person. The office provided her with an iCommunicator™ during her sophomore year; but the error rates for the speech-to-text readout were too high and she rejected it. This most recent summer e-mail includes a request for Viable Realtime Transcription (VRT) service. When the secretary in the office read the e-mail, she quipped: "What will she want next?" How should the Disability Services Officer respond?

Suggested Best Practice   While it appears that this student is too demanding of the Office of Disability Services, it is also encouraging to see students play an active role in determining their access needs. This young woman, like her hearing and deaf peers, is well aware of the rapidly advancing technological changes that impact our daily communication. The rate of change and its infiltration into society is unprecedented (Gladstone, 2002; Nelson, 2002). The Office of Disability Services has shown a progressive attitude thus far in providing the aforementioned technologies. Most likely, its investigation into VRT will similarly yield another "field trial" that will either prove valuable or be rejected. Also, it is possible that the purchase of the VRT, like the purchase of the iCommunicator™, will be contingent upon a successful trial period. Shared funding of this technological support service is also quite likely with the interagency agreement the university has with the Department of Vocational Rehabilitation Services. Viewing her request as yet another opportunity to try the latest technology seems appropriate. The officer in charge of approving these opportunities (possibly alongside a VR counselor) is actually gaining valuable insights about the rapid advances in technology and their application in the postsecondary setting.

Departure Questions for Discussion

1. At what point should the Office of Disability Services tell this student that enough is enough?
2. How does all this technology affect the oral transliterators? Shouldn't they have something to say about what's going on?
3. What if the university doesn't have an interagency agreement with the Vocational Rehabilitation Office? Isn't there a limit to how much money they should have to spend?
4. Who defines "reasonable" accommodations?

Summary

This chapter has presented several administrative issues relevant to educational interpreting: characteristics of the administrator, the interpreter's position description and contract, procedural policies, interpreter competencies, evaluation procedures, teaming, inservice training, and mentoring. Several difficult situations have also been presented with recommended best practices for resolving them or reducing the tensions that can escalate when resolutions are not found. Departure questions that enable further deliberations and additional searches for answers point to the volatility these issues can provoke. Administering an educational interpreting program is challenging, especially when administrators have little previous experience with educational interpreters and consumers of educational interpreters. The information presented in this chapter should prove helpful to administrators who work to meet these challenges, as well as to interpreters and teachers who may rarely see issues from the administrator's perspective. Interpreters who work to educate their administrators (by sharing copies of this book, for example) in a nonassuming and nonthreatening manner should eventually see the benefit of their efforts in strong administrative support.

REFERENCES

Anderson, J. L. (1988). *The supervisory process in speech-language pathology and audiology.* Boston: College-Hill.

Antia, S. D., & Kreimeyer, K. H. (2001). The role of interpreters in inclusive classrooms. *American Annals of the Deaf, 146,* 355–365.

Beaver, D. L., Hayes, P. L., & Luetke-Stahlman, B. (1995). In-service trends: General Education teachers working with educational interpreters. *American Annals of the Deaf, 140,* 38–46.

Bublitz, S. (2002). Overview of the NCI performance and interview examinations. *RID Views, 19,* 10–11.

Budding, C. M. (2001). Virginia interpreters respond to Educational Interpreting Performance Assessment (EIPA). *RID Views, 18,* 14–17.

CED/RID Ad Hoc Educational Interpreter Committee (1993). *Competencies for the certification of educational interpreters: Approved version.* Rochester, NY: NTID.

Clark, T. S. (1995). *Mentorship: A sign of the times: A guide to mentoring in the field of sign language interpretation.* Stillwater, OK: National Clearing House of Rehabilitation Training Materials.

Conference of Interpreter Trainers (1994, October). *Proposed standards for interpreter education.* Paper presented at the CIT Convention, Charlotte, NC.

Doerfert, K., & Wilcox, S. (1986). Meeting students' affective needs: Personality types and learning preferences. *RID Journal of Interpretation, 3,* 35–46.

Florida Department of Education. (1998). *Competencies of Educational Interpreters.* [Online]. Available: http://www.fsdb.k12.fl.us/eit/98competencies.html

Gladstone, V. S. (2002). Tapping into technology. *The ASHA Leader, 7,* 3, 11.

Hurwitz, T. A. (1980, May). *The tutor/notetaker as a support service for hearing impaired students: Overview of the NTID tutor/notetaker program.* Paper presented at the annual meeting of the Association on Handicapped Student Services Programs in Post-Secondary Education, Denver, CO.

Hurwitz, T. A., & Witter, A. B. (1979). Principles of interpreting in an educational environment. In M. E. Bishop (Ed.), *Educational mainstreaming: Practical ideas for teaching hearing-impaired students.* Washington, DC: Volta Bureau.

Linehan, P. (2000). Educational interpreters for students who are deaf and hard of hearing. *Project Forum at NASDSE.* U.S. Office of Special Education Programs.

Nelson, J. (2002). The state of the wireless industry. *NADmag, 2,* 20–21.

Ramsey, C. L. (1997). *Deaf children in public schools: Placement, context, and consequences.* Washington, DC: Gallaudet University Press.

Registry of Interpreters for the Deaf, Inc. (1995). Code of Ethics of the RID, Inc. *RID Membership Directory.* Silver Spring, MD: RID Publications.

Salend, S. J., & Longo, M. (1994). The roles of the educational interpreter in mainstreaming. *Teaching Exceptional Children, 26,* 22–28.

Schick, B., & Williams, K. (1994). Evaluating educational interpreters using classroom performance. *Interpreter Views, 11,* 15–24.

Schwenke, T., Hoffman, L., & Nessanbaum, H. (2002). NYC Metro RID's mentoring program: A team approach. *RID Views, 19,* 6.

Seal, B. C. (1995). Evaluating the educational interpreter. *RID Views, 12,* 17, 38.

———. (1997). Educating students who are deaf and hard-of-hearing. In L. Power-deFur & F. Orelove (Eds.), *Inclusive education: Practical implementation of the least restrictive environment* (pp. 259–272). Gaithersburg, MD: Aspen Publishers.

———. (2000). Guidelines for inservicing teachers who teach with educational interpreters. In (RID, Inc.) *Educational interpreting: A collection of articles from Views: 1996–2000.* Silver Spring, MD: RID Publications.

Stewart, D. A., Schein, J. D., & Cartwright, B. E. (1998). *Sign language interpreting: Exploring its art and science.* Boston: Allyn & Bacon.

Stuckless, E. R., Avery, J. C., & Hurwitz, T. A. (Eds.) (1989). *Educational interpreting for deaf students: A report on the national task force on educational interpreting.* Rochester, NY: NTID/RIT.

Teagle, H. F. B., & Moore, J. A. (2002). School-based services for children with cochlear implants. *Language, Speech, and Hearing Services in Schools, 33,* 162–171.

Turner, E. (2001, Winter/Spring). Roles in educational interpreting. *Odyssey, 2,* 40–41.

Warren-Norman, H. (2002, August). *Parameters for interpreter services in public school settings.* Paper presented at the National Educational Interpreters Conference, San Antonio, TX.

Zachary, L. J. (2000). *The mentor's guide: Facilitating effective learning relationships.* San Francisco: Jossey-Bass.

3 Best Practices in Educational Interpreting in the Primary Grades Setting

The provision of interpreting services for preschool and primary-school deaf and hard-of-hearing children raises many questions. This chapter is organized around those questions frequently asked by interpreters assigned to early childhood classrooms. This chapter also includes valuable information for school administrators, teachers, and parents as they sort out their expectations of the educational interpreter and interpreting services.

Question 1: What is expected of the educational interpreter in the primary grades?

The needs of a deaf or hard-of-hearing student in preschool, kindergarten, or first grade, and in many cases even up through the second and third grades, are quite different from the needs of that same student and other students in later grades. Changes in a child's cognitive, linguistic, and social development require commensurate changes in the responsibilities of the interpreter. Critical to the interpreter's optimum performance is a working knowledge of child development and the changes that are expected to occur during these important learning years.

The first year of a child's life is an extremely important foundation year for language learning. The child's ability to attend selectively to communication information presented through audition, vision, and touch accelerates rapidly following birth, *if* that sensory input meets a functioning neurological system. The baby with a profound hearing loss may go through normal eye gaze development. If so, he first looks at his caretaker as she nurtures him. Then, weeks later, he looks at objects (diectic gaze); weeks later, he ensures that his caretaker is also looking at the same object (joint attention); and, weeks later, he extends a pointing gesture to request that object (Bloom, 2000; Owens, 1996). All of this happens during the first six to nine months of life. This same infant also learns to follow his mother's eye gaze, discriminate her facial expressions, and match her symbolic responses (words and signs) to his own early gaze and gestural communication. And then the baby engages in practicing the symbolic responses offered by his caretaker, her "motherese." His canonical babbling ("ba-ba-ba" for spoken language and "A-A-A" for sign language) is perceived by Mom and Dad as a true word (bottle) or as a true sign (MILK)[1] (see Marschark, 1997, and Masataka, 2000, for more on sign babbling); and by about 12 months of age, the baby's success at gaining MILK with a repeated A-hand marks the onset of what we call language.

Within the second year of life, the same child goes through a phenomenal period of word and/or sign acquisition. The first 50 words or signs develop as single words and single signs, but by 18 to 24 months, these 50 are joined to make simple two- and three-word or -sign sentences. Between 30 months to 6 years, the hearing child learns about 3.6 words per day; between 6 years to 8 years, 6.6 words per day; and between 8 to 10 years, 12.1 words per day (Bloom, 2000). This learning leaves a normally developing 6-year-old hearing child with a vocabulary of about 20,000 words (Miller & Gildea, 1987). While we have no research on the longitudinal sign learning of a normally developing deaf child, we have every reason to expect that this same child would have acquired about 20,000 *sign equivalents* by the age of 6 years. We also know that vocabulary size is highly variable among hearing and deaf children, but several correlations are commonly acknowledged by language acquisition scholars. A child's vocabulary size is correlated positively with his parents' vocabulary size, with his later literacy development, and with intelligence (Bloom, 2000).

Vocabulary learning also correlates with syntactic learning. That is, between 3 and 5 years of age, as the child pivots and sequences his growing vocabulary into growing sentences, he basically acquires the necessary rules of grammar and the complex rules of discourse that characterize his parents' language (Owens, 1996). Both deaf and hearing children who acquire the native language of their parents during this period demonstrate an impressive talent for absorbing language. Indeed, this period is referred to as the "critical language learning period," a period in which the order of language acquisition is predictable across all cultures (Bloom, 1970; Brown, 1973). Another way to look at this language acquisition is to recognize that the average 3-year-old who acquires language unremarkably from his parents is about 75% intelligible to other adults who share the same language. The average 4-year-old is about 85% intelligible to other adults who use this same language; and the average 5-year-old is about 95% intelligible to others who share his parents' language. Although language learning continues over the next few years (and, to some degree, throughout all stages of our lives), these earliest years are special in that children are most successful—perhaps even neurologically programmed to be successful—in acquiring the language or languages of their environment and/or culture.

---

[1]As is conventional, signs are glossed in all caps.

A child's cognitive development also accelerates during these critical early years. From birth until about age 2, children develop knowledge of their world from their sensory-motor experiences with the world. From about 2 to 7 years of age, children develop in a preoperational cognitive stage. During this stage, the acquisition of a symbol system is best realized in the development of language. Play dominates children's activities, with dramatic play representing or symbolizing the events of their daily lives. As a child's language and communication skills advance, he or she moves from solitary play (alone) to parallel play (side-by-side) to associative play (interacting) and, finally, to cooperative play ("I'll be the mommy and you be the little girl.") with peers. Socially, this period is marked by the onset of leave-taking and increasingly prolonged separations from parents. During this stage children come to accept other adults as surrogate caretakers and may even refer to them on occasion as "Mommy" or MOMMY.

The implications of this language-cognitive-social learning can be overwhelming for educational interpreters employed in early childhood or primary settings. In fact, one of the arguments against having educational interpreters at this level involves the definition of interpreting. Elizabeth Winston (1994) explained that interpreting involves moving across languages, and that without an already existing language, interpreting cannot truly occur. This argument is meaningful for many deaf or hard-of-hearing children who come to school without a solid language foundation. Few children, however, including those who are diagnosed with severe and profound hearing losses, enter their formal school years without some level of language learning. The degree to which that level matches the language learning of their peers is dependent on two intricately linked factors: (1) the nature of the intervention in the years prior to schooling and (2) the nature of the neurological development of the child. Both of these benefit from early diagnosis.

The incidence of hearing loss in infancy has increased in recent years. Most likely, the increase is due to advances in audiological testing that permit relatively accurate diagnosis of hearing loss even hours after birth. Where congenital hearing loss was diagnosed at an average age of about 24 months in the early 1990s, Universal Newborn Hearing Screenings now identify hearing loss within the first few months of life. The earlier the diagnosis, the earlier the intervention and the better the outcomes (Yoshinago-Itano, 2000).

Medical advances are responsible for another growing population of deaf and hard-of-hearing babies. Those who would have died in the 1980s are surviving at increasingly lower birth weights and with increasingly more involved medical needs. Some of these needs are more overt than others. Certain low-incidence genetic syndromes, for example, may present with malformations (microtia and/or atresia) of the outer ear; but most present with no observable physical signs of hearing loss. The prevalence of pervasive developmental disorders (including autism and Asperger's syndrome) and attention deficit disorders (with and without hyperactivity) is up across every socioeconomic level in the United States (see Samar, Parasnis, & Berent, 1998, for information on ADD and learning disabilities in deaf students). Many of these children, at least 10%, have significant hearing loss.

Medical advances are also responsible for another rapidly growing population of deaf babies. In 1990, the U.S. Food and Drug Administration (FDA) approved the surgical implantation of electrodes into the cochleas of deaf children ages 2 through 17 years. In 1998, the age was lowered to 18 months, and, in 2001, FDA approval extended to children 12 months of age, if they have a hearing loss of 90 dB or more. Prior to the most recent FDA approval, children could be considered for implants only upon verifying they did not benefit from traditional amplification. In the decade of the 1990s, approximately 1 in 10 preschool children received a cochlear implant (CI) (Boswell, 1999). Rapid gains in implant technology, increased coverage for the surgery by insurance carriers (Kluwin & Stewart, 2000), and general acknowledgement of gains in the spoken language development of these CI candidates (e.g., Tye-Murray, Spencer & Woodworth, 1995) are probably responsible for today's prognostic indicator: By 2010, at least one in three deaf preschoolers will be implanted (Boswell, 1999).

A wide range of communication levels, a wide range of hearing levels, and a wide range of learning abilities characterize these very young deaf and hard-of-hearing children. Some children with implants show near-normal spoken language development while others show improvements in their comprehension of spoken language, but limited intelligibility of their speech and reduced scores on vocabulary measures (Connor, Hieber, Arts, & Zwolan, 2000). Current trends in intervention tend to place young children who are implanted into either strictly oral programs or total communication programs, and no empirical evidence currently exists to suggest that either one of these programs is advisable for all CI children (Carney & Moeller, 1998). We estimate that about half of our youngest implanted children enter preschool programs without a sign language background and about half enter with a signing background. Among those in total communication programs are those who use mostly sign, those who use mostly speech, and those who use both sign and speech simultaneously (Geers, Spehar, & Sedey, 2002). Children who are implanted, whether they use sign language or spoken language or both, are also more likely to enter educational mainstream or inclusion programs than deaf children who are not implanted (Niparko, Cheng, & Francis, 2000). When the signing child is placed in an inclusion program with hearing peers and teachers who do not sign, the educational interpreter can be an important link in guiding general education teachers to understand the student's communication and to facilitate its development level.

Wide variability is also common to the population of preschoolers who are not implanted. Those with multiple disorders, those from homes where neither English nor ASL constitutes the native language of the parents (see Chapter 1 for demographics), those with and those without functional residual hearing, and even those who appear to have normal neurological development will show a wide range in their rate of vocabulary acquisition, their styles of communication, and their general dispositions in working with an interpreter. The interpreter assigned to a deaf preschooler diagnosed with autism will likely struggle to adjust to his lack of directed eye gaze and to differentiate his signs from his idiosyncratic hand movements (Tinsley, 2001). The interpreter assigned to a kindergartener with a moderate hearing loss will likely struggle to adjust to her lack of visual attending, in determining how much she takes in auditorally when she is not looking at the interpreter. The interpreter assigned to a second grader with ADHD will likely struggle with his distractibility and failure to attend.

We currently have no research on the effects of missing or reduced eye gaze on the educational interpreter's performance, but we know from observation and experience that interpreters tend to lower their hands, employ fewer facial expressions, and generally provide a less dynamic interpretation when our consumers are not watching. In contrast, research on "sign motherese" (Erting, Prezioso, & O'Grady-Hynes, 1990; Masataka, 1996, 2000) reveals that deaf mothers who use sign language with their young children will attempt to gain and maintain their attention through touch, and by waving their hands and moving their signs within the child's visual field. They also exaggerate their facial expressions and certain features of their signs, with larger signs articulated slower and with lots of repetition or redundancy in their signing. The impact of this knowledge while working in primary settings with special-needs deaf and hard-of-hearing children points to the complicated role interpreters have in facilitating communication and language learning.

The argument can easily be made that any adult who communicates with a child during these language learning years is a language model, and, to one degree or another, a language teacher. The argument can also be made that only the teacher is hired to teach; that only the teacher has the training, the credentials, and the skills to teach; and that all other supplemental aides and resource staff (the teacher aide, the librarian, the interpreter, as examples) serve to support the teacher. This attitude represented the prevailing view of teaching and learning 30, 40, and 50 years ago—that teachers were responsible for identifying discrete learning material and were responsible for teaching that material through fragmented lessons and drills. Today's preschool and primary educators are more likely to view language learning as a process that encompasses all activities of the school day. Today's language teaching is more likely to be developmentally and philosophically "whole," with the process for teaching or intervening guided by findings from natural language learning.

Several principles are fundamental to the *whole language* philosophy: (1) every facet of communication (isolated speech sounds, a dramatic mime, a crayon drawing, a fingerspelled word, a written autobiography, as examples) contributes meaning in an integrated, not fragmented, way to the whole learning of the child; (2) learners in natural environments are actively, not passively, engaged in their own learning through meaningful interactions within the physical and social environment; (3) learning involves incorporating and integrating new information into existing knowledge; and (4) language is a tool for all learning (e.g., Norris & Damico, 1990). In today's primary classrooms, then, every interaction and every opportunity for interacting are viewed as critical to language learning. In these classrooms, the educational interpreter is very much a language teacher. That is, the educational interpreter communicates regularly with the student, interacting meaningfully with knowledge of the student's existing language and with the ability to integrate new information into this existing knowledge. The interpreter who interacts with a deaf or hard-of-hearing student, even in representing the language of others, is a language teacher, not necessarily in the textbook fashion that some may think of as teaching, but in a cooperative fashion that recognizes communication as the best context for learning.

Although interpreter training programs frequently require their students to take a course in child development (Dahl & Wilcox, 1990; Shroyer & Compton, 1994), a single course may not provide the educational interpreter with sufficient knowledge of language development, particularly in the child who is deaf or hard-of-hearing, and particularly if that child has an implant, or comes from a home where a language other than ASL or English is used, or has medical and psychological needs that extend beyond the hearing loss. Because the educational interpreter has a background in deafness and understands the impact that hearing loss can have on language development, however, he or she brings to the interpreting role a broader grasp of the "whole needs" of the child than an interpreter whose knowledge and experience base is limited to a single survey course and to interpreting for adults. The combination of a strong developmentally oriented teacher with a knowledgeable interpreter can be a winning combination for deaf and hard-of-hearing students whose cognitive, social, motor, and language skills are developing.

Sorting the various roles of the interpreter in the primary setting (Luetke-Stahlman, 1992), then, requires careful insight into the needs of the primary-aged consumer. The variety of roles the interpreter plays at this level are, in many ways, more challenging than the responsibilities that upper grade levels present to the same interpreter. Imagine, for example, the point at which the interpreter functions as an aide—helping a student put her coat on or take it off, helping a student put toothpaste on his toothbrush, or get on and off the bus. The educational interpreter assigned to a deaf student indeed may be the best person to "help" the child in these physical activities because she or he communicates the language that accompanies the activities.

As the interpreter operates within this helping model, she or he may take on a "shadowing" role, actually duplicating the language that the teacher uses, but reproducing it in first person. Of course, the use of first person is practiced in interpreting for adults, too (Frishberg, 1990). The difference for interpreters who interpret in first person for preschool and primary students is that at some point during this developmental period the student learns that the person interpreting is not the same "I" as the "I" who is talking. (This subject—the age or stage at which young deaf or hard-of-hearing students come to know that their interpreters are representing the language of others—emerges again in Chapter 7.) The interpreter in the primary setting, then, cannot function only as the hands of the classroom teacher in signing or cueing the words the teacher used. The interpreter in the primary setting actually reproduces the language in such a *helping* way that the child "learns" the language that accompanies the activities. Interpreters who grimace at the thoughts of functioning in a helper model with adult consumers should easily see the philosophical difference in functioning as a professional helper with primary-aged students.

The notion of the *helper model* emerged from the early work of volunteers (often family members) who attempted to "fix" the communication between hearing and deaf persons. These interpreters who engaged in helping often played patronizing and controlling roles, making the deaf consumer appear helpless—unknowing and unable to make decisions without the help of the interpreter. Janice Humphrey and the late Bob Alcorn, in their book, *So You Want to Be an Interpreter* (1994), described a conversation between a deaf patient and his interpreter in the waiting room of a doctor's office. In their example, the helping interpreter not only drove the patient to the doctor's office, but also advised the patient on how to inform his wife of the possibility of cancer, on the importance of writing a will, and on the potential benefits of a black-market medication.

Educational interpreters in primary settings may laugh at this extreme example, secure in their own knowledge and skills that they would never violate their ethical standards to *help* like this interpreter did. Educational interpreters would not volunteer to drive a student to and from school, would not advise parents on how to discipline their child, would not volunteer to serve as the babysitter in after-school hours. The questions for educational interpreters in primary settings, then, are more realistically these: How can I meet the demands of my role? meet the needs of my consumers? function in a helping role, without setting myself up to be viewed as the student's helper? without making the student or teacher helpless? I would answer that helping is a critical part of the role, that helping is not only appropriate but also important to the success of all those involved. I would also qualify the concept of helping by suggesting that it is intertwined in the natural events of the communication day, that the interpreter does not seek to help in order to make the student or teacher feel helpless, but seeks to help because it is natural and appropriate to the activity and the communication surrounding the activity.

This view of helper expands the role of the interpreter as one who is an expert in the language and communication of the deaf student, and, as an expert, is the person most likely to interact with the student in a way that *teaches* language. This model views helping in a professional, instructional manner that is consistent with the activities and demands of the classroom environment, and appropriate to the function of an interpreter in that setting.

A final word about the interpreter's role in *helping* young students gain communication access and language: Learning involves the interpreter's skill level and earlier discussion about "motherese." Early childhood teachers use a communication style, referred to as Child Directed Speech, that is comparable to motherese. Brenda Schick (2001) discussed the prosodics of a hearing teacher's Child Directed Speech as changes in her pitch, intensity, and the duration of her voice, as organizational units of her utterances, as emotional content of her message, and as extralinguistic information (which words are important or what she expects the student to know). Interpreters at all levels, but especially at this level, must be able to represent these dynamic features of the source language in their interpreted target language. Early childhood interpreters cannot be without affect. Equally important, early childhood interpreters must be able to "read" the child's communication, and not just the signs he forms, but the *way* he signs, his prosodics. "The interpreter's ability to clearly interpret the child's message is critical to the child's development of language and thinking skills. This is true with all children, hearing and deaf, who use interpreters, whether or not they are developing language skills in a typical manner (p. 11)."

Question 2: What is the interpreter's role in working with an educational team?

Critical to the role of any team member is the ability to share information relevant to the student's learning with the other members of the educational team. This sharing may occur incidentally or it may occur under more formal circumstances. The exact nature of the sharing is likely to be determined by the members of the educational team and their contact with the student. The educational team may itself be constituted formally. An Individualized Education Program (IEP) team, for example, is a very important decision-making team. Members of this team may include the classroom teacher, the principal, the speech-language pathologist, the educational audiologist, the teacher of the hearing-impaired, the school psychologist, and the student's parents. The interpreter's role in sharing information with this team will likely be very formal. The interpreter may be invited to join the team at certain junctures of the school year, or the interpreter, by virtue of the position description, may be included in all activities of the team. The psychologist may need to consult with the interpreter prior to formal testing to determine how directions will be administered, how nonverbal test items will be modeled, and so on. Similarly, the speech-language pathologist may rely on the interpreter's expertise in determining how to collect a language sample, how to interpret the language used during the sample, and so on. The interpreter's role in these cases is undeniably critical to the functioning of other members of the team. The interpreter must help these other team members in their understanding of and intervention with the student.

Other educational teams exist outside the constituency of the IEP team. The *teaching team* is an equally important team. The teaching team is likely to include the teacher, the librarian, the speech-language pathologist, the art teacher, the physical education teacher, the teacher of the deaf, and others. These individuals have more frequent contact with the deaf or hard-of-hearing student than perhaps other IEP team members whose contacts may be annual or as needed. Sharing information with members of this team is also likely to be more incidental than formal. Imagine the interpreter observing Johnny as he looks at the new monthly calendar on a Monday morning and telling the teacher: "Johnny just signed to himself 'FOUR BIRTHDAY PARTIES' as he checked out the new calendar." This type of interpreting, much like "inform talk" (Luetke-Stahlman, 1991), which an interpreter uses to fill in a deaf student on conversations occuring in the periphery, is critical to the teacher whose knowledge and skill in sign language or fingerspelling or cued speech is limited. The primary teacher takes in information that represents a student's learning all day long, every day of the school year. Having access to that same information from the deaf or hard-of-hearing student may only occur because of the interpreter's ability to inform, to collaborate, to share, to *help* the teacher and all others who are involved in the student's learning to understand the student's language.

Being a member of a collaborative team—either a formally appointed team or the teaching team—requires certain expectations. Some of these expectations come about through a demonstration of the services that the interpreter provides. As teachers, teacher aides, speech-language pathologists, librarians, physical educators, and others observe the interpreter's work, they are likely to develop the sense that the student needs the interpreter's services, and that, they, in working with the same student, also need the interpreter's services. This sense of mutual need is quite possibly the most important expectation that members of a collaborative team can have of each other. Once that sense is established, the interpreter is then expected to perform as other members, sharing knowledge and recommendations with regard to the student's learning. Many of the guidelines suggested for speech-language pathologists who work collaboratively with teachers are equally applicable to educational interpreters. These include (1) providing high-quality services, (2) developing good communication with other professionals, (3) educating other professionals about the services being provided, and (4) respecting professional boundaries.

The provision of high-quality services is sometimes misrepresented to naive onlookers. Most interpreters have experienced praise from naive observers who "just love to watch the interpreter." Comments about the rate at which the interpreter signs, the interpreter's ability to "keep up," the interpreter's ability to process all that is being heard, and so on, are generally not meaningful to educational interpreters who aspire to be equal members of a collaborative team. But even these comments can be responded to with a professionalism that acknowledges the observer's interest in the service. Responses—such as, "If you've never been exposed to interpreters before, it's only natural that you're drawn to the process"; "You'll soon acclimate to what's happening"; or "I find it easy to keep up in Mrs. Jones's class; she organizes her activities in a logical way, and she always shares what I can expect well ahead of time"—are important responses for interpreters who receive naive comments about the quality of their services. No response to naive praise, however, can ever match the contribution that providing truly high-quality services makes to an interpreter's perceived effectiveness. Interpreters who fail to provide optimum services will only be impressive to members of a team for a short while. Interpreters' contributions ultimately are evaluated by how they communicate with the other team members and how well they educate these team members to what interpreting actually entails. Providing "clear, concise, and relevant information," minimizing jargon that others may not understand, and providing accurate information about the services being provided and the needs of the student are recommended by Hedge and Davis (1995, p. 142) as important practices in collaborating with other professionals.

The American Speech-Language-Hearing Association and the Council on Education of the Deaf joined forces to interpret the Individuals with Disabilities

Education Act—Part H, as Amended (the IDEA—Part H), as it applied to children who are deaf and hard-of-hearing from birth to 36 months. Several skills and knowledge areas were recommended in their report (Joint Committee, 1995) for members who work on a "multidisciplinary" team:

1. Skill in involving families as equal partners of the multidisciplinary team;
2. Knowledge of first language acquisition and the effects of hearing loss;
3. Knowledge of hearing loss and/or other conditions and their effect on early development of cognition, communication, speech, motor, adaptive, and social-emotional development;
4. Knowledge of how a child who is deaf or hard-of-hearing and/or has special needs affects relationships within the family and community;
5. Knowledge that assessment and management is a dynamic, ongoing process requiring a variety of skills and techniques;
6. Skill in sharing, consulting, joint goal setting, and planning with all members of the team;
7. Skill in using appropriate counseling strategies;
8. Knowledge of the various roles of members on the multidisciplinary team;
9. Skill in integrating and implementing the knowledge and recommendations of other team members;
10. Knowledge of resources available for deaf and hard-of-hearing children and their families, including local, state, and national organizations;
11. Knowledge of the range of services appropriate to meet the individual needs of the child and family;
12. Knowledge of Deaf culture and issues of cultural diversity as they affect children who are deaf or hard-of-hearing and their families;
13. Skill in summarizing and integrating assessment information into an educational report and program plan (p. 66).

Members of the collaborative team will have varying levels of competence in these 13 knowledge areas and skills. Some members may demonstrate only a few of the competencies, while others may demonstrate all the competencies. Various educational interpreters can also be expected to have varying degrees of competence in these knowledge areas and skills. The greater the interpreter's knowledge base and skills, however, the greater his or her contributions to the team.

Question 3: Are there problems with confidentiality when the interpreter is expected to share information about the student with others?

Many individuals struggle to understand how issues of confidentiality are violated when the educational interpreter shares information about a student with other members of a student's educational or teaching team. Part of this struggle has been brought on by well-meaning interpreters who themselves interpret their

Code of Ethics as a confining dictum. The Code of Ethics established and maintained by RID was never intended to be used as such (Rudser, 1986). The interpreter who refuses to answer a substitute teacher's question about a student's performance in reading group because it violates the student's confidentiality is potentially violating the Code of Ethics herself by not "functioning in a manner appropriate to the situation." Interpreters who refuse to share appropriate information with members or substitute members of the educational team in the name of ethics are likely promoting a code of ethics that does not belong to other professional interpreters, especially other educational interpreters.

By the same token, it is possible that an educational interpreter may fail to follow ethical conduct in all situations. Providing personal opinions that are not professionally founded, for example, is inappropriate for any member of the educational team. Likewise, it is "inappropriate for the interpreter to assume any of the instructional responsibilities in the classroom, such as executing a test, assisting in grading papers, modifying curriculum, counseling, or disciplining students" (Witter-Merithew & Dirst, 1982, p. 402). Most school systems have adopted the RID Code of Ethics (in the Appendix) to guide their interpreters and those who work with interpreters in judicious actions. Other schools have written their own interpretation of RID's Code with school-specific language. The tenets of this revised Code (see Table 3.1) are consistent with the highly regarded RID Code of Ethics.

Educating team members about the interpreter's Code of Ethics may be necessary as part of the getting-to-know-you process. Direct instruction may not be as effective, however, as experiences involving the interpretation of ethical standards. Interpreters who function by a code of conduct or set of ethical standards are generally more successful in imparting their code or standards to others than

---

TABLE 3.1 Educational Interpreter's Code of Conduct

1. The educational interpreter shall hold all school-related information confidential. As a member of the educational team, the interpreter shall function in a manner that is appropriate to the team, sharing information that relates directly to the work of other professionals in their contacts with the deaf or hard-of-hearing student in a professional and judicious manner.

2. The educational interpreter shall strive to equalize the source language and target language by using language that is compatible with the student's developmental level.

3. The educational interpreter shall not counsel or advise students or other professionals in a manner that is inconsistent with his or her role as an interpreter.

4. The educational interpreter shall present a professional appearance and demeanor appropriate to the educational environment(s) in which he or she works.

5. The educational interpreter shall develop professionally through continuing education, including education that is relevant to the role(s) for which the interpreter is hired.

those who talk about them. In fact, talking about ethical standards rarely occurs unless some violation (real or perceived) has also occurred. All teachers, all members of a school program, all professionals who provide services to students are expected to function within a set of acceptable standards. These standards may be unwritten, generally accepted rules of behavior or performance, or they may exist as a written document that has been prepared by a committee or administrative representative for the entire school. Educational interpreters who apply their standards with other professionals who expect and promote ethical standards for themselves should not have to worry about breaching confidentiality.

Question 4: What should the interpreter do during free play and other activities that are designed to promote social interaction?

When Public Law 94-142 was first implemented, the fear of many deaf educators about "least restrictive environment" centered around social development. As a result of this fear and in response to the subsequent and widespread mainstreaming of preschool hearing-impaired children, many early childhood development and deaf education researchers investigated the social interactions of deaf children who were placed in hearing preschools and primary school programs. Some of the research focused on the best conditions for promoting social interactions among deaf and hearing children (e.g., Luetke-Stahlman, 1991; Ross, Brackett, & Maxon, 1982; Spencer, Koester, & Meadow-Orlans, 1994), and some focused on the communication used by deaf and hearing students when they interacted (e.g., Antia, 1982; Arnold & Tremblay, 1979; Spencer, Koester, & Meadow-Orlans, 1994). What has emerged from this and more recent research (e.g., Antia, 1998) is knowledge that social development is highly related to communication development. Those with better communication skills are more likely to interact with a larger number of peers (Marschark, Lang, & Albertini, 2002). Increased interactions with multiple peers tend to enrich communication skills that, in turn, strengthen social skills. In contrast, those with poor communication skills are likely to interact with fewer individuals, and, in some reported cases, just the interpreter (Shaw & Jamieson, 1997). Implications of this knowledge suggest another role of the interpreter in the primary setting, that of a facilitator. The following vignette should illustrate:

> As a 4-year old, Sean was relatively comfortable using some speech, some signs, and lots of gestures with his hearing peers, particularly Jack, who shared his passion for the Lego table. One morning before Jack arrived, Sean worked diligently to make a Lego vehicle and a road. He aligned the road on one side of the Lego table, and each time students approached that side, he directed them away, to leave it alone. When Jack arrived, however, Sean eagerly welcomed him to play. After just three or four minutes, as Sean was lengthening the road, Jack began taking apart the vehicle. Sean became upset and tried to stop Jack's dismantling by taking the vehicle away. Jack pulled away and an altercation began. Sean did a

quick head turn, isolated his interpreter, and approached her with a loud MINE while he pointed to Jack holding the Lego car.

The interpreter's response simply was: COME ON, I'LL INTERPRET FOR YOU. The two approached Jack and the interpreter voiced as Sean signed: THAT'S MINE. GIVE IT BACK. Sean proceeded to give the car to the interpreter. She handed it back to Jack and said, "Watch Sean, Jack. What's he saying?" She then directed Sean to TELL HIM AGAIN. This time, Jack responded to Sean, "But I'm going to make it bigger."

By then, the teacher had arrived. She kneeled to the level of the boys and, with arms extended around both, asked "What's going on?" Jack responded first that he wanted to make Sean's car bigger. Sean, in quick retort, reported that the car was his and Jack was trying to break it. At this point, the interpreter (who was also bent to the teacher's level) successfully interpreted the teacher's suggestion that they "build lots more cars, some smaller and some bigger." Within minutes, both adults were standing at a distance watching Jack and Sean (and Sahid, Benjamin, and Henry) make more cars.

The educational interpreter who functions as a facilitator in primary settings is likely to make numerous contributions during free play, group time, recess, and other events that include social exchanges. Many of these contributions "extend beyond mere renditions of other participants' utterances" (Metzger, 1999, p. 2). The facilitator is aware of the environmental conditions that enable or impede communication (including lighting, noise, and proxemics or distance between communicators), the linguistic conditions that enable or impede communication (including the different languages, linguistic codes, communication modes), and the different levels of linguistic competence demonstrated by those involved. In the scene just described, the interpreter demonstrated knowledge of the linguistic conditions and different levels of linguistic competence demonstrated by her consumers. She also offered a consumer lesson to the two boys when she agreed to interpret for Sean, when she directed Jack to attend to what Sean was telling him, and when she directed Sean to repeat himself. Each of these contributions facilitated another communication exchange between the boys. The only caution interpreters might consider in this same situation is not to exclude the teacher from those exchanges. Directing Sean to his *teacher* with COME ON, I'LL INTERPRET FOR YOU might be more facilitative in some classrooms, especially where teachers may unknowingly use their interpreters to avoid engaging with their deaf students directly (Ramsey, 1997).

Finding the appropriate distance from the student who may seek out the interpreter to tell another student that the car is his may require some experimenting. At the same time, the interpreter who facilitates communication in social contexts may need to be removed from the context to enable communication exchanges to occur. Wegner and Swartzman-Waters (1994) compared the communication interactions of a deaf preschooler with her 22 hearing peers on those days when the interpreter was present to the interactions that occurred on those days when the interpreter was absent. They reported that the interpreter facilitated more interactions that included more initiations, more communication turns, and with more varied communication partners than those observed during her absence. In contrast, Hulsing, Luetke-Stahlman, Loeb, Nelson, and Wegner (1995) reported that their deaf 5-year-olds relied on their interpreters as partners to communicate but did *not* use them to facilitate interactions with their peers. Once again, the heterogeneity of communication styles among deaf and hard-of-hearing students requires the preschool and primary educational interpreter to be aware of different communication behaviors among different students in different social circumstances. This interpreter is likely to recognize the need to observe and report social communication as it occurs both with and without an interpreter.

Collaborating with the classroom teacher, the speech-language pathologist, the teacher of the deaf, and possibly other individuals, is important in planning and carrying out observations that focus on a student's social communication. Classroom teachers who value discourse as a means to teach and to learn (and, for some teachers, as a means to evaluate their students' learning) are interested in understanding the discourse skills their students bring to the classroom—for all communication, not just for social communication. Included in these discourse skills are the student's ability to attend to a speaker (or to the interpreter), to take a communication turn, to maintain a topic with a communication partner, to repair communication when a partner fails to understand, to request repairs when he or she fails to understand a partner or other communicator (Creaghead & Ripich, 1994). The classroom teacher may not be able to determine (or can only partially determine) these discourse skills in a deaf or hard-of-hearing student without input from the educational interpreter. Furthermore, a student who has successful discourse skills with one or more peers may not have the same success with other peers. A student who understands the teacher's personal communication directed to him or her without the interpreter may not understand the teacher's classroom communication when it is directed to the whole class unless the interpreter is available. As a consequence, the educational interpreter and classroom teacher may find that systematic and careful observations are necessary to find those contexts—social and academic—in which the student's best discourse skills are promoted.

The speech-language pathologist may also be involved in collaborating with the classroom teacher and the educational interpreter for information on the student's social communication skills. The interests of the speech-language pathologist, however, may go beyond what is observed with and without the interpreter's intervention to what is observed following or as a result of the speech-language pathologist's intervention. In spite of the growing trend of treating students in their classrooms, speech-language pathologists still most often see their deaf or hard-of-hearing students two or three times a week in pull-out sessions (in their speech offices or rooms) where they work individually on the student's speech, speechreading, and listening skills (Otis-Wilborn, 1992; Seal, 2000).

Speech-language pathologists who are unable to work in the classroom should benefit from the educational interpreter's observations of the student's transfer of practiced skills from the speech room to the classroom. For example, the educational interpreter may observe and report on the student's intensity when playing with other students in the housekeeping area. The interpreter may also observe for and report on the student's use of certain social phrases that were practiced in the speech room. The interpreter may observe and record spoken utterances that occur with sign language and those that occur without accompanying signs. Indeed, any number of skills that focus on the student's communication may be observed and reported to the speech-language pathologist as evidence of successful carryover or, in contrast, as evidence of the need for continued work or a change in the approach. When educational interpreters were asked about their work with speech-language pathologists (Seal, 2000), 42% responded that they had collaborative relationships that included these tasks: interpreting during the therapy session, facilitating carryover from the session to the mainstream classroom, working on pragmatic goals, providing the speech-language pathologist (SLP) signs for a communication wallet, and co-teaching sign language to the hearing students and teachers (pp. 22–23). Figure 3.1 offers an observation checklist with sample communication skills that may be customized for individual students and provide an additional focus of collaboration between speech-language pathologists and educational interpreters.

FIGURE 3.1 Observing a Student's Interaction Skills

Date of Observation: _____

Nature of the Interaction: _____

Interaction	Never	Sometimes	Frequently	Comment
Transitions into and out of conversations with peers	_____	_____	_____	_____
Introduces a topic with peers	_____	_____	_____	_____
Maintains a topic with peers	_____	_____	_____	_____
Answers questions from peers	_____	_____	_____	_____
Interrupts peers appropriately	_____	_____	_____	_____
Introduces a topic with teacher	_____	_____	_____	_____
Maintains a topic with teacher	_____	_____	_____	_____

FIGURE 3.1   (continued)

Interaction	Never	Sometimes	Frequently	Comment
Answers questions from teacher	_____	_____	_____	_____
Interrupts teacher appropriately	_____	_____	_____	_____
Expresses feelings appropriately	_____	_____	_____	_____
Requests repairs appropriately	_____	_____	_____	_____
Attempts to repair when misunderstood by peers	_____	_____	_____	_____
Attempts to repair when misunderstood by teacher	_____	_____	_____	_____
Seeks interpreter when communication is unsuccessful	_____	_____	_____	_____
Attends to interpreter when teacher is addressing the class	_____	_____	_____	_____

Comments:

Question 5: Should the educational interpreter be expected to teach sign language (or cued speech or fingerspelling) to other students and adults?

Answering this question takes us back to the implications of the first question: Is the interpreter a language teacher? Much like the previous discussion of the role of the interpreter in modeling language, this answer focuses on an interpreter's knowledge of language learning in young children. Many children, hearing or deaf, who observe an educational interpreter with any sense of routine, "pick up" signs or cues. Their mere exposure to a different language or different modality may provide natural *lessons* in that language or modality. This natural acquisition of signs by hearing students and adults will likely need additional formal instruction, and even then, interpreters should not assume that the children's signing will be fully comprehensible or used appropriately (Ramsey, 1997). Preschool and kindergarten students are generally accustomed to finger plays and musical lyrics that require gestures, and whole-body and limb movements. These students also typically enjoy, and learn equally well, signs that are appropriate to their daily communication.

One of the most important vocabulary sets for a preschool or primary classroom involves the selection of name signs for the students and teachers. The educational interpreter, in collaboration with the classroom teacher, can help select name signs that are motorically simple and conceptually appropriate. Avoiding "cutesy" or awkward signs that frequently take on stigmas is important. I recall the preschooler whose name sign was "T" signed like TOILET. His hearing parents were alarmed when they learned, much too late in the school year, that he was sometimes teased because of his name sign. A forward-thinking interpreter should be able to instruct the students in selecting name signs and other sign vocabulary in a way that results in positive, not negative, communication interactions. (For more information, see Supalla, 1995, *The Book of Name Signs*.)

Name signs might need to extend beyond the classroom, too. Name signs for other teachers, cafeteria workers, the secretaries, the principal, and others, are important to the student's comprehension and interaction. The following excerpt from a first-grade class should illustrate the value of name signs on a broad scale:

All the pencils down now, markers down. Everybody's eyes up here. I see 2, 4, 6, 8, 10, 12, 14 eyes, 16, 18, 20, 22, 24, 26, 28, 30, 32, 34, 36, 38 eyes. Why do I need to see 38 eyes? Sarah? Because everyone has two eyes and 19 students times two eyes is 38 eyes. (Hannah, close that for right now, OK, while I go over something.)

Mr. Shell asked us to go over these rules before we go to the cafeteria [*holding up a chart of rules*]. These are rules of things he saw that he wants changed. He wants us to remember them when we go to the cafeteria. One thing that will be changed—you will not take your tray up until it's time to leave to come to the classroom. So, Mrs. Walker won't ask you to take your tray up before time to line up. You'll then take your tray up to Mr. Kline and then you'll line up to come back to the classroom. So, that will be a little different. Jonathon, how will it be different today than yesterday? [*Jonathon mumbles something.*]

OK, here are some other rules that you must follow when you go to the cafeteria. You are to remain seated, stay in your seat, until it's time to take your tray up. You'll only go up one time now, instead of two times. Keep all your food on your tray. Don't pass food back and forth. Don't throw food around. If you're not gonna eat it, Shelley, leave it on your tray. Don't give it to someone else. And don't bother anyone else's tray, Brian. Our third rule, keep your hands and feet in your own space. Someone else's tray is not in your space.

You may talk quietly to those who are close by if you can do so without turning around. (Sit down please, Jonathon.) I'm sitting across from Missy. I can talk to Missy, here I can talk to Missy. And I can talk to Michael, and I can talk to Paul, but I can't talk to Jessica. Why, Sarah? In order to talk to Jessica, what do I have to do? [*Sarah answers.*] That's right. I'd have to turn around. You can talk to people next to you or across from you. Michelle? [*Michelle asks something.*] No, Michelle, you can only talk to the teacher if you're able to without turning your whole body around. OK?

Now, we need to wash our hands quickly. Another thing Mr. Shell asked us to do is to make sure we are at lunch on time. Yesterday we were three minutes late for lunch. That makes the next class three minutes late because they're still serving our class when Mrs. Shepherd's class is coming in. So, we need to make sure we're there on time. To do that, I'm going to call your name and when I do that you can come and wash your hands and line up and get your lunch boxes. Girls first. OK, Lindsey, Sarah, Jennifer, and Michelle, go wash your hands.

Another important sign vocabulary that should be taught to teachers who interact with the deaf or hard-of-hearing child is a vocabulary for personal greetings, emotional assurances, and praise. An interpreter who invests a few teaching minutes each day with a teacher who invests an attitude of desire in learning to communicate with the student on a one-to-one level is a generally successful combination. Signs for GOOD MORNING, PRETTY, GOOD, WOW, EXCELLENT, SORRY, PLEASE, THANK YOU, YOUR TURN, and any other pet phrases used routinely by the teacher, are important for the teacher's rapport with the student. As the teacher models to other students in the classroom this newly acquired ability to communicate, she demonstrates that the student who does not hear is important. The hearing students will likely follow her lead and find their own interest in learning to sign or cue to be successfully nurtured.

Barbara Luetke-Stahlman (1991), in "Hearing-Impaired Preschoolers in Integrated Child Care," reported that teachers should reward hearing children for speaking, cueing, or signing to their deaf classmates. I would suggest that the combination of positive rewards for interacting and positive modeling on the teacher's part by interacting with the deaf or hard-of-hearing children are a powerful combination. I would also suggest that the educational interpreter has the same potential in his or her interactions with hearing students in the classroom—modeling for the deaf or hard-of-hearing student how communication can and does occur. In the world of best practices, the classroom teacher and interpreter working together should find themselves an important team in encouraging communication among all members in the educational setting.

A caveat about vocabulary learning and teaching is appropriate before leaving this question. This caveat focuses on how we humans come to learn the vocabulary of a language, especially a language that may not be used as the native language in the learner's home. George Miller and Patricia Gildea (1987) provided a provoking discussion of this process in their article, "How Children Learn Words." Paul Bloom (2000) offered a more recent discussion in *How Children Learn the Meanings of Words.* "The reading vocabulary of the average high school graduate should consist of about 40,000 words. If all the proper names of people and places and all the idiomatic expressions are also counted as words, that estimate would have to be doubled" (Miller & Gildea, 1987, p. 94). The acquisition of 80,000 words over a period of 17 years breaks down to about "5,000 words per year, or about 13 per day" (p. 94). The process of this learning is not yet fully understood, but by the accounts of most authorities, the acquisition of a lexicon, whether spoken, cued, written, or signed, occurs, for the most part, *without* formal instruction. In fact, we acquire our words or our signs most easily by interacting with others who use those words or signs. During the primary years, this interaction can occur in the context of interpersonal communication and it can occur in the context of literary communication. In either case, communication is the operative word. Educational interpreting is about communication.

Question 6: What is the interpreter's role during story reading?

Story reading, poetry reading, and group singing are common experiences in the preschool and primary classrooms. The teacher's role in these activities, particularly as a story reader, is viewed by educators and researchers as similar to the parents' role in reading to their babies and toddlers—children who are read to become children who read to themselves; children who read to themselves become adults who read to themselves; and adults who read to themselves are likely to become parents who read to their children. Literacy is a value unsurpassed in educated societies. As Miller and Gildea (1987) put it, "a teacher's best friend in this endeavor is the student's motivation to discover meaning in linguistic messages" (p. 98).

Interpreters meet with various challenges in preschool and primary classroom settings, as well as in library settings, where book sharing occurs. These challenges include at least the following:

- Finding the most appropriate position in relation to the reader and the deaf or hard-of-hearing child to make the story accessible
- Negotiating how and when to interpret and how and when to direct the child's attention to a picture or title or word or other visually salient bit of information
- Engaging the deaf or hard-of-hearing child during interactions that are elicited by the reader (e.g., "and now, Johnny, what do you think is going to happen to Max?")
- Making poetry, music, and other auditorally challenging material visually effective

No single method works for all interpreters in meeting all these challenges. One commonality, however, that appears worthy of sharing is that good interpreters learn to *read* their story reader. Educational interpreters must learn the different voices that a reader takes on to represent different characters and different dialects in their stories. Effective interpreters must learn to hear the *rhythm* of poetry and prose so that their bodies (not just their limbs and faces) take on or represent that rhythm. Talented educational interpreters learn to hear the rhetorical questions in their story readers and can differentiate those from questions that require a directed response from the students. Finally, skilled interpreters learn to prepare—no story, no poem, no song should ever be interpreted without sufficient preparation.

Sometimes, regardless of the interpreter's preparation and skill level, the interpreter may sense that the student for whom she is interpreting does not comprehend the story. In these cases, the interpreter may need to suggest to the teacher (or to the appropriate members of the student's team) that she suspects that comprehension is affected by the length of the story, the nature of the story's dialogue, the subtle meanings that were implied in some of the story's lines, the overall disposition of the student during the story, and so on. Sometimes, the interpreter's knowledge of or feel for the student's comprehension during a story is intuitive, based not so much on differences in the student's attending skills (although attending skills can be a wonderful sign that a student is or is not comprehending), but based more on the interpreter's knowledge of the student's language. In these cases, the interpreter is advised to discuss that intuition, the observations, or suspicions with the teacher. She is also advised to examine her own skill at building a mental representation of a story. Susan Mather and Elizabeth Winston (1998), in their research on spatial mapping and ASL storytelling, identified several effective strategies that "provide an equivalent of the written English story in ASL" (p. 193). Each of these strategies involves spatial mapping or setting up space to represent various referents within the story and using that space prosodically for phrasing and chunking. Mather and Winston suggested that skill at effectively recreating the meaning of a story requires considerable time and effort and is not easily achieved by all, even those who are experienced teachers of the deaf and certified interpreters. On-going research that investigates the strategies deaf parents use in book sharing with their young signing children is likely to advance our interpreting skills in this important arena.

Question 7: What is the role of fingerspelling in a primary educational setting?

The learning of fingerspelling, like the learning of written spelling, is developmentally bound (Padden, 1991). The acquisition of fingerspelling by young deaf children is similar to the spelling acquired by children who are learning to write (Groode, 1992; Wilde, 1989). That is, some spelling-like movements will occur as a young deaf child attempts to represent a referent with something other than a single sign. The child then moves from this arbitrary spelling stage to a more purposeful stage when *invented* spellings can be expected to occur. Once invented spellings occur, the refinement to actual or correct spellings can be expected to follow. Movement across these stages and acquisition of fingerspelling for loan signs, for nominalization, and as a decoding strategy for reading may be dependent upon early and abundant exposure to fingerspelling (Padden, 1991).

The interpreter's use of fingerspelling with preschool and young primary children has parallels to the use of synonyms and pronominalization. The semantic referent is critical in conveying a symbol for a concept or idea or thing. Imagine interpreting a teacher's spoken phrase: "Tomorrow, boys and girls, we are going to the Metropolitan Zoo." The interpreter's use of fingerspelling for the word M-E-T-R-O-P-O-L-I-T-A-N (and possibly for Z-O-O) would be followed by a name sign, perhaps an initialized M shaken in the neutral space for Metropolitan (and possibly a sign for zoo). Every time the word *Metropolitan* occured in the teacher's language, the interpreter would fingerspell and then use the initialized name sign. Continued reference to the name could occur when it was used in print and when it was used in spoken language. The student, through the repeated exposure of the fingerspelled word and its name sign, learns that this particular lexical item is represented by at least two, possibly three, and possibly four, symbols. The name can be (1) fingerspelled, (2) signed, (3) spoken, and (4) written. Through time, the young preoperational student learns that all words conveyed by the interpreter can be represented with a variety of modalities. Through time, the young student learns to use these same modalities in his or her own communication.

As a result of this perspective that fingerspelling develops, that it is not just taught as an end but is acquired over developmental stages as a means to language competency and literacy, the educational interpreter again can be viewed as a language teacher. In selecting name signs, for example, the interpreter who spells a child's name and follows it with a name sign provides the deaf child, and the hearing children who are watching, with the knowledge that what I can sign I can also spell. This philosophy, "what I can say, I can also write; what I can write, I can also read; what I can read can be read by others" is a philosophy long held by those who approach language teaching and language learning from a *holistic* or gestalt perspective. This philosophy is also frequently espoused by those who support whole language. Ownership of this philosophy by the educational interpreter who works with young deaf and hard-of-hearing students is valuable.

Educational interpreters are also likely to use fingerspelling when reading instruction is phonologically based. Imagine the interpreter's use of fingerspelling in representing the instructional language used by this kindergarten teacher:

> OK, everyone, let's think about the sounds of this sentence: The man has a dog. How would we write this sentence? I'll write the first word "The" [she proceeds to print 'The' on the board]. Now, what letter should I write first for the word "man"? Jabar? [Jabar answers.] It's the "m" sound, right. The letter "m." The next letter, Katie? "m-a a-a-a"? [Katie answers.] No, not the "e" sound but a short "a" sound [writing "a" beside the "m"]. What's next, Lateesha? "ma—n" [Lateesha answers.] Yes, the "n" sound and the letter "n."

Primary educational interpreters frequently find a favorite way to distinguish letters and their sounds by experimenting with different strategies: holding the targeted letter next to the mouth while articulating its corresponding sound; placing the targeted letter in a prominent spatial location (with classifiers to spatially represent the "board") and offering it sustained eye gaze while mouthing its corresponding sound; and pointing to the mouth to draw attention to a sound's shape and simultaneously pointing to the ear and signing the corresponding letter. Some sign language interpreters use cued speech to represent the sounds letters make. Consistency in strategy, once a successful strategy is identified, is appropriate in facilitating these prereading skills. As Barbara Schirmer (2000) explained, kindergarteners are expected to enter first grade with the ability to recognize and name all uppercase and lowercase letters, and with the knowledge that letters in a written word represent the sounds of a spoken word. Research in literacy development also seems to point to an advantage in those deaf students who use phonological processing (Marschark, Lang, & Albertini, 2002). Educational interpreters who succeed in representing the sound-letter match in their interpreting are likely to be important links to this literacy development.

Question 8: Should signs be invented in the preschool and primary setting?

The student whose IEP calls for American Sign Language may indeed be exposed to more fingerspelling than the child whose IEP calls for Signed English. Certainly the books that have been developed for preschool sign language users (Bornstein, Saulnier, & Hamilton, 1973–1984) have a predominance of *invented* signs that represent English words common to the preschool and primary setting. Determining the need for inventing signs may be a decision for the child's IEP team. In some schools, philosophies about inventing signs are maintained throughout a child's school years. In others, the interpreter is left to use his or her own judgment as to whether the concept of the source language should be represented with an invented sign in the target language. There are obviously times when invented signs are practical—as in the case of "Metropolitan Zoo" just described. Appropriate execution of these invented signs leads a child to recognize their transiency.

Again, words and concepts can be represented with different symbols. Some words have signs that are colloquial or belong only "in house." The interpreter's use of these invented or in-house signs should be conveyed as such. The facial expressions, arbitrariness of their execution, and so on, especially if followed or preceded by the corresponding fingerspelled word, are important procedures for teaching the deaf or hard-of-hearing child that language symbols are frequently used by one group or class or at one time but that these same symbols are not used in other groups or classes or at other times. In this approach, the interpreter teaches the notion of *codes,* that both formal and informal codes exist in all communication, and that invented signs represent a different code from those signs that exist inside the formal code.

The interpreter who teaches (again, through interacting and modeling) that different codes or registers exist for different interpreted material also is likely to feel comfortable with different sign vocabulary of individuals who are involved in the student's life. For example, hearing parents who sign a particular word or concept with a particular sign are sometimes confused when their child comes home using a different sign or signing style. I recall one instance when a hearing mother was so worried that her daughter's teacher was using signs that were different from those she and her husband had learned that she threatened due process to have her daughter's teacher replaced by someone who was a better signer. While this story did not involve an educational interpreter, it does lead to a philosophy—*semantic flexibility is important in language learning*—that is critical for educational interpreters to embrace.

Educational interpreters should be comfortable with different signs used by different people. In fact, the interpreter who offers multiple signs to a student for a particular concept or word increases that student's exposure to semantic flexibility. Confusion occurs when a student is restricted to a set of rigid language symbols, only later to learn that rules for rigid language symbols are subject to being broken. Spoken language is full of inconsistencies, full of parallel meanings, and full of words that lend themselves to multiple interpretations. The same is true for signed languages. The educational interpreter who is comfortable with multiple interpretations and multiple language codes exposes the deaf or hard-of-hearing student to these multiple interpretations and multiple codes. The young student becomes a more competent language user as a result of these exposures.

Question 9: Should interpreters use their perspective or their student's perspective when interpreting number lines, calendars, and other spatial propositions?

We currently are without research-based recommendations on how interpreters should place or proposition their number equations, classifiers, and other referents in space. Cynthia Roy (2002) reported that most interpreters "sign equations in space, from *their* left to *their* right. When a student watches this unfolding equation, it begins at the student's right and moves to the left. This movement and representation is backward from the direction of all the other representations that the student is seeing" (p. 13). Think about how the interpreter should set up or proposition her number line in this second-grade math class in which the teacher has taped a number line on the blackboard and all students, including the two deaf students, have the identical number line taped across the top of their desks:

> OK, let's subtract 4 from 6. Now, I will write that number sentence as 6 take away 4 [*writing the equation on the board vertically*]. So where do we start, Brittany? On the 6 or on the 4? [*Brittany answers.*] Right, we start on the 6 and we hop backwards how many? Cody, how many? [*Cody answers 4.*] OK, here we go: Hop 1, hop 2, hop 3, hop 4, and where do we land? Chelsea? [*Chelsea answers*] Everybody agree? Raise your hand if you agree that 6 take away 4 is 2. You all are so smart! OK, let's do one more.

Interpreters who face their students, with their backs to the board, are inclined to position their number lines in front of them, show a place for the 6 and "hop backwards 1, 2, 3, 4," moving as they count from their right to their left, going against the direction of their students' perspective and against the direction of the teacher's work on the blackboard and against the students' same view of the desktop number lines. Why do we do this? And, should we?

Answering this question takes us back to the development of directed eye gaze mentioned in the beginning of this chapter. Children who develop normally (neurologically, that is) show an early attention to their caretaker's visual perspective. Between 6 and 9 months of age, they show the ability to look at what someone else is looking at. The *inability* to do this, a characteristic common to children with autistic disorder, represents a deficit in "theory of mind" development or an inability to figure out what people are thinking when they use facial expressions or words (Baron-Cohen, 1995) or signs. One-year-olds also show pretense, "as when pretending that a banana is a telephone" (Bloom, 2000; p. 63), and they can determine from the responses of their communication partners whether or not they accept that the banana is a pretend telephone. Theory of mind development, the ability to "read" the minds of others, to know intuitively that others have minds that actively engage during communication events, is quite possibly the foundation for all language learning (and some would argue that early sign language communication actually promotes its development). It is also quite likely the basis for taking on the perspective of an interpreter. The ability to look at what someone else is looking at, in this case, a pretend number line, may be problematic for students when the interpreter is inconsistent in her spatial propositions or in directing her own eye gaze to these referents. Determining whether your right is my left is in the eyes. And, perhaps like the reading of fingerspelling, these early experiences with spatial propositions of number lines and directed eye gaze lead to the later establishment of contralateralization, or the knowledge, demonstrated at about 10 years of age in children with normal neurological development, that your right is my left and my right is your left (Corballis, 1983). Providing the child with experiences that lead to this normal developmental milestone is, at least until research proves otherwise, our best practice.

Question 10: What are the best practices for handling difficult interpreting situations in preschool and primary settings?

The following cases are offered as representative of some of the hundreds of cases that confront educational interpreters every day. Some of the cases may have more application to particular interpreters than to others. The suggested practices offered for each of the cases may be more appropriate for some interpreters than for others. With each case, though, the interpreter should think through the variables that impact on the situation and determine what *best practices* could be offered in handling the same situation.

The Case of the Positioned Interpreter

Miss Litten welcomed her sign language interpreter—gave her a desk space for her books and materials, a closet shelf for her personal belongings, and a seat in which she could interpret. Miss Robinson, the interpreter for this kindergarten class, was appreciative of the welcome, but shared with Miss Litten that she may not need the chair, that she would "feel out" Miss Litten's movements within the classroom and position herself as appropriate for

Kyle, the deaf child's, best learning. Miss Litten's response took Miss Robinson by surprise: "I prefer for you to sit here."

The first week of the school year made it clear to Miss Robinson that the seat in the front near the blackboard was *not* the most appropriate place for her. Kyle was frequently on the floor with the other students—in reading circle, in math activities, in calendar work, and in sharing time. Every time she attempted to move near the learning locus, however, Miss Litten asked her to please stay in her interpreting seat so that all the children could learn who the interpreter was and who the teacher was. The tension brought on by this insistence was growing in Miss Robinson. What should she do?

Suggested Best Practice   Miss Robinson has several options for action, some direct, some indirect. A comment that might be appropriate follows: "Oh, Miss Litten, the students don't have any trouble identifying you as the teacher; you are definitely in control as the teacher. I, on the other hand, am clearly the interpreter because I sign what you say." If Miss Litten's sense of proprietorship is not lessened with these words, a conference might be in order: "I see that my moving around in the classroom bothers you, Miss Litten. Perhaps we can discuss this next Friday when the supervisor is in the building. She might have some suggestions that would work for both of us."

If neither of these approaches satisfies the positioning problem, Miss Robinson or the supervisor may have to educate Miss Litten that visual access to the interpreter is critical to the success of the interpreted message (Frishberg, 1990). It may be important to point out that interpreters for older students are more likely to stay seated during a 50-minute class, but that such a restriction contradicts what is best for an interpreter who works with a dynamic teacher who moves frequently and expects the children to move within the classroom space.

Certain responses to resistant teachers can actually be more counterproductive than no responses at all. Frances Block (1995), in her chapter, "Collaboration: Changing Times," provided alternative responses to resistant statements. I have adapted her examples to make them applicable to interpreters:

TEACHER: I don't want you to do that.

INTERPRETER: What precisely are your objections?

TEACHER: This is *not* the way we did it last year.

INTERPRETER: What activities that were done last year might be appropriate for this year?

TEACHER: The other teachers wouldn't do this.

INTERPRETER: Let's ask the other second-grade teachers and see what they recommend.

The supervisor's input on this matter may well troubleshoot future incidences. Sharing a class, sharing a room, sharing attention is sometimes difficult for those who have never worked with an interpreter. The supervisor's orientations should attend to these possible surprises so that their presence does not set up a negative relationship between teacher and interpreter that may never be rectified.

Departure Points for Discussion

1. What if Miss Litten's attitude toward Miss Robinson's placement continues to be negative?

2. Shouldn't the orientation of the classroom teacher to having an interpreter and a deaf student involve information about positioning and movement within the room?
3. How long should an interpreter attempt to "win over" resistant teachers before abandoning the cause as lost?
4. Can an interpreter and a teacher have a poor working relationship without impacting on the students' education?

The Case of the Inattentive Child

Robbie had not been diagnosed with ADHD but Mrs. Chew, his first grade teacher, and Carolyn, the interpreter, both agreed that his activity level was hyper and, at best, borderline disordered. He tended to disrupt the other students with his high energy level, impulsivity, and intrusions in their space, and he required lots of prompts to PAY ATTENTION. These prompts are the most recent issue.

After the workshop at the opening of the school year, Carolyn felt that Mrs. Chew had a good handle on her role in disciplining Robbie. One day after what seemed to Carolyn to have been a hundred attempts to direct Robbie to look at her, she decided to approach Mrs. Chew. Carolyn was really surprised at Mrs. Chew's reaction to her request that she take a more active role in disciplining Robbie. Mrs. Chew responded that Robbie's inattention was not a discipline problem; it was an interpreting problem, that he was obviously not mature enough to work with an interpreter. Mrs. Chew said she thought Robbie would be better off in the deaf class with other children who have additional learning needs and where the teacher could communicate with him directly. She indicated that she hadn't said anything prior to this discussion because she didn't want Carolyn to lose her job. How should Carolyn respond?

Suggested Best Practice   Robbie's needs are the central issue here, not Carolyn's job, not Mrs. Chew's read on his behaviors, and not Carolyn's read on Mrs. Chew's reaction. Both adults, however, should reassess their respective roles in responding to Robbie's needs. Mrs. Chew, as his teacher, should be concerned about his inattention to the interpreter because the interpreter represents Mrs. Chew's communication to Robbie and the rest of the class. Carolyn, as Robbie's interpreter, should be concerned about her ability to interpret if his inattention interferes with his comprehension and her ability to do an effective job.

Robbie's IEP team may have input on Robbie's placement, but they will need to be informed about the concerns expressed here. Carolyn and Mrs. Chew both see Robbie as a child with exceptional needs. Working in tandem to inform the IEP committee of their perceptions, and ensuring appropriate follow-up is recommended.

Departure Questions for Discussion

1. Why should the interpreter be responsible for flagging the student to attend? Why can't the teacher be responsible? Doesn't the teacher monitor all hearing students' attending behaviors?
2. How many times should an interpreter flag a young student who isn't attending? What constitutes *normal* inattention from *disordered* inattention? What differentiates a behavior disorder from a disciplinary problem?

3. What if Robbie is diagnosed with ADHD and prescribed medicine to subdue his hyperactivity? Should he then remain in the inclusion class or be placed in the special education class with other deaf students who have multiple needs?

4. Isn't Robbie's learning also an issue? No one mentioned his performance. Are we to assume he's on grade level?

The Case of the Brer Rabbit Stories

Jack's employment as an educational interpreter in a second-grade class with two deaf children met all his expectations. He found that he enjoyed the variety of roles he played, enjoyed the children (deaf and hearing alike), and was extremely satisfied with his position and the challenges it brought him. There was, however, one exception to his list of positive features, and Jack found the exception more and more frustrating: The librarian's weekly stories for three consecutive weeks had involved Brer Rabbit stories. Jack told her after the first week that if she planned to use the Uncle Remus book again, he would need to prepare, that the different voices were difficult for him, and that he had to struggle to follow her. Jack also shared that he didn't think the two deaf children had comprehended the dialect stuff, at least not like the hearing children. The librarian seemed somewhat surprised but indicated that she would try to choose something else the next time.

Unfortunately for Jack, the second week proved equally difficult with yet another Brer Rabbit story and lots of strange-sounding words that he just couldn't interpret. Once again, he spoke to the librarian and asked that if she intended to read from the book again, he would like to borrow a copy or be able to read with her, in order to figure out the language. Again, she agreed to stay away from the stories, only to read from the book the very next week. In the third week, however, she did tell Jack before the story began that she had tried to find another copy of the book but was unable to do so and that the children had showed so much interest in the stories that she was planning to continue using it for the duration of the spring. After hearing this, Jack found himself ready to explode. What should he do?

Suggested Best Practice   Exploding is not recommended as one of Jack's choices of action. In fact, responding to the librarian with anger would probably be more damaging to all involved than remaining composed and doing the best possible job he could do with the material. An issue exists, however, on the role of the interpreter in representing different, and sometimes difficult, dialects. Skilled interpreters who enjoy these challenges are generally adept at changing postural and facial expressions to represent a variety of speakers with a variety of dialects. Jack's discomfort with the task might be more of a concern than the librarian's continued persistence in reading the stories. In fact, Jack's involvement with second graders will probably meet with many more story challenges—Dr. Seuss books, Shel Silverstein books, and others. Six- and seven-year-olds love the play with language that dialects, limericks, and other "silly sounding stuff" provide. The educational interpreter needs to approach this play-with-the-sounds-of-language as play-with-the-*looks*-of-language. If this means securing an extra copy of a book or borrowing a book overnight, then, by all means, the work is well worth the effort. The child who is deaf or hard-of-hearing needs visual access to the information that hearing children have auditory access to. It is not always easy, but equalizing the target language and source language is what interpreting is all about—at any grade level and with any material.

Departure Points for Discussion

1. What if Jack does explode, actually "loses his cool" with the librarian? Should the teacher report Jack for his outburst?
2. What if the librarian reports Jack for his behaviors? Should the classroom teacher support Jack or support the librarian or stay out of it altogether?
3. What kinds of strategies should Jack use to make the dialects accessible?

The Case of the Aggressive Student

Albert was an aggressive student on the first day of kindergarten, on the second day, on the tenth day, and again today, Monday of the last week of this first six-week period. Albert's aggression included kicking, hitting, pushing, spitting, and biting; his parents were well aware of his daily outbursts because they saw the same behaviors at home. His parents were insistent, however, that as an intelligent young child, Albert belonged in the regular kindergarten class, not in a special class with other special children. Their insistence had resulted in several IEP rejections when the IEP team had recommended a smaller student–teacher ratio that was only possible by a placement in the special education classroom. Albert's enrollment in the kindergarten class had been agreed upon only if it indeed proved to be the least restrictive for him (and the least disruptive for the other children) after the first six-week trial period.

Here's where the interpreter, Beth, comes in. Beth had witnessed all the physical aggression Albert inflicted on other children and even on the teachers who attempted to settle him. Beth herself had never been a victim of his aggression; in fact, she seemed to be the only one capable of quieting Albert when he began his tantrums. For a couple of weeks now, Beth felt she was "reading" Albert better than she had earlier, that his outbursts were almost always attached to his inability to communicate his wants and needs directly with others. If Jeremy was on the swing, for example, and Albert wanted the swing, he simply pushed Jeremy off. He appeared to have no sense that he could make a request to another child, even in his sign language, and have that request honored.

The IEP team was to convene again Friday afternoon. Mrs. Logan, the kindergarten teacher, had documented 55 aggressive outbursts over the first five weeks of school, and even though a downward trend was apparent (17 outbursts the first week, 14 the second week, 10 the third week, 8 the fourth week, and 6 this past week), Mrs. Logan was eager to have Albert removed from her classroom. Beth's knowledge of the data, her increased sense that Albert's problems were communication-based, and her own success at settling Albert put her in an awkward situation. She wanted to go against Mrs. Logan's recommendation and suggest that he be continued in her class for a second six-weeks. She knew, though, that Mrs. Logan would reject her suggestion and that going against Mrs. Logan would probably jeopardize their relationship and possibly even work against Albert's successful integration into her class. What should Beth do?

Suggested Best Practice   Beth's dilemma appears to be a no-win situation. Her advocacy for Albert could be challenged by the IEP team members as inappropriate for her role as interpreter. Her challenge of Mrs. Logan's request could also be viewed as inappropriate for her role as interpreter. Beth obviously needs to discuss her opinions and dilemma with someone, preferably her supervisor. She may want to request confidentiality in sharing her thoughts with the supervisor. At the same time, she needs to be prepared for the supervisor to support Mrs. Logan and the other IEP team members if indeed they believe that Albert's placement is restrictive to him (and other children).

On the other hand, Beth may provide the supervisor with information that could be taken to the IEP meeting without involving Beth as an antagonist. As a product of their conversation, the supervisor may be willing to point to Albert's weekly improvement and match it with other evidence that shows growth in his language development. The supervisor may be able to present the information in such a way that the team agrees to support Albert's placement. The supervisor may even be able to suggest strategies for Mrs. Logan to use when working with Albert. As example, the supervisor might suggest that Mrs. Logan learn a few of the "settling" signs that Beth uses with Albert. Beth's role, then, to teach Mrs. Logan some signs, could possibly make their relationship even stronger, especially if Mrs. Logan experiences success in calming Albert and reducing his tantruming. Beth's best choice, then, is to be discreet in how she communicates her thoughts with the supervisor and to hope that the supervisor has the wisdom to support her thoughts without implicating her in a role conflict.

Departure Points for Discussion

1. Would this case have been handled differently if Beth had been a member of the collaborative team that determined Albert's placement?
2. At what point is it appropriate for the interpreter to advocate for her deaf student?
3. What if Beth's supervisor convinced the team to maintain Albert in his placement for yet another six weeks, and what if his behaviors become more aggressive, even with the interpreter?

The Case of the Parent Conference

Justin's parents are deaf. Parent–teacher conferences are scheduled for next Thursday night. Ms. Freemont, the first-grade teacher, received a note which she showed the interpreter, Mrs. Talbert. The note was from Justin's parents; they indicated that they would be at the conference and would need an interpreter. Ms. Freemont asked Mrs. Talbert if she was planning to interpret the conference, but Mrs. Talbert said she had plans to go to a conference with her own children's teachers and would not be available. The next day, Mrs. Talbert received a note from the principal indicating that she was expected to interpret the conference with Justin's parents and Ms. Freemont, and that she should make plans to arrive at 6:45 and stay through the evening (until 9:45) or until Justin's parents had finished their conference. Mrs. Talbert read the note with surprise, but thought that she could easily call Justin's parents and ask them to come early so she could interpret their conference, and still make her conferences with her own children's teachers. When she suggested this to Ms. Freemont, however, Ms. Freemont recommended that Mrs. Talbert make other arrangements for her own conferences and that she remember that she is just like the other teachers who have children in the school system—she is there as a professional, not as a parent. What should Mrs. Talbert do?

Suggested Best Practice   Mrs. Talbert's role as an educational interpreter may indeed include serving as interpreter for parent–teacher conferences. The assumption that she is to be the interpreter for parents of the child for whom she is employed is probably no more erroneous than her assumption that she would not be the interpreter for Justin's deaf parents. While some deaf parents may prefer to have an interpreter who is unrelated to their child's educational experiences, others may want to experience the same interpreter that their child experiences. Justin's parents, in asking Ms. Freemont to assure them that an interpreter would be present, were not asking that Mrs. Talbert, in particular, serve as the interpreter. At the same time, though, they did not ask that Mrs. Talbert *not* serve as their interpreter.

Mrs. Talbert would be well advised to review her policy manual and any formal documentation that might address her role outside the school day. Setting up an appointment with her supervisor or another administrator to discuss the expectations her principal and Ms. Freemont may have in this and other potential meetings with Justin's parents is important. Working out the logistics of these interpreting assignments should benefit Mrs. Talbert and other interpreters who find themselves in an awkward situation because of assumptions.

Departure Points for Discussion

1. What if the policy manual doesn't mention the interpreter's role outside the school day? Does Mrs. Talbert have cause for filing a grievance against the administration?
2. What if the parents ask Mrs. Talbert to interpret for them as they seek to conference with the P.E. teacher? the art teacher? the speech-language pathologist? Is Mrs. Talbert's assignment extended beyond the conference with Ms. Freemont? Would she be in trouble if she refused to interpret for other conferences?
3. What if Mrs. Talbert's salary is fixed, not hourly? Should she bill these additional hours to the school?

The Case of the Phone Call

Jennifer had just walked in the door when the phone rang. Mrs. Smith introduced herself as Thomas's mother and reminded Jennifer that they had met at the company picnic, in July just two months earlier. Jennifer responded that indeed she did remember her and that she was very much enjoying working with Thomas, that he was a bright and energetic first grader who brought her many smiles each day. Mrs. Smith went on to say that her reason for calling was to find out how Thomas was doing in the classroom, that she hoped he was behaving himself and following directions. Again, Jennifer responded that he was just wonderful, worked hard, cooperated with the teachers, and seemed to follow directions as well as any of the hearing children. Mrs. Smith asked if Jennifer had any trouble communicating with Thomas, if their sign systems were compatible; and again, Jennifer responded that Thomas was very easy to communicate with, that she occasionally used a sign that was different from his, and that he was quick to correct her. They both laughed, Mrs. Smith thanked her for her time, and they hung up.

Jennifer rushed through her evening chores and crawled into bed with another pleasant thought about Thomas and his mother. She wished she had remembered to tell Mrs. Smith about what he said that day to Loren when Loren wouldn't eat her grapes— Thomas had informed Loren in a very authoritative manner that grapes were good for her and she should eat them all. Loren had no trouble understanding Thomas's wise words. In fact, all the children communicated well with Thomas. His spoken language was particularly easy to understand and he signed in such a clear manner that the kids were picking up new signs everyday. Jennifer's next thought was that she would tell her about Thomas and

Loren the next time Mrs. Smith called her to ask about him. Then, like a bolt of lightening, it hit her: *Mrs. Smith had called her, the interpreter, to ask about Thomas.* Shouldn't she have called Mrs. Petruci, the teacher? Should Jennifer have referred her to Mrs. Petruci? What if Mrs. Smith did call Mrs. Petruci? Would she have told Mrs. Petruci that she had just talked with her? Should Jennifer have been so willing to talk about Thomas? Had Jennifer breached her contract? Had she violated her code of ethics? How in the world could she have been so casual? What should she do now?

Jennifer had a restless night, tossing and turning about her conversation with Mrs. Smith. She replayed it in her mind a hundred times, thinking that she should have referred Mrs. Smith to Mrs. Petruci. She practiced how she was going to tell Mrs. Petruci about Mrs. Smith's call. She hoped Mrs. Petruci would not be offended that she didn't refer Mrs. Smith to her. She hoped Mrs. Petruci would understand her spontaneity in talking about Thomas. She hoped Mrs. Smith hadn't called Mrs. Petruci, too, and already shared with her the conversation Jennifer had had with her. She worried all night about the best way to handle what she now felt was poor judgment on her part. What should she do now?

Suggested Best Practice   Some lessons are harder to learn than others. No doubt, many professional interpreters have found themselves in situations in which they were too quick to disclose, especially when the information being disclosed was pleasant. The fact remains, though, that Jennifer may have been out of line in talking to Mrs. Smith about Thomas. Mrs. Smith also may have been out of line in calling Jennifer to query her about Thomas, but only Jennifer's actions are to be judged here. Whether she breached her contract and violated her code of ethics is the question. Even if no harm was done, the fact that Jennifer is now struggling emotionally with her own behavior indicates that she has done some-thing wrong. How she rectifies the situation may not be nearly as important as the lesson she learned by finding herself in the situation.

Clearing her conscience is obviously important to Jennifer. She needs to address the issue with someone, and obviously she will talk to Mrs. Petruci about the phone call. Before she talks with Mrs. Petruci, though, Jennifer should benefit from talking to a mentor. Jennifer, like all interpreters, is human. Humans make errors in judgment—some more critical and serious than others, but all humans make errors in judgment at some point in their lives. No one is perfectly right in all decisions, in all actions, in all judgments. Linda Siple (1991), in "The Functions of Mentoring," discussed the psychological functions a mentor relationship enhances. She detailed these functions as the responsibility a mentor takes on in providing guidance to an interpreter who is less experienced. These functions include acceptance, confirmation, protection, coaching, and counseling. Jennifer, like all inter-preters, needs a relationship with someone to whom she can disclose her errors, someone who provides her with acceptance and feelings of protection in her need for confidentiality, and someone who can counsel and coach her through her experience so that she becomes a better interpreter as a result of the experience.

A breakfast meeting with or an early morning phone call to her mentor may provide Jennifer with the direction she needs to rectify her error. Jennifer's mentor would likely advise her that she should let Mrs. Petruci know she had a phone call from Mrs. Smith and that she is troubled by the conversation the two shared. Her mentor would likely share with her that she understands how something like this could happen and that she trusts in Jennifer's wisdom to learn from the situation. Her mentor would likely support her by reaf-firming her belief in her and by reminding her that as a professional, she recognizes and takes advantage of opportunities to learn and develop. Her mentor would be genuine in providing her with the colleagueship she needs at this time.

Jennifer's error in judgment may very well go no farther than the sleepless night, the helpful conversation with her mentor, and a conversation with Mrs. Petruci about the phone call. Mrs. Petruci may agree to follow up with a phone call to Mrs. Smith, a call in which she offers her an opporunity to talk about Thomas. Mrs. Petruci may, by virtue of calling Mrs. Smith herself, provide a subtle message that she is the person to whom Mrs. Smith should address her concerns about Thomas. Mrs. Petruci may even ask Mrs. Smith if she would like a formal conference with her, or with her and Jennifer. Mrs. Smith would hopefully infer from Mrs. Petruci's call that future phone calls or requests for conferences should be directed to her. Mrs. Smith would also hopefully infer that Jennifer's relationship with Mrs. Petruci is bonded by a professional collegiality, and that the two together have a commitment to Thomas. If these lessons are learned, then all parties—Jennifer, Mrs. Petruci, Mrs. Smith, the mentor, and Thomas—will have benefited.

Departure Points for Discussion

1. What was "wrong" with Jennifer's behavior?
2. Is it possible to rectify or fix mistakes once they've been made?
3. Would sharing this story benefit other interpreters who might also find themselves vulnerable to parents' phone calls?
4. But, would sharing Jennifer's story expose Jennifer in a way that violates her right to confidentiality?

Summary

This chapter focuses on the interpreter's role in early childhood settings. Young deaf and hard-of-hearing students present many challenges to educational interpreters. Their developmental needs require an interpreter whose knowledge of normal cognitive, social, and linguistic development is strong. At the same time, interpreting for children with cochlear implants and children with additional medical and psychological needs often raises issues that challenge even a confident interpreter's sense of what is normal cognitive, social, linguistic development. Likewise, the curriculum demands in a preschool or primary educational setting are such that the educational interpreter frequently plays multiple roles—helper, language teacher, communication facilitator, observer, and reporter. These roles may be awkward for some interpreters and teachers. Working through awkward situations, such as those provided here as difficult case stories, should strengthen the interpreter's knowledge, skills, and attitudes and enable the interpreter to be a strong member of the student's educational teams. Discussing decisions about fingerspelling, inventing signs, teaching signs, interpreting stories, and what perspective to take in setting up spatial propositions with selected members of the teaching team, may also be important to the success of the interpreter and the student in these primary grades.

REFERENCES

Antia, S. D. (1982). Social interaction of partially mainstreamed hearing-impaired children. *American Annals of the Deaf, 127,* 18–25.

———. (1998). School and classroom characteristics that facilitate the social integration of deaf and hard of hearing children. In A. Weisel (Ed.), *Issues unresolved: New perspectives on language and deaf education.* Washington, DC: Gallaudet University Press.

Arnold, D., & Tremblay, A. (1979). Interaction of deaf and hearing preschool children. *Journal of Communication Disorders, 12,* 245–251.

Baron-Cohen, S. (1995). *Mindblindness: An essay on autism and theory of mind.* Cambridge, MA: M.I.T. Press.

Block, F. K. (1995). Collaboration: Changing times. In D. F. Tibbits (Ed.), *Language intervention: Beyond the primary grades* (pp. 61–136). Austin, TX: Pro-ed.

Bloom, L. (1970). *Language development: Form and function in emerging grammars.* Cambridge, MA: M.I.T. Press.

Bloom, P. (2000). *How children learn the meanings of words.* Cambridge, MA: M.I.T. Press.

Bornstein, H., Saulnier, K., & Hamilton, L. (1973–1984). *The signed English series.* Washington, DC: Gallaudet College Press.

Boswell, S. (1999). Wired for sound: Cochlear technology takes off. *The ASHA Leader, 4,* 1, 6.

Brown, R. (1973). *A first language: The early stages.* Cambridge: Harvard University Press.

Carney, A. E., & Moeller, M. P. (1998). Treatment efficacy: Hearing loss in children. *Journal of Speech, Language, and Hearing Research, 41,* 561–584.

Connor, C. M., Hieber, S., Arts, H. A., & Zwolan, T. A. (2000). Speech, vocabulary, and the education of children using cochlear implants: Oral or total communication? *Journal of Speech, Language, and Hearing Research, 43,* 1185–1204.

Corballis, M. C. (1983). *Human laterality.* New York: Academic Press.

Creaghead, N. A., & Ripich, D. N. (1994). Introduction to school discourse problems. In D. N. Ripich & N. A. Creaghead (Eds.), *School discourse problems* (2nd ed.), (pp. 1–6). San Diego: Singular Publishing Group.

Dahl, C., & Wilcox, S. (1990). Preparing the educational interpreter: A survey of sign language interpreter training programs. *American Annals of the Deaf, 135,* 275–279.

Erting, C. J., Prezioso, C., & O'Grady-Hynes, M. (1990). The interactional context of deaf mother-infant communication. In V. Volterra & C. J. Erting (Eds.), *From gesture to language in hearing and deaf children* (pp. 97–106). Berlin, Germany: Springer.

Frishberg, N., (1990). *Interpreting: An introduction.* Silver Spring, MD: RID Publications.

Geers, A., Spehar, B., & Sedey, A. (2002). Use of speech by children from total communication programs who wear cochlear implants. *American Journal of Speech-Language Pathology, 11,* 50–58.

Groode, J. L. (1992). *Fingerspelling: Expressive and receptive fluency* (video). San Diego: Dawn Sign Press.

Hedge, M. N. & Davis, D. (1995). *Clinical methods and practicum in speech-language pathology* (2nd ed). San Diego: Singular Publishing Group.

Hulsing, M. M., Luetke-Stahlman, B., Loeb, D. F., Nelson, P., & Wegner, J., (1995). Analysis of successful initiations of three children with hearing loss mainstreamed in kindergarten classrooms. *Language, Speech, and Hearing Services in Schools, 26,* 45–57.

Humphrey, J. H., & Alcorn, B. J. (1994). *So you want to be an interpreter: An introduction to sign language interpreting.* Salem, OR: Sign Enhancers.

Joint Committee of the American Speech-Language-Hearing Association and the Council on Education of the Deaf. (1995). Technical report: Service provision under the Individuals with Disabilities Education Act—Part H, as Amended (IDEA—Part H) to children who are deaf and hard of hearing, ages birth to 36 months. *American Annals of the Deaf, 140,* 65–70.

Kluwin, T. N., & Stewart, D. (2000). Cochlear implants for younger children: A preliminary description of the parental decision process and outcomes. *American Annals of the Deaf, 145,* 26–32.

Luetke-Stahlman, B. (1991). Hearing-impaired preschoolers in integrated child care. *Perspectives in Education and Deafness, 9,* 8–11.

———. (1992). Sign interpretation in preschool. *Perspectives in Education and Deafness, 10,* 12–15.

Marschark, M. (1997). *Raising and educating a deaf child: A comprehensive guide to the choices, controversies, and decisions faced by parents and educators.* New York: Oxford University Press.

Marschark, M., Lang, H. G., & Albertini, J. A. (2002). *Educating deaf students: From research to practice.* New York: Oxford University Press.

Masataka, N. (1996). Perception of motherese in a signed language by 6-month-old deaf infants. *Developmental Psychology, 32,* 874–879.

Masataka, N. (2000). The role of modality and input in the earliest stage of language acquisition: Studies of Japanese Sign Language. In C. Chamberlain, J. P. Morford, & R. I. Mayberry (Eds.), *Language acquisition by eye* (pp. 3–24). Mahwah, NJ: Lawrence Erlbaum Associaties.

Mather, S., & Winston, E. (1998). Spatial mapping and involvement in ASL storytelling. In C. Lucas (Ed.), *Pinky extension and eye gaze: Language use in deaf communities* (pp. 183–210). Washington, DC: Gallaudet University Press.

Metzger, M. (1999). *Sign language interpreting: Deconstructing the myth of neutrality.* Washington, DC: Gallaudet University Press.

Miller, G. A., & Gildea, P. M. (1987). How children learn words. *Scientific American, 257,* 94–99.

Niparko, J. K., Cheng, A. K., & Francis, H. W. (2000). Outcomes of cochlear implantation: Assessment of quality of life impact and economic evaluation of the benefits of the cochlear implant in relation to costs. In J. K. Niparko, K. I. Kirk, N. K. Mellon, A. M. Robbins, D. L. Tucci, & B. S. Wilson (Eds.), *Cochlear implants: Principles and practices* (pp. 269–288). Philadelphia: Lippincott Williams & Wilkins.

Norris, J. A., & Damico, J. S. (1990). Whole language in theory and practice: Implications for language intervention. *Language, Speech, and Hearing Services in Schools, 21,* 212–220.

Otis-Wilborn, A. (1992). Developing oral communication in students with hearing impairments: Whose responsibility? *Language, Speech, and Hearing Services in Schools, 23,* 71–77.

Owens, R. (1996). *Language development: An introduction* (4th ed.). Boston: Allyn & Bacon.

Padden, C. (1991). The acquisition of fingerspelling by deaf children. In P. Siple & S. Fischer (Eds.), *Theoretical issues in sign language research: Volume 2: Psychology* (pp. 191–210). Chicago: University of Chicago Press.

Ramsey, C. L. (1997). *Deaf children in public schools: Placement, context, and consequences.* Washington, DC: Gallaudet University Press.

Registry of Interpreters for the Deaf. (1995). Code of Ethics of The Registry of Interpreters for the Deaf, Inc. *RID Membership Directory.* Silver Spring, MD: RID Publications.

Ross, M., Brackett, D., & Maxon, A. B. (1982). *Hard of hearing children in regular schools.* Englewood Cliffs, NJ: Prentice Hall.

Roy, C. B. (2002). An interpreting puzzle: Math equations. *RID Views, 19,* 13.

Rudser, S. F. (1986). The RID Code of Ethics, confidentiality, and supervision. *RID Journal of Interpretation, 3,* 47–52.

Samar, V. J., Parasnis, I., & Berent, G. P. (1998). Learning disabilities, attention deficit disorders, and deafness. In M. Marschark & M. D. Clark (Eds.), *Psychological perspectives on deafness, Vol. 2* (pp. 199–242). Mahwah, NJ: Lawrence Erlbaum Associates.

Schick, B. (2001). Interpreting for children: How it's different. *Odyssey, 2,* 8–11.

Schirmer, B. R. (2000). *Language and literacy development in children who are deaf.* Boston: Allyn & Bacon.

Seal, B. C. (2000). Working with educational interpreters. *Language, Speech, and Hearing Services in Schools, 31,* 15–25.

Shaw, J., & Jamieson, J. (1997). Patterns of classroom discourse in an integrated, interpreted elementary school setting. *American Annals of the Deaf, 142,* 40–47.

Shroyer, E. H., & Compton, M. V., (1994). Educational interpreting and teacher preparation: An interdisciplinary model. *American Annals of the Deaf, 139,* 472–479.

Siple, L. A., (1991). The functions of mentoring. *RID Views, 8,* 28–29.

Spencer, P., Koester, L. S., & Meadow-Orlans, K., (1994). Communicative interactions of deaf and hearing children in a day care center. *American Annals of the Deaf, 139,* 512–518.

Supalla, S. (1995). *The book of name signs: Naming in American Sign Language.* San Diego: Dawn Sign Press.

Tinsley, K. A. (2001). Educational interpreting for special needs students. *RID Views, 18,* 1, 6.

Tye-Murray, N., Spencer, L., & Woodworth, G. (1995). Acquisition of speech by children who have prolonged cochlear implant experience. *Journal of Speech and Hearing Research, 38,* 327–337.

Wegner, J., & Swartzman-Waters, P. (1994). Communicative interactions with and without an interpreter. Paper presented at the American Speech-Language-Hearing Association Convention, New Orleans.

Wilde, S. (1989). Looking at invented spelling: A kidwatcher's guide to spelling, Part 1. In K. S. Goodman, Y. M. Goodman, & W. J. Hood (Eds.), *The whole language evaluation book* (pp. 213–226). Portsmouth, NH: Heinemann Educational Books.

Winston, E. (1994). An interpreted education: Inclusion or exclusion? In R. C. Johnson & O. P. Cohen (Eds.), *Implications and complications for deaf students of the full inclusion movement.* Gallaudet Research Institute Occasional Paper 94-2. Washington, DC: Gallaudet University.

Witter-Merithew, A., & Dirst, R. (1982). Preparation and use of educational interpreters. In D. G. Sims, G. G. Walter, & R. L. Whitehead (Eds.), *Deafness and communication: Assessment and training* (pp. 395–406). Baltimore: Williams & Wilkins.

Yoshinaga-Itano, C. (2000). Successful outcomes for deaf and hard-of-hearing children. *Seminars in Hearing, 21,* 309–326.

4 Best Practices in Interpreting in the Elementary- and Middle-School Setting

The scope of issues surrounding educational interpreting for elementary- and middle-school students is extensive. The questions and answers presented in this chapter should provide interpreters and their educational colleagues with a meaningful exploration of some of these issues.

Question 1: What is expected of the educational interpreter in elementary- and middle-school settings?

The elementary- and middle-school years pose many interesting challenges for educational interpreters. Just as the preschool- and primary-aged student presents an ever-changing development, so does the pre- and early-adolescent student present a changing profile that varies both within the individual and between individuals at any given period. The educational interpreter who has an appreciation for the changing profile that characterizes this age group is probably an interpreter who is experienced with this particular age group. Interpreters who have no experience, either personally or professionally, with third, fourth, fifth, sixth, seventh, and even some eighth graders, will probably learn early in their work with this age group that a critical part of the changing profile involves the development of social competence.

A growing body of literature attests to the recognition that a child's social competence from 8 to 12 or 13 years of age is defined by relationships. Several categories of relationships can be found in the educational setting: peer relationships that exist between and among students who are deaf, hearing, and hard-of-hearing; teacher-student relationships; teacher-interpreter relationships; teacher-student-interpreter relationships; and the broader category of relationships that exist within educational communities.

Interpreters in the middle- and upper-elementary school grades, must be sensitive to and knowledgeable of the dynamics involved in each of these relationships. Tanya Gallagher (1993) addressed language competence and its effect on peer relationships during these changing years. She described two kinds of peer friendships: *friendships of popularity* that occur when one is liked or accepted by one's peers, and *close friendships or chumships* that occur when mutual needs for intimacy are met.

The first friendship, friendship of popularity, is evidenced in group behavior. Students in the elementary- and middle-school age group are likely to want to dress *like*, look *like*, and have things just *like* their peers whom they perceive as popular. Being different, especially different enough to have an interpreter, may challenge the student's sense of self-esteem and impact negatively on the student's relationships with peers. Gallagher (1993) reported that during the upper-elementary school grades, "when self-presentation and peer group inclusion are highly valued," students with limited language skills "could become the focus of negative peer attention" (p. 203).

I recall three different stories of young deaf girls who, each at about the fourth to fifth grade, experienced emotional struggles over their differences. In the first story, the mother of a very bright, attractive, and financially advantaged girl, was devastated when her deaf daughter told her and her father that they could no longer sign to her when they went out to dinner—because, as she indicated, she wanted to pretend to be hearing. In the second story, the mother of a very popular deaf girl was worried when her daughter was feeling left out because her two best friends since first grade had become very talkative on the telephone in the afternoons. Her daughter wanted to become hearing so she, too, could talk on the telephone. In the third story, the mother of a very capable young girl who moved comfortably between sign language and spoken language indicated that their compliant and sweet daughter was becoming defiant and resistant, both at home and at school. There were indications that the daughter was becoming increasingly rude and inconsiderate to her interpreter, a woman she had previously adored.

An educational interpreter who recognizes the need for the deaf or hard-of-hearing student to be acclimated in the larger group probably experiments to find the most appropriate avenue for interpreting social exchanges. As the interpreter gains familiarity with different communication behaviors in the classroom, especially those behaviors that constitute "side" conversations, the interpreter should become more proficient in representing the different communication behaviors—even the slang, sarcasm, and slander that are common to these side conversations. Certainly, a hands-off role is most appropriate for intimate communication behaviors or when social exchanges involving the deaf student are successful *without* the interpreter. Indeed, the fourth grader who treated her interpreter with growing obstinacy actually became quite competent in letting her interpreter know when she needed her. The student grew to handle her own in-group exchanges during in-class and out-of-class activities that are so rich for social development. Right or wrong, her growing obstinacy appeared to be the only way she knew to declare her independence from the interpreter in situations that were to shape or define her social competence.

The interpreter's role in facilitating or enabling peer relationships may well become the standard for his or her role in all the other relationships found in the classroom. Just as the successful interpreter experiments to find the best approach for side conversations and personal exchanges, so does the successful interpreter take time to learn to *read* the teacher's communication style and the communication styles of the deaf student(s), hearing students, and various other teachers who also may be part of the classroom or educational environment.

Jon Nussbaum (1992) described communicator style as bound by the "individual's particular style of communication, by the course content, level of the class, size of the class, and so on" (p. 147). Courtney Cazden (1988) referred to the communication of a classroom as bound by a tripartite: "the language of curriculum, the language of control, and the language of personal identity" (p. 3). The successful interpreter takes a few days to learn how to represent the communication of the classroom, particularly the communication styles of the teacher and the individuals with whom the teacher communicates. Within a short time, the successful interpreter learns to anticipate signals, even subtle changes, which represent changes in an individual's communication style. Some of these signaling devices may require direct interpretation; others may require a hands-off approach so that the student's attention is fully directed to the teacher or another communication source. Although probably not an exhaustive list, Table 4.1 lists signaling strategies that should be developed by the interpreter within the early days of the school term.

TABLE 4.1   Signaling Strategies Useful in Interpreting Communication Style

- Signaling time to attend
- Signaling the importance or perceived lack of importance of announcements and assignments
- Signaling time to put away, to get out, and transitions from one activity or lesson to another
- Signaling interruptions, especially student interruptions that may also signal confusion or lack of attention
- Signaling communication control and the relinquishing of control
- Signaling humor, anger, and emotionally linked changes in communication mood
- Signaling language of negotiation and compromise, of behavior control and manipulation
- Signaling positive feedback, negative feedback, and feedback that is emotionally neutral
- Signaling questions and their intent: procedural, introducing, eliciting, probing, redirecting, expanding, clarifying, justifying, closing

Most of these signaling devices occur nonverbally or nonmanually—that is, facial expressions, hand waving (Bienvenu & Colonomos, 1985–1988), postural changes, rate variations, and intensity changes (largeness and smallness) of the interpreted message serve to cue additional meaning to the linguistic message that is interpreted. Effective interpreters, like effective teachers, are also consistent in their own communication style so that the deaf or hard-of-hearing student, as well as *all* other students and the teacher(s), become acclimated to the signals, to the standard that defines communication exchanges. Once the signals are established, once the standard is set, once everyone is comfortable with the communication style of the others, the classroom then takes on its own communication style. Imagine the following classroom scene:

> MRS. R: The geological structure of the Piedmont differs from the geological struc-
> ture of the Tidewater in several ways. We discussed three of these ways yesterday.
> Who can tell me three differences between the geology of the Piedmont and the
> geology of the Tidewater?

Ten or 12 hands go up immediately, with nonverbal grunts, whole body moves, and facial expressions that say "I know-I know!" In the 10-second wait for the teacher to select a respondent, the deaf student's hand goes up—as high as all the others—and the teacher calls on the deaf student to respond.

The interpreter's style in this scene first should represent the teacher's style: formal, deliberate, authoritative, a deliverer of important information. The interpreter's posture in matching the teacher's style should take on the formality, the deliberateness and importance of the topic. As the question is asked, however, and the hands fly up, the interpreter should change her communication style with a change in facial expression that signals the students' eagerness to respond. A shift in body posture and eye gaze should reflect hands up, with points to those hands that are raised. Then the interpreter must return to the teacher's role, signaling the silence or the wait, the surveying that the teacher demonstrates as she chooses a student to respond. During this wait, and immediately after the teacher calls on the deaf student to respond, the interpreter must determine how she or he will interpret the teacher's choice, whether to:

1. Fingerspell or cue or sign the deaf student's name as the teacher calls it;
2. Point to the deaf student and mouth his name to signal that he has been selected to respond; or
3. Remain posed as the teacher is, seeing that the deaf student has read the teacher's call on him without the interpreter's involvement.

As the deaf student begins to respond, the interpreter must make yet another decision. This time perceived intelligibility of the student's response, personal desire of the student (especially of older students), teacher's responsiveness to the deaf student's response, and perceived responsiveness of the classmates are all factors in selecting the right choice from among the following three possible choices:

1. To take on the student's voice, delivering the response to the teacher (and class), reflecting the same sense of confidence or caution in the response that the student shows while answering;
2. To assume a silent posture, waiting for the student to respond in whatever communication mode is most comfortable, and possibly repeating the response *if* the teacher shows difficulty understanding; or
3. To assume a silent posture, waiting for the student to respond in his most comfortable communication mode, and depending on the teacher to echo the student's response for all students to understand.

Although the interpreter's choice is important in setting the precedent for later expectations, it is also important for the interpreter to recognize that neither of these three choices will always be right. The *comprehensibility* of a deaf student's spoken language is influenced by many variables (Barefoot, Bochner, Johnson, & vom Eigen, 1993), especially the listeners' familiarity with the topic, the listeners' familiarity with the speaker, and the listeners' experiences in making judgments or observations about the intelligibility of the student's response. Barefoot and his colleagues reported that the comprehensibility of their students' communication was positively and significantly related to the English language proficiency demonstrated by the students and to their speech intelligibility. The interpreter's responsibility, then, includes an awareness of the comprehensibility of the deaf student's communication to all others in the classroom environment, and awareness of a change in the comprehensibility of the student's communication as others in the classroom become familiar with the student's communication.

Courtney Cazden (1988) described classroom vignettes like this one involving the geology of the Piedmont and Tidewater, as a three-part sequence—teacher initiation, student response, teacher evaluation. She reported that this sequence is "the most common pattern of classroom discourse at all grade levels" (p. 29). She also explained that as humans we search for repeated patterns and draw from them the discourse "rules" that we grow to depend on. Once we decipher the rules and learn to abide by the rules (including those that are unwritten and never discussed), we demonstrate a type of communication competence. The classroom example just described is likely to be repeated hundreds of times within a typical school week. Every time this Initiation-Response-Evaluation, or IRE, sequence is repeated, students in the classroom become more comfortable in expecting certain behaviors from their teacher, from each other, and from the interpreter. Within a few days and a few hundred practices, everyone in the classroom learns the standards or rules of expected communication behaviors. Knowing the rules and abiding by them leads to communication competence. The cycle continues: Communication competence leads to the building of relationships, especially relationships that indicate group or peer acceptance. Once relationships are built, social competence develops. The interpreter's role, then, is important to the student's successful development of social competence.

Before leaving this topic of social competence, a look at instructional groups is important. Grouping within the class (intraclass groupings) is a common procedure for students in or approaching the middle school grades. Several characteristics of the 10-, 11-, and 12-year-old support peer grouping within the class. Chris Stevenson and Judy Carr (1993) explained that in the preadolescent years, students are "inclined to describe themselves in terms of what they can do. Being a worker, being a producer, and being known by others and for those traits become increasingly important to healthy identity development" (p. 14). Teachers who recognize the power of social relationships in facilitating healthy identity development also "recognize their responsibility in helping children acquire the social skills needed for getting along with others and for becoming effective group members" (Shepherd & Ragan, 1992, p. 107). These teachers frequently organize their instructional activities in one of three types of groups: *skill* groups, *interest* groups, and *project* groups (Shepherd & Ragan, 1992).

Skill groups are generally homogenous, with students who have a particular cognitive or physical skill or readiness for a task grouped together to perform that skill or task. For example, students who are skilled in written language might be grouped together to create a poem following a fieldtrip to a museum; students who are skilled in drawing and painting might be grouped together to paint a wall collage about a history theme. In contrast, interest and project groups are generally more mixed or heterogenous in their members' skills and knowledge. During an ecology unit, for example, students who are interested in studying solid waste management using the computer might be grouped together; students interested in interviewing members of the city council regarding the volunteer recycling program might be grouped together; those interested in studying the soil, zoning, and public water maps of the city might be in another group; and those interested in measuring and graphing their own roadside trash collection efforts might work in a different group.

The communication that occurs in each of these three types of groups will differ from the communication that occurs in the larger group or in the whole class. The "limitations and rigidities characteristic of most teacher–student interactions" (Cazden, 1988, p.134) are lifted in peer group interactions. We could assume that this *lifting* of teacher influence would enable all students in the group to speak or sign and interact freely. A different type of communication hierarchy is likely to emerge, however, depending on who constitutes the group. Speaking roles in groups most likely reflect the students' perceptions of which group members are best at a particular skill or have the most knowledge about a particular topic. High-status and low-status perceptions will dictate communication patterns in intraclass groups. One or two students in a group of five or six will dominate the talk or sign time. Other students will respond with various levels of passivity or activity, contingent on how the high-status members attempt to and succeed at engaging them.

The interpreter's influence on facilitating positive perceptions or inhibiting negative perceptions of the student who is deaf or hard-of-hearing is an interesting area to ponder. Some educational interpreters may find themselves playing a more active interpreting role in interest and project groups than in skill groups, especially if the communication skills of the skill group's members are rather horizontal or homogenous. In homogenous groups, the hearing and deaf students may interact more willingly and more often without the interpreter than with the interpreter present. The interpreter's sensitivity to group interaction patterns, then, is critical in making decisions about close or remote availability. The interpreter may need to be within ear shot of the group in order to interpret as needed, or the interpreter may need to be within eye shot—be able to see the group and its individual members—but able only to hear the collective buzz that is created by all the groups. The interpreter may also need to rove with the teacher so that any bid for the teacher's intervention would signal a bid for the interpreter's intervention.

In contrast, in heterogenous or mixed groups, the interpreter may need to be a member of the group in order to interpret. Finding the best location within the group may depend on several factors. We might assume that the interpreter should find a position that opposes the deaf student's position for the best visual access to the interpretation and all the members represented in the interpretation. In some groups, however, the interpreter might be better positioned near the member(s) who is(are) likely to have the highest perceived status within the group, and, consequently, the most talk or sign time.

Teachers who change groups routinely, either with seating assignments or project assignments, are likely to experiment to find the best possible group match. Similarly, educational interpreters are advised to experiment with groups to find the best possible match in meeting the communication and social competence needs of the deaf and hard-of-hearing student. The following vignette represents such a case where experimentation is appropriate:

> Four deaf boys, ages 11 to 12, attended homeroom with another 18 hearing students in their local middle school. On Thursdays, homeroom was extended 40 minutes for critical thinking activities, and an educational interpreter came in. On the day observed, each of the four deaf students was assigned to a different group at a different table that held a stack of newspapers. The assignment was to sort through the newspapers and locate headlines that represented **world**, **national**, **state**, and **local** news. One of each of the four headlines was then to be cut out and taped onto a single sheet of paper, with each student's signature to indicate full participation in the activity.
>
> The interpreter accompanied the teacher to the first table where a deaf student sat holding a newspaper and watching the other three hearing students talk about the activity. She interpreted the teacher's question: "How's it going?" One of the hearing students answered, "We've already found a national headline. This one works, doesn't it?" The teacher affirmed their choice and then asked, "What about you, Derek, what are you searching for?" And Derek, the deaf student, responded, "I don't know."
>
> The same sense of isolation appeared to occur at one of the other tables where the sole deaf student sat observing without any interaction. At the third table, a hearing girl was using lots of fingerspelling as she attempted to engage her table's deaf student. And at the fourth table, the deaf student who used relatively intelligible spoken English seemed to be telling the other students what to do.

The interpreter's role in this classroom is clearly complicated by the group membership, and her frustration at feeling ineffective is understandable. To her credit, the observation needed by this teacher who made the assignments is probably facilitated by the interpreter's presence at her side. Had the interpreter taken upon herself a separation from the teacher, moving from one table to the next and the next and back again to interpret, the teacher could be misled that all is well. In contrast, the teacher realized the awkwardness of the group memberships and suggested that they try different groupings over the weeks to come.

Question 2: How should the interpreter deal with textbook language in the curriculum?

Prior to about the third grade (for some children, the second grade), the student is taught language as an end. That is, the curriculum that teaches reading, writing, mathematics, social studies, and so on, is a curriculum that attempts to provide the student with educational tools that can be used from that point in matriculation on. A first-grade student is taught to read, but a sixth-grade student is expected to use his or her reading skills in order to be taught—taught different writing styles, different languages, different social structures, different math formulas, different problem-solving strategies, different content in a multitude of different subjects. The student who enters a third-grade class, then, enters with a preparation to use what was previously learned to learn much more. Both the educational process and the product change.

Most of the changing curriculum that occurs from about third or fourth grade on involves textbooks. Indeed, many school subjects or curricula are centered around a particular textbook series or publisher's series of books. An estimated 75% of classroom time is focused on textbooks, the "single most available and widely utilized curriculum document" (Shepherd & Ragan, 1992, p. 217). Sandra Tattershall (1994) explained that even children who do well in the primary grades with word decoding and story reading often experience difficulty when their learning is later bound to the more complex language of textbooks. From grade to grade, these books are written with increasingly more complex sentence structure and increasingly more abstract vocabulary. Their "story grammar" is different, with more "reporting, summarizing, comparing, clarifying, classifying" (Shepherd & Ragan, 1992, p. 349) than books classified as literature. Textbooks are filled with descriptions, lists, and expository text that become increasingly less personal, less predictable, and less pleasurable to read than books used in the primary grades. Cynthia King and Stephen Quigley (1985), in their book *Reading and Deafness*, discussed four variables that influence text difficulty: vocabulary, syntax, discourse structure, and format. A look at these and their impact on interpreting follows.

Vocabulary is particularly difficult when frequently occurring words, or high-frequency words, are replaced with low-frequency synonyms, when new vocabulary words are placed in important propositions, and when vocabulary is highly figurative. Educational interpreters understandably are challenged by difficult textbook vocabulary. The search for synonyms to use in interpreting the vocabulary of textbook language is never-ending. (The notion of semantic flexibility that was discussed in Chapter 3 is critical here, too.) Some interpreters, in preparing for difficult vocabulary, rely on the textbook's index or glossary of terms. Interpreters frequently refer to their own pocket thesaurus as a resource for synonymous vocabulary. When the synonymous sign is used to define another word or concept, however, the skilled interpreter must rely on a supplemental interpretation (fingerspelling or cueing or oral interpreting) to discriminate the terminology.

Imagine, for example, the interpreter's choice of signs for this propositional sentence: *Pioneers were early settlers who traveled to a new area in hopes of establishing a home for their families.* Synonyms offered for PIONEER include SETTLER and IMMIGRANT. Using the same sign for two words when one is defining the other can be very confusing unless the spoken language or fingerspelling or cued speech supplement clarifies that the terms are interchangeable. Successful interpreters find strategies that identify synonymous forms or that signal that one sign is used to represent words that are synonymous.

Successful interpreters are also diligent in their search for signs that may already exist. The National Technical Institute for the Deaf (NTID) began a technical signs project in the early 1970s. Their project resulted in the documentation of thousands of technical sign videotapes that are available for purchase and for loan through Captioned Films/Videos for the Deaf, Modern Talking Picture Services (1988). In using the vocabulary list from the NTID Technical Signs Project (TSP), I was able to locate signs for SOLUTION, DENSITY, FORM, and BASE, which appear in this seventh-grade science project:

> When two liquid solutions are mixed together and a solid appears in the container, you have a precipitate which has formed. A precipitate has a greater density than the liquids and can be centrifuged to the bottom of a tube with the use of centripetal force. Some liquids will precipitate only in an acid solution, some only in a base solution and some will precipitate in both acid and base solutions. The formation of precipitates is dependent upon the type of ions in the solutions.

Clearly, the vocabulary in this paragraph presents several low-frequency words that are not likely to be in the everyday vocabulary of most interpreters. Relying on technical sign resources such as those provided by NTID, newly emerging web-based sign dictionaries and CDs, and traditional sign dictionaries, such as *Signs for Science and Mathematics: A resource book for teachers and students* (Caccamise & Lang, 2000), is important. Abundant fingerspelling is also appropriate when these resources fail to yield a sign-word match and when creating initialized signs to represent the most prominent words. In fact, Carol Padden and Claire Ramsey (2000) reported a strong relationship between skills in fingerspselling, identifying initialized signs, and reading achievement in their fourth- and seventh-grade subjects.

Discussion of vocabulary learning in Chapter 2 suggested that a hearing 6-year-old's vocabulary contains about 20,000 words. Between 6 and 10 years of age, we expect this vocabulary to double, with students learning 6 to 12 new words a day. Another 20,000 to 40,000 words are also added between the ages of

10 and 17 (Bloom, 2000; Miller & Gildea, 1987). Paul Bloom, in discussing this mysterious acquisition, stated: "All we can say with certainty is that word learning typically reaches its peak not at 18 months but somewhere between 10 and 17 years" (p. 45). Marilyn Nippold (1998) shared some of these words for us to con-template: Most fourth graders know the words *dodge, locket, tangle,* and *widow;* most sixth graders know *adhesive, bridal, campus,* and *grit;* and most eighth graders know *amend, fluorescent, horoscope,* and *lingerie* (p. 14). Their knowledge of these words is highly dependent upon their exposure to them in school. Direct instruc-tion ("A *widow* is a woman whose husband has died. How do you think the black widow spider got her name?") is used by many teachers, but even the best teach-ers are unlikely to teach their students 4,000 to 5,000 new words a year. Exposure to most new words comes from the textbook where literate students *and literate interpreters* rely on context ("Double-sided tape has *adhesive* on both sides.") and grammatical analysis ("The First *Amend*ment to the Constitution guarantees free-dom of speech.") to learn their meanings.

Growth in word knowledge during this middle childhood period also involves acquiring new meanings for previously learned vocabulary (Nippold, 1998). Words with multiple meanings are especially common to the language of mathematics and its extensive use of prepositions: The stock market is *up;* our time is *up;* count *up* to 60 (p. 22). Words that modify, particularly adverbs of likeli-hood *(apparently, probably, definitely)* and magnitude *(considerable, somewhat, rather)* emerge during these years (p. 25). Words that refer to metacognitive and metalin-guistic functions (particularly verbs of thinking—*be sure, figure, imply*) are used with increasing accuracy in this same developmental period (Nippold, 1998, pp. 27). Successful sign language interpreters who provide *meaningful* access to these words are likely themselves to have broad vocabularies (in both ASL and English), broad facility in adding adverbial nonmanuals and directional verbs (Winston, 1989), and broad flexibility in moving between English-based signing (finger-spelling, selective initializing, and inventing signs) and ASL.

Syntax complexity, another variable that impacts on the readability of a textbook, is frequently discussed in terms of sentence length and grammatical structure. King and Quigley (1985) reported that sentence length is not necessar-ily a measure of difficulty. Imagine, to illustrate, interpreting the sentence: *To be or not to be, that is the question.* The use of an infinitive verb "to be" and its negated alternative "not to be" as a subject phrase that is further represented by a pronoun "that" makes this rather short sentence difficult to interpret. The experienced educational interpreter may negotiate four or five versions in providing the most appropriate interpretation for Shakespeare's language. In fact, interpreting this sentence with multiple versions may indeed make the meaning more accessible, rather than more vague, to the deaf or hard-of-hearing student. Being sensitive to language complexity is an important catalyst in making selections that are con-ceptually accurate and physically meaningful to the text being studied.

The educational interpreter's knowledge of the grammar of English, as well as the grammar of the visual language (especially if that language is American Sign Language [ASL]), cannot be overstressed. Interpreters are language experts.

They come to their expertise by negotiating the grammar of the language in order to represent it in equivalent forms. The task can be difficult but becomes increasingly easier for those who work at it.

The syntax of mathematics frequently presents interpreters with interesting challenges. Take a look at the following problems from fourth-, fifth-, sixth-, and seventh-grade assignments:

1. One-third of Ryan's paycheck is spent on rent; another two-sixths is spent on groceries. Do the rent and groceries take up the same amount of his paycheck? How did you figure that?
2. Thirty children were divided into smaller groups for a field trip. Three of the groups had seven children each; one group had six children. How many children were in the other group?
3. The perimeter of a square is four times the length of one of its sides. The perimeter of the square is 68 inches. Find the length of one of its sides.
4. Rob was given $1.75 by his brother Trent and $2.60 by his sister Jennifer. Rob bought their mother a pen for $5.95. How much did Rob contribute to the gift?
5. Zac has taken 15 fewer piano lessons than Emile. Emile has taken 2 lessons a week for the past 17 weeks. How many lessons has Zac had?

Interpreters who capitalize on their expert knowledge of the language and its grammar are likely to subscribe to the spatial manipulations that belong to ASL in negotiating some of the ambiguities of these problems. Setting up a space for Ryan's "whole check," for example, and representing one-third of that space for rent and another two-sixths of that space for food should add to, not detract from, a sign language interpretation that is provided in English syntax. Similar use of spatial manipulations and classifiers in problems 2 and 3 could be helpful in improving the interpretation. Using pronominal forms and directional signs should also improve the readability of the passive voice in problem 4 and the comparative relationships in problem 5. Skilled interpreters work with the linguistic forms of the target and source language to expose their simplicity, not to complicate their complexity.

Finally, King and Quigley (1985) discussed text cohesion; the organization of information; and formatting of illustrations, pictures, headings and subheadings as important to the readability of a text. I would suggest that these same variables are important to the interpretability of a text or any instructional material that is textbook bound. Interpreters who learn to use their own connectives between concepts, paragraphs, pages, and sections enhance the readability and comprehension of the material, whether that material is presented during an oral reading or referred to in a lecture.

Skilled sign language interpreters make use of their space to mark information that can later be connected to information in another designated space. Skilled sign language interpreters, oral interpreters, and cued speech transliterators demonstrate facial expressions that mark new information and connect it to old information. Talented interpreters reference page numbers and sections by point or by visual gaze to increase the student's access to implied relationships that might otherwise be lost in a context that appears void of boundaries. A look at the following excerpt should illustrate the point:

> Mrs. Logan visited us at 3:00. She had been to see her cousin in the country. She brought back enough fresh corn for everyone. We each had one ear for dinner. Mine was a little tough, but I thought it best not to say anything to hurt her feelings. Mom gave me a double helping of cake because I was so polite.

On first reading, the educational interpreter might find this paragraph to be easy to interpret. Sentence length is certainly manageable, and even if a teacher or student reads it at a rapid rate, the paragraph is short enough and contains enough commonly used language so that holding it in memory should not be difficult. Deeper analysis of the paragraph shows that it includes several figurative expressions: "one ear," "thought it best," "hurt her feelings," and "double helping." The paragraph also contains at least two words that can be interchangeable in sign language: SEE and VISIT. The sentences have no visible connectors, but implied or inferred connectedness is embedded in several bits of information that can be taken from the paragraph: (1) Mrs. Logan brought corn back from the country; (2) fresh corn means the visit occurs in summer; (3) not saying anything to hurt her feelings implies that Mrs. Logan stayed for dinner; and (4) here, *polite* refers to remaining silent.

My experiences with this paragraph led to lots of mental negotiations about how my interpreting of this apparently easy text could have been improved to make it more meaningful, more comprehensible to the fourth grader with whom I was working. Several strategies could have made this, and other deceptive texts like it, more meaningful. Some of these strategies are concept or ASL based: adding signs and classifiers for clarification (e.g., WOMAN and person CL to Mrs. Logan); adding transition or connector signs (e.g., BEFORE, PREVIOUSLY) between sentences one and two; embedding questions in sentences three and six (e.g., BROUGHT-BACK WHAT?); setting up spatial referents (e.g., a place for the country and a place for "us"); and using nonmanual markers to modify utterances (e.g., facial expressions to modify A LITTLE TOUGH, negative head nod to modify NOT TO SAY ANYTHING). Several English-based strategies are also appropriate to interpret this passage meaningfully: offering an oral shadow or mouthing of the figurative expressions (e.g., ear of corn, thought it best, double helping of cake), fingerspelling P-O-L-I-T-E before offering a sign synonym, and generally following the syntactic order of the English as it is written and read.

Other strategies are likely to be found by the ambitious interpreter who strives to make the target and source languages compatible. Current research suggests that successful educational interpreters demonstrate a necessary mix of speech-driven (English) and sign-driven (ASL) strategies (Kelly, 2001; Siple, 1998; Sofinski, Yesbeck, Gerhold, & Bach-Hansen, 2001; Winston, 1989) in their voice-to-sign product. Indeed, the judicious interaction of ASL interpreting and

English transliterating rarely needs apologizing when interpreters are striving for academic literacy (Akamatsu, 1998; Marschark, Lang, & Albertini, 2002).

At least two important points need to be made in summarizing the interpreter's role in interpreting content that is derived from or bound to textbooks: (1) Interpreters need to have their own set of books; and (2) interpreters need to do their homework. Educational interpreters should be given (and, if not, should request) their own personal copies of textbooks. Having these books available during the course being interpreted and to take home or to use during a planning period for preparation is important to the interpretation process. Interpreters cannot interpret what they do not understand (Cokely, Baker-Shenk, Isham, & Colonomos, 1992). The notion of comprehension in order to interpret has obvious implications if the interpreter is expected to practice any of the strategies just discussed. But should the educational interpreter know the Magna Carta, the Pythagorean theorem, the conjugations of past progressive verb forms, the genus and species of the insect kingdom, how to spell every multisyllabic word that appears in a textbook? The answer includes both a yes and a no: *Yes*, the educational interpreter must have a working knowledge of what he is interpreting in order to interpret; but, *no*, the level of comprehension needed to interpret successfully is not the same as the level of comprehension needed to demonstrate learning.

Question 3: What is the interpreter's responsibility with other curriculum situations that are not textbook bound?

Many content areas in the elementary- and middle-school setting are taught without textbooks. These include physical education, music, and art, as the most common examples; drama, computer science, and creative writing, as perhaps less common examples. While handbooks, workbooks, and resource materials may supplement or augment the instruction, these content areas are not as likely to be bound to a textbook that dictates the scope and sequence of instruction. Interpreters come to these other curriculum areas with varied expectations and concerns. These courses or subjects are frequently viewed as "breaks" within the interpreter's physically and cognitively demanding day. At the same time, however, some interpreters may find calisthenics more demanding to interpret than a lecture on the executive branch of government taken from the fourth chapter of a civics book.

A seventh-grade art class might provide a glimpse at some challenges during the interpreting process. Most art teachers, and an increasing number of social studies, science, and mathematics teachers, prescribe to an experiential or hands-on philosophy in offering students different learning experiences. In a drawing unit, for example, students might be exposed to the concept of "vantage" and "perspective"—two vocabulary items that may be interchanged as synonymous forms. As the teacher lectures or describes the concept of "perspective," he or she might illustrate through a demonstration. The interpreter then faces an important decision: how to interpret the verbal instruction and draw the student's eyes to the demonstration at the same time. The interpreter must position himself close enough to the speaker (and demonstrator) so the student has visual access to both. Virginia Swisher's research (1991) on 8- to 12-year old deaf students revealed developmental improvements in their ability to identify signing in their peripheral vision while focusing on another target in their central vision. That is, as deaf students mature, they get progressively better at watching two things at the same time. The degree to which this skill enables learning is still suspect. Ideally, the demand for taking in both the language of the demonstration and the demonstration itself can be handled with careful timing. Teachers who *learn* to sequentially talk and demonstrate, and offer substantial pauses between the two, are held in high regard by educational interpreters.

Interpreting in computer labs, or even in the regular classroom where students might venture off to the computer at various times during the school day, poses another challenge for interpreters who must negotiate competing visual referents. Interpreters who are accustomed to positioning themselves close to the source language are often thrown when the teacher sits beside the student at a computer terminal. Adding a seat next to the teacher only removes the student's gaze farther from the computer screen, where the focus of the instruction is expected. Imagine the best strategies for interpreting this computer-focused instruction:

> Mr. K: OK, Kristen, show me what you've got [*looking at the screen as he talks*]. Well, this web site has quite a bit about Harriet Beecher Stowe. Now, scroll down and highlight the text you want to copy. I want to see your report, too, so you'll have to minimize this and bring up the document you're working on. Did you try to copy her picture? Click on it and then go up to your toolbar and click on Paste and let's see what happens.

Where to stand or sit in order to direct eye gaze between the screen and the teacher and student, where to place the hands in order to show movement on the screen, what to sign, what to point to, what to fingerspell, what to classify—all of these decisions are critical to the successful interpreting of this common instructional scene.

Interpreting captioned videotapes is yet another challenge for educational interpreters, but one that is often not fully confronted until these elementary and middle school years. Mark Marschark, Harry Lang, and John Albertini (2002) reported that the recommended captioning rate for children's television is 60 words per minute, but the rate of available programming often exceeds 140 words per minute (p. 210). Students' comprehension of captions is even more compromised when their visual attention is split between the captioning and the events unfolding on the monitor. Educational interpreters may be more comfortable interpreting (or attempting to interpret) captioned tapes and programs in lower elementary grades than at upper elementary and higher grades. They may find their struggle to interpret fast-paced captioning is even more complicated by their older student's resentment of the interpreting, particularly if it exposes the student's difficulty in reading. This dilemma, whether to interpret for increased comprehension or to find an alternative to interpreting captioned media, should be discussed with teachers who offer this accommodation in naive anticipation that it solves all access problems.

Question 4: What about interpreting for field trips, assemblies, musicals, and other special learning experiences?

Just as the interpreter who interprets course material without a textbook must negotiate many events before and while processing the language, so must the interpreter who accompanies a class on a field trip or to an assembly or special program be prepared to negotiate anticipated events of the assignment. If a visit to the site is impossible, a phone call, letter, or e-mail is appropriate in requesting information about the site and the learning that the students might be expected to accomplish during the experience. The following script was mailed to a coordinating interpreter after her phone call to the Grand Caverns. Imagine her pleasure in being able to share this script with four other interpreters. Their group study and preparation prior to the field trip were fundamental in the successful interpretations during the field trip. They were even able to prepare for those points on the tour when the lights were going to be turned out, as in "showing total cave darkness." The paragraphs that follow represent three paragraphs of a 47-paragraph script during the two-hour field trip:

> Grand Caverns was discovered in 1804 by a young trapper named Bernard Weyer. He was out on this hill checking his traps one day. He discovered that one of them was missing and he went to look for it. He found it lodged behind a crack in the rock. It proved to be the entrance to the cave. The caverns were opened to the public in 1806, under the name Weyer's Cave, making this the oldest commercial show cave still in operation in the United States. The cave kept the name of Weyer's Cave until 1926; then the name was changed to Grand Caverns. In 1974, the Cave officially became part of the Upper Valley Regional Park Authority.
>
> One type of formation you will find in the cave are stalactites. These are formed on the ceiling of the cave by water seeping through the cracks in the limestone rock dissolving calcium carbonate or calcite as it comes through and depositing it on the ceiling of the cave. If the water flows fast enough, it will drip to the floor of the cave, depositing the calcium carbonate there in the form of stalagmites. If the two should come together, they will form a column. It takes approximately 100 to 125 years, under optimum growth conditions, to form one cubic inch of formation. The water you see, feel, and hear all around you means this cavern is very active and still growing.
>
> This is the Cathedral Hall, one of our larger rooms. It is 280-feet long, 60-feet wide at its widest point, and the ceiling ranges from 40- to 70-feet high. *(ASK YOUR*

GROUP TO GUESS HEIGHT OF THE STATUE.) The statue is eight-and-a-half feet tall. It is an optical illusion, because we are standing on an incline and are about 200 feet away. (Courtesy of Grand Caverns National Park, Weyer's Cave, Virginia)

Like field trips, musical performances and plays present interesting challenges for educational interpreters. A visiting orchestra may have a performance that cannot be interpreted. Perhaps a review of the score or consultation with the conductor or music teacher in describing the score would be sufficient in equalizing the target and source language in this case. When musical performances involve words that represent another language, as in songs from an Italian opera, the interpreter may want to seek out a translation of the words in order to interpret the words. (This topic comes up again in the next chapter in dealing with interpreting in foreign language classes.) Some interpreters operate on the principle that using translated words, rather than the original score, goes beyond the goal of equalizing target and source language.

Some interpreters would argue that if the hearing students do not have access to the translated words, then the deaf students also should not have access to the translated words. I have difficulty understanding what symbol system would be used in the interpretation, however, if a translation is not available. I recall a couple of personal experiences in interpreting Latin and Hebrew lyrics. With the translation, I was able to render translated words into signs. Regardless of attitude or approach, however, rehearsing with the choir or the orchestra or the actors is especially important if such rehearsal is feasible. In each of these circumstances, again, preparation is the key to successful interpretation. Failing to prepare can be the equivalent of preparing to fail, with this important caveat: When the interpreter fails to prepare, the student may fail to learn. The following e-mail from a colleague shares his satisfaction after substantial rehearsal for a play:

> There was a powerful scene where Joan of Arc was being tried for heresy. She was brought on stage, and I was standing directly beside her. She began a moving speech about seeing visions that told her what to do, how she wanted to believe her church, how she trusted God, and then described how they were burning her for these beliefs. At the same time, I was interpreting this beside her. Now think of signing with a fire starting at your feet and then going up your body to your head as you look up in the sky in prayer. Several members of the audience said it was quite dramatically powerful. I know the feeling!

Question 5: What is the interpreter's role in interpreting tests?

Educational settings are well known for their testing activities. Even in nontraditional classrooms, evaluation is important in monitoring a student's learning, development, and progress. Teacher-made tests and commercially made tests may be used routinely and require nothing more from the interpreter than his or her availability for questions or comments. By the third or fourth grade, students are generally comfortable with test-taking routines: The teachers administer them, the students take them, the teachers retrieve them and return them graded or marked at a later date. Administration generally involves announcements or directions that may or may not be repeated on the test itself. The interpreter's role, of course, is to make the target language equal to the source language in delivering the directions; drawing the student's attention to the directions on the test itself; and being available to interpret comments, questions, or other interruptions that might occur during the test taking. In some cases, the interpreter may be asked by the educational team to interpret the written version of the test. While this is not a common experience, it is possible that students who have difficulty reading English benefit from having the language of the test interpreted into ASL. Decisions about the interpreter's role, if that role is to be extended beyond interpreting directions and incidental interruptions, should be made by the child's educational team.

One particular type of test that deserves special discussion is the *spelling test*. In elementary grades (and in some primary grades), students frequently are expected to take a weekly spelling test. The spelling words may be derived from a spelling text or workbook, may be derived from a basal reading series, may be thematically selected (holiday words at holiday times, as an example), or they may be chosen by the teacher for reasons that are not always obvious. The interpreter's role during the administration of a spelling test can be awkward, especially when finger*spelling* is used to represent the words being studied. Some interpreters actually use rapid fingerspelling when interpreting words administered orally during a spelling test. Some interpreters cue the student to a particular word by mouthing the word or providing an oral transliteration and the initial letter(s) of the source word. Some interpreters accommodate spelling lessons and the subsequent tests with invented signs, initialized signs, and with cued speech. Finally, some teachers who administer oral spelling tests are agreeable to testing spelling in other ways. One suggestion that should be determined by the child's educational team would involve having the students identify incorrect spelling words within their linguistic context, most likely a written language context.

Tests that are administered outside the curriculum are of particular interest to interpreters. Standardized tests are frequently given to students at particular intervals within their matriculation through school, often beginning in third or fourth grade and then repeated at designated years. Some SEAs and LEAs require minimal competency tests to be administered each year until the student passes the tests. These high-stakes tests may even determine a student's graduation or acceptance to another program (refer to The Case of the Vocational Test in Chapter 5). The interpreter's responsibilities during these formal group-administered tests should resemble those that have been documented by the Educational Testing Service (1994). They include:

1. interpreting directions and instructions before the start of the test;
2. interpreting comments from the test administrator, such as, "Five more minutes";

3. interpreting clarifying directions that pertain to a specific portion of the test;
4. interpreting directions about handing in test booklets, remaining seated, etc., at the end of the test (p. 2).

ETS also recommends that the interpreter's presence during the test possibly reduces stress that occurs in deaf students who would otherwise not have equal access to the communication provided by the test administrator, and provides a sense of safety and access to emergency notifications.

Question 6: What is the role of the interpreter with students who present with a mixed communication profile?

Defining a *mixed communication profile* involves describing students who are deaf or hard-of-hearing and who use at least two languages or two communication modes in their educational and personal lives. These students include: (1) the hard-of-hearing student who hears and speaks in certain environments but also benefits from a visual interpretation in other environments, (2) the profoundly deaf student who uses an English-based sign system in the school environment but ASL with his or her deaf parents at home, (3) the deaf or hard-of-hearing student whose parents are hearing and use a predominance of fingerspelling and home signs to communicate with their child, (4) the deaf or hard-of-hearing student whose hearing parents speak a language different from English. Each of these children brings to the educational interpreting situation a different communication profile, a profile that is mixed because of language, modality, and culture.

In the early 1980s, the Amy Rowley case presented a dilemma for the schools and courts in determining whether she needed an educational interpreter. Amy's "significant residual hearing" (*Newssounds,* 1982, p. 6) provided her with some access to spoken language, but her hearing loss prevented full access to the language of the classroom, and as a child whose deaf parents used sign language in the home, Amy's communication profile was mixed. Amy's progress from kindergarten (where an interpreter was tried but discontinued) through the third grade indicated that she performed better without an interpreter than half of her hearing peers. The U.S. Supreme Court ultimately ruled in favor of the school, that a sign language interpreter was not appropriate for Amy's educational success.

In the years since Amy's case surfaced, the number of children who have been recommended to have educational interpreters has increased, not decreased. As mentioned in Chapter 1, as many as 24,000 students currently work with educational interpreters in their early, middle, and high school placements; thousands more in their residential school placements; and thousands more in post-secondary placements. Many of these students have clear, unquestioned need for an interpreter. Others, however, those like Amy Rowley, have mixed communication profiles that require their interpreters to become proficient at moving from one language or modality to another within the different demands of the curriculum and school day. My own experiences with students who are hard-of-hearing (moderate-to-severe hearing loss) lead me to make this statement: *Interpreters must be able to assess the student's interpreting needs and respond to those needs with the most appropriate interpreting mode, code, or recommendation for an alternative communication system.*

The interpreter who truly "reads" the student and is sensitive to the student's native language will adjust his or her interpretation mode (oral, manual, nonmanual) and code (instructional English, social ASL) as frequently as the demands of the day require, and as thoroughly as his or her knowledge of the languages permit. Fifty years ago, the United Nations Educational Scientific and Cultural Organization (UNESCO) reported that a child learns more quickly through his or her "mother tongue" than through an unfamiliar linguistic medium (as cited in Brice, 1994). A look at the following case should make that point clearer.

> Tommy was diagnosed with a moderate-to-severe bilateral hearing loss as a preschooler. He lived in a rural mountain community where his mother was the only deaf resident; she had attended the state school for the deaf as a young girl and considered ASL her native language. She returned to her mountain home, had Tommy, and was raising him on her own. She became concerned about Tommy in the second grade when his report card showed failing grades; she requested a full-time ASL interpreter for him in the third grade.
>
> As a consultant to the school system, I was asked to make an assessment of Tommy's need for an interpreter for the upcoming third grade. Because the school year had ended, I had to schedule a summer visit. I worked with him in the library of his school. I also met with his mother and determined early on that although she used ASL with me, her communication with Tommy was not the ASL that I expected. She communicated with Tommy through fingerspelling and gestures. Tommy responded to her with exaggerated speech, more gestures, and lots of fingerspelling.
>
> My one-on-one evaluation of Tommy's communication skills involved a battery of informal assessment materials, all representing the type of material he had just had in the second grade and new material that he would be expected to learn at the beginning of the third grade. I presented half of the assessment materials in a simultaneously presented English sign system (after observing several Signed English markers in his telling of a story he had just read using his sign language) and the other half in spoken English alone, without the benefit of signs. The two halves were matched for difficulty level, question type, and information load. At the end of the three-hour session, I reviewed the videotape of the session and prepared for a detailed analysis of Tommy's communication.
>
> The results of the analyses indicated that Tommy relied more on the visual and auditory features of spoken language than on the visual features of the supplemental sign language. His comparative scores revealed better performance in following directions, in comprehending a story, in answering questions, and in tested responses to the material when sign language was not used. My recommendation not to provide a sign language interpreter was guarded, however, with another recommendation for the hearing-impaired specialist or learning disabilities specialist to

work with Tommy in his difficult subjects (mathematics and spelling) in a remedial or tutorial capacity.

Two years after the recommendation, I ran into Tommy's supervisor at a conference. She shared with me that Tommy had flourished in the third and fourth grades—that his social confidence had soared, along with his football and baseball skills; and that his report card placed him on the honor roll almost every six weeks. Tommy's aural/oral communication in the academic environment did not negate his use of a visual-based communication system in his home environment with his mother. Indeed, a sign language interpreter was provided routinely for parent conferences, but the use of a sign language interpreter during the academic day was neither necessary nor appropriate.

Tommy's story easily could have taken a different direction. Had I found him to have been an ASL signer, I would have likely recommended an ASL interpreter for him, in spite of his reported hearing and speech. Had he demonstrated more native-like strengths in an English signing system, I would have likely recommended a transliterator. Had he demonstrated a propensity toward speechreading, I probably would have recommended a cued speech or oral transliterator for him. The important point here is that Tommy's preferred communication—the system that he was most comfortable using—was the best indicator among the choices. We can never be sure that a deaf student's previous linguistic experiences are indeed ASL or Signed English or cued speech used consistently enough for the student to have developed a mother tongue in one communication system. We must be especially vigilant in determining the student's communication needs according to those most consistently provided by the student himself or herself.

Some may even question why I would suggest that the interpreter has a role in this assessment process. I return to the notion that the interpreter is a language expert. Speech-language pathologists and/or teachers of deaf and hard-of-hearing students should work together with the interpreter to analyze the communication skills of a student who presents a mixed profile (Seal, 2000). Observing the student in class activities, in social activities, and in personal situations (especially with parents or siblings) should support choices when language, modality, code, or system are at question. Similarly, the speech-language pathologist and hearing-impairment specialist should work with the interpreter in determining when changes in choices are needed. Language is dynamic; it changes across time.

Monitoring changes in communication needs is particularly important for students who wear cochlear implants. Two groups of CI students are currently enrolled in elementary, middle-school, and high-school settings: (1) those who received an implant in their preschool or early primary years, and (2) those who are new implant candidates. Age at implant is an important variable in both groups. Among those in the first group are students who may have worn their implants since they were 5 years of age (those born before 1990) and those who may have worn their implants since they were 2 years of age (those born after 1990 but before 1998). Children implanted before age 5 typically show greater gains in speech perception than children implanted after age 5 (e.g., Carney &

Moeller, 1998). Neither group, even those who have "excellent results with an implant [can] be said to have 'normal' hearing. Their performance on appropriate tests is typically similar to that of a child with a severe hearing loss" (Boothroyd, 1998, p. 110); and wide variability exists in students with a severe hearing loss. Some show a high reliance on their combined hearing and speechreading and only an occasional need for interpreters, and some show limited use of their combined hearing and speechreading and a strong reliance on their interpreters.

Students in the second group, the new candidates for implants, have an *age disadvantage* in developing independence with their hearing, but a *technology advantage* in receiving the latest multi-electrode implants. Their outcomes are difficult to predict (refer to the case in Chapter 2). We do not know if their greatest gains in using the implants will occur within the first 6 to 12 months, as is typical with adults, or after 18 months, as is typical with children implanted after age 5 (as reported in Carney & Moeller, 1998). We do know that some of these children will show no gains at all. We also know that the educational interpreter can play an important part in the ongoing assessment of the communication needs of students with implants who have previously worked with interpreters.

This need for a functional assessment across time is also seen in the deaf or hard-of-hearing student whose parents speak a language other than English. The increasing number of hearing students who must learn English as a second language is matched by an increasing number of deaf students who come to language learning from a different cultural and linguistic orientation (refer to Chapter 1). These students, much like the hard-of-hearing student whose parents use ASL and much like students with implants, present mixed communication profiles and require careful evaluations in determining their language competence and communication needs. A look at the bilingual-bicultural evaluation process (Daimco, 1991; Kayser, 1989) reveals that the process for making recommendations for children of limited English proficiency (LEP) backgrounds includes four stages: (1) observing, (2) interviewing, (3) testing, and, (4) collecting and comparing baseline data on the student's communication competence. Educational interpreters are likely to be important contributors at each of these four stages.

Question 7: What is the interpreter's role in teaching the deaf or hard-of-hearing student to become an effective consumer of interpreting services?

An assumption may be implied here that deserves questioning. Do deaf and hard-of-hearing students who have interpreters need to be taught or trained to use their interpreters? An absolute answer is not appropriate. Just as all students bring different language levels and experiential backgrounds to the classroom or educational environment, so do all students bring different levels of experiences in using educational interpreters. To whom, then, does the responsibility belong when a student does not know how to use the interpreter, or worse yet, when a student *ab*uses or *mis*uses his or her interpreter?

Before deliberating on an answer, it is important to establish some factual information about the cognitive skills of students from about age 7 through 12. These students think differently from those in the primary grades and those in the secondary grades by virtue of their concreteness. Students at this age are referred to as *concrete operational* thinkers; they problem solve by focusing on the specific, practical, here-and-now—the concrete variables involved in the problem. They are unable to project abstractly; they are unable to think about the consequences of their problem solving or the consequences of their thinking. (Interested readers should refer to a developmental psychology book for more information on the cognitive characteristics of students at this age.) Inherent in this cognitive stage is the importance of rules. Between the second and seventh or eighth grade, students enjoy playing games; and all games have rules that are regulated by a mutually agreed-upon *code*. Right and wrong are defined by conformity—if everyone agrees that some act is right, then, the act is right. Anyone who disagrees is wrong.

In their book, *Language Intervention in the Classroom,* Donna Merritt and Barbara Culatta (1998) discussed the nature of school scripts. Students must learn the "necessary talking routines or scripts needed to engage actively in learning. . . . [they must] learn routines that regulate who to talk to, where to talk, what to talk about in class, and when to talk during the course of interacting and for different purposes. Violations of these scripts is often interpreted as problems in behavioral compliance" (p. 7).

Applying these developmental hallmarks and expectations to student consumerism raises some interesting thoughts. If students are to be trained, or taught, to use interpreters, then this period is probably the best period in which to do so. Orientations, inservices, and lessons on the rules—the dos and don'ts—may be better internalized during the concrete-operational period than the same orientations, inservices, and lessons at a later cognitive period that is often characterized by philosophical challenges to previously learned rules. Furthermore, the training is probably most appropriate and successful when it involves the larger group. If the instruction is delivered to the entire group and everyone learns that a certain procedure or script is right, then, violations of that procedure or script are obviously wrong—not just wrong in the eyes of the interpreter or teacher, but wrong in the eyes of everyone. The code belongs to all. Breaking codes or rules of the group is less likely to happen during this concrete-operational period than during the previous preoperational period or during the latter period, the formal operational period. Developmentally, then, instruction on how to use an interpreter is likely to be most successful if it occurs during these elementary- and middle-school years, and if it is presented to the entire class, not just to individuals.

Students who had interpreters as "helpers" in the primary years may view their interpreters as helpers as they advance in grades, especially if the same interpreter serves the same student from year to year. In contrast, a student who is mainstreamed in the primary years without an interpreter and receives an educational interpreter for the first time, let's say around the fourth grade, may view this person as a fortunate resource or necessary link to the auditory environment and increasing academic demands of the classroom. At the same time, the student who has managed without an interpreter in primary years may resent the intrusion that an interpreter represents in the elementary years, and be more inclined to misuse the interpreter as a consequence. Students who move from residential or self-contained programs where everyone uses the same sign language or system, to inclusion programs, where only a few people, or perhaps even one person, can communicate in the same language or system may also resent the change and struggle to use the interpreter. One of my deaf colleagues lectures against the term "using" an interpreter and recommends the term "working with" an interpreter. She also conducts workshops and inservices on teaching students how to work with interpreters. Among her recommendations are some basic courtesies, some functional pragmatics, and some cautionary points regarding ethical dilemmas.

Back to the original question, then. To whom does the responsibility belong when a student is about to work with an interpreter for the first time? I would suggest that the teacher of the deaf, a hearing-impairment specialist, or a responsible administrator in the school system set up orientation meetings or inservice meetings for the class (or grade or school). I also would suggest that a deaf adult, who has worked with educational interpreters, conduct the meetings. Within this training, I would suggest covering the basic courtesies, functional pragmatics, and potential ethical concerns that could spoil or solidify the working relationship as it becomes established.

If we borrow from information on the types of inservices provided to teachers who work with educational interpreters (Beaver, Hayes, & Luetke-Stahlman, 1995), we find that typical inservices occur only once per school year and are conducted by the teacher of the deaf. These inservices generally focus on the roles and responsibilities of the interpreter, the teacher, and the communication methods used. Although these topics are appropriate for a general orientation or inservice, they should not take the place of the three topics mentioned earlier: basic courtesies in working with an interpreter, functional pragmatics, and ethical issues. An inservice or series of lessons that focus on these areas, in my judgment, are more practical in teaching consumerism for interpreter services than the more superficial topics generally used. In cases where the speech-language pathologist or communication skills specialist is agreeable to input from the educational interpreter (and I suggest this should be a commonality, not a rarity), goals may be established for the students that focus on consumer issues.

Patrick Schloss and Maureen Smith (1990) provided many activities that focus on pragmatic communication skills. Among their suggestions are use of certain situations that lend themselves to role play and focus on asking and answering questions, giving and receiving compliments, and initiating and responding to small talk. Other suggestions are offered in Table 4.2. Additional topics under *Ethical Concerns* are available from some of the cross-cultural challenges Brenda Cartwright (1999) and her colleagues (Stewart, Schein, & Cartwright, 1998) have provided.

TABLE 4.2   Inservice Topics for Students Working with Interpreters

Category:	**Basic Courtesies**
Topics:	How to exchange social courtesies (greetings, closings, compliments) with an interpreter
	How to use an interpreter to exchange social courtesies with others
	How to interrupt an interpreter, how to avoid interrupting an interpreter
	How to interrupt an interpreter without interrupting the source language
	How to interrupt an interpreter to interrupt the source language
	Others?
Category:	**Pragmatic Concerns**
Topics:	How to maintain attention and minimize fatigue
	How to rest when fatigued
	How to ask questions, respond to questions, and interact with the teacher during lecture and demonstration
	How to ask questions, respond to questions, and interact with classmates during discussions and small-group work
	How to ask for clarification when there is a misunderstanding
	How to provide clarification when there is a misunderstanding
	Others?
Category:	**Ethical Concerns**
Topics:	How to identify ethically challenging situations
	How to handle ethically challenging situations brought on by the interpreter
	How to handle ethically challenging situations brought on by the teacher or classmates
	Others?

Question 8: What are the best practices for handling difficult interpreting situations in elementary- and middle-school settings?

The selection of difficult interpreting situations at elementary- and middle-school levels that I have chosen to share in this chapter represent only a handful of the interesting cases I have experienced or learned about over the past few years. The whole concept of difficult interpreting situations continues to grow as my experiences with interpreters in educational settings grow. Determining the best practices for these and other difficult situations is always a matter of judicating the most ethical, most professional, and most educationally sound practice from among the many choices interpreters frequently face.

The Case of the Difficult Teacher

Mr. Reeks proved to be difficult from the first day of class. He watched the clock as the minute hand moved to 12 and began calling roll that second. The four or five students who walked in during roll call were chastised never to be late again, that math started at 11:00 promptly, not 11:01, 11:02, 11:03, or later. Sarah, the deaf student, was among those who straggled in late. She recognized her interpreter, Mrs. Jordan, and found a seat near her. Mrs. Jordan, in interpreting Mr. Reeks reprimands, was also chastised by Mr. Reeks: "Is this necessary? Well, it's going to drive me crazy having you flap your hands like that all the time!" Sarah was embarrassed, Mrs. Jordan was embarrassed, and in spite of the few giggles, most of the students who knew Sarah from elementary school (this was the first day of middle school) were embarrassed for her. *All* the students appeared to be scared of Mr. Reeks.

By the second week of the term, Mrs. Jordan, Sarah, and the rest of the class had Mr. Reeks's idiosyncracies figured out. No one was ever late and no one was ever unprepared to answer when he questioned homework answers, answers to in-class assignments, answers to any question Mr. Reeks presented. Mr. Reeks believed, as he put it, in the fair exchange between teacher and student: "Questions–answers" was the name of his educational game. One problem was becoming increasingly apparent in his routine, however. He had yet to ask Sarah a question. Day 9, day 10, day 15, week 3 passed. Sarah finally mentioned to Mrs. Jordan that Mr. Reeks called on each of the other students at least once during each and every class, but he never called on Sarah. Mrs. Jordan, also well aware of the difference Mr. Reeks made in his approach with Sarah, responded to Sarah that perhaps she should ask *him* a question, to "break the ice" and show him that she could indeed communicate, even if it was through an interpreter.

Sarah did not respond favorably to the suggestion. Instead, she asked Mrs. Jordan if she would be willing to talk to him after class. Mrs. Jordan offered to interpret for her if she wanted to talk to him after class, but indicated that she would not talk to him personally, even if she did have her lunch break at the same time as his. Nothing happened on day 16. Day 17, 18, week 5 passed. The same flagrant neglect to ask Sarah questions occurred every day. Sarah's homework assignments were being returned with favorable grades; her quiz grades were also good, but Mr. Reeks did not include her in his daily question-answer exchanges. As the students took the six-weeks test, Mr. Reeks approached Mrs. Jordan and said, "How much of her work are you doing for her? Isn't she capable of learning this material without you?" Mrs. Jordan was shaken by the insinuations and responded that she was not doing any of Sarah's work, that Sarah was doing her own work, and that she was merely providing Sarah with the sign language interpreting she needed to have access to Mr. Reeks' teaching. Mr. Reeks retorted with a sarcastic "Sure!" and walked away.

After class, Sarah asked Mrs. Jordan what Mr. Reeks had said to her during the test. Mrs. Jordan shared the conversation. Sarah started crying. Mrs. Jordan, too, felt like crying; she felt like she had let the whole situation get too far out of control. What should she do?

Suggested Best Practice Mrs. Jordan probably has let things go too far. Her lack of assertiveness in this case can be explained by her desire and belief that Sarah should own the responsibility of making a change here, but Sarah, as a new sixth grader in the middle school, is obviously not able to take on the ownership of that responsibility. Much like the interpreter of primary-aged students, Mrs. Jordan has a role to play on the educational team that services Sarah. It is frustrating to think that six weeks could go by without some report of Mr. Reeks's behavior to other members of that team. It is also interesting that Sarah's parents have not shown some sense of responsibility in addressing Mr. Reeks. Sarah's silence with her parents and her other teachers or support services may represent a fear of Mr. Reeks that could stay with her for a long time. The bottom line is that the differential treatment Mr. Reeks has shown to Sarah and to Mrs. Jordan is inappropriate and requires action. But who must initiate action here?

Mrs. Jordan is responsible for facilitating communication in Mr. Reeks's classroom. Because Mr. Reeks does not communicate with Sarah in the same manner that he communicates with the other students, Mrs. Jordan is unable to perform her role. Mrs. Jordan needs to report the situation to her immediate supervisor. The supervisor may assume the responsibility for explaining to Mr. Reeks the role of the interpreter. It is possible no one bothered to share the nature of Sarah's placement with Mr. Reeks and the nature of the interpreter's assignment in his classroom. If, on the other hand, he was made aware of the situation and proceeded to reject Sarah and Mrs. Jordan, or what he may feel is their intrusion on his teaching style, then his immediate supervisor should be made aware of Mr. Reeks's performance and attitude so that action can be taken immediately.

Mr. Reeks is not only singling out Sarah and Mrs. Jordan as unwanted; he is also sending a strong message to all the students in his class that he will not communicate with the deaf student and her interpreter. This message is wrong. Corrective action needs to be taken with the student body at once. An inservice or a class meeting to discuss Sarah's use of an interpreter may be appropriate, especially if the inservice is conducted by a knowledgeable administrator, deaf advocate, or the hearing-impairment specialist.

If Mrs. Jordan's reporting of the situation to her supervisor does not set into action the dominoes that are expected to follow, then Sarah's IEP committee may need to be convened to review the placement issue. Unless changes are made in the communication environment, Sarah's enrollment in Mr. Reeks's class cannot be viewed as least restrictive.

Departure Points for Discussion

1. Why shouldn't Sarah be expected to take action here? As a student, shouldn't she be advised that she has rights, and that her rights are being violated?
2. What if Mrs. Jordan's reporting the circumstances to her supervisor doesn't change the situation? What if Mr. Reeks continues to discriminate against Sarah? Should she merely be pulled from his classroom? Shouldn't the punitive actions be directed toward him, not her?

The Case of the "Redneck" Jokes

The "Redneck" jokes are everywhere—in the hallway, in the classroom, on the playground, in the lunchroom. Juarez, a fifth grader with a moderate hearing loss, is a boisterous and fun-loving student by nature. He frequently teases and "hams it up" with several of the boys in his class. Mr. Halloway is generally good-natured about Juarez's sense of humor, even though the interpreter, Belinda, thinks he sometimes lets things go too far. Following a winter holiday, for example, one of the boys in the room came back to school with a book of "you know you're a redneck if . . ." jokes. Everyone wanted to see the book; many of the students memorized two or three of the jokes and told them relentlessly to anyone who would listen. Juarez laughed good-naturedly when anyone told him a joke.

At the end of class, however, he approached Belinda and asked her to explain the jokes to him, and said that he didn't really understand redneck jokes. Belinda was surprised. She thought he was following along without difficulty. What should she do?

Suggested Best Practice   Belinda's assumption that Juarez was following the jokes presents more of a concern here than Juarez's asking for an explanation. Because jokes reflect cultural attitudes toward differences (as in making someone the butt or victim of cultural prejudice), students who are not part of the mainstream culture can be expected to have difficulty comprehending the humor intended by the joker. Juarez, with his hearing loss, and possibly with a cultural background different from that of the majority of his peers, is likely to have problems comprehending the humor. His quick laughs may be attempts at covering up his lack of understanding, or he simply may be amused by the spirit of the joking. In either case, Belinda must respond to Juarez's request to explain the jokes.

Belinda may agree to interpret (and explain) the jokes, but chances are pretty good that her interpretation will not have the impact on Juarez that he expects. Imagine, for example, Belinda's attempts at explaining this one: *"You know you're a redneck if today's supper moved too slow on the road yesterday."* Describing "roadkill" and the implication that it is eaten by rednecks may not be funny. In fact, jokes that need explaining are, by design, not funny.

Belinda might also view Juarez's request as an opportunity to share with Mr. Halloway (or her supervisor or the hearing-impairment specialist) that Juarez has questioned the meaning of the jokes. A sensitive teacher might take advantage of the teachable moment to do a study on ethnic jokes, teaching all the students the subtle differences between appropriate joking and inappropriate joking. If Mr. Halloway has a culturally mixed group, he might also take advantage of the mixture and have students who are not part of the mainstream culture bring in a joke from home. Chances are good that several of the culturally different jokes will be "not funny" to others in the class, possibly leaving Juarez with a deeper understanding of cultural humor.

John Luckner and Sherry Humphries, in their article, "Helping Students Appreciate Humor" (1990), reported that a wise teacher takes time to capitalize on funny, spontaneous things that happen in the classroom, and uses them to improve classroom communication. They also suggested that reading joke books, riddle books, and funny stories enhances a student's thinking processes by expanding comprehension, vocabulary, and use of context. Because of the literal and figurative play on words that might be critical in helping students "get" the jokes, they recommended explaining key words and words with dual meanings and how those meanings interact to make the joke funny. Belinda's role as the interpreter, then, includes explaining jokes in a way that facilitates comprehension. Also, as a member of the educational team, she is responsible for bringing Juarez's need for the jokes to be explained to the attention of his teacher (or other professionals) who can have an impact on the situation. Attempting to honor Juarez's request to explain the jokes that he brings to her and educating Mr. Halloway (or other teachers responsible for Juarez) about Juarez's interest in learning about the jokes are both professional activities that fulfill the facilitative and cultural mediator role of the interpreter.

Departure Points for Discussion

1. How could teaching the language of jokes be up to the interpreter, not the teacher?
2. Wouldn't it be more appropriate for Belinda to "inform" interpret here, rather than transliterate or try to interpret the jokes (i.e., shouldn't she just inform Juarez that the students are making jokes, give an example of one, and ignore the rest of the situation)?

3. What messages might she give Juarez if she chose to ignore the situation and let it be someone else's problem?

The Case of Weekly Religious Education

Becky was hired as an interpreter for two deaf students in the fourth grade in a rural community school. Becky had lived in the South only a few months when she saw the advertisement for an educational interpreter in the newspaper. She called about the opening, felt good that the system was interested in her, and decided to go for it.

In the second week of the school year, the teacher announced to the class that all the students would be walking across the field for Bible in the weekly religious education (WRE) trailer. Becky was surprised at the announcement, but followed along with the group and set herself up as the interpreter for Mrs. Canner.

Mrs. Canner kept the students for about 40 minutes. She introduced the lesson on "Jesus is your Savior" with a prayer, then followed with some readings from the New Testament; and then she asked the children each to tell about their church or religious activities or why they did not attend a church. Mrs. Canner dismissed the students with another prayer and good wishes until they met again the following Wednesday morning.

Becky was overwhelmed by the whole experience. She interpreted as professionally as she knew how to do, but was shocked, offended, and angered at the thoughts of returning to the trailer on a regular basis. Even though she had signed a contract, she knew she would quit before she would subject herself to the experience again. As a Jewish woman, living in the rural South was proving to be more than she had bargained for. Interpreting was one thing, but interpreting WRE was something else. What should Becky do?

Suggested Best Practice   This situation could be awkward, to say the least. Separation of church and state continues to be a politically hot topic in many rural southern schools where the majority of students are Christians. Sensitivity to the issue and religious orientation are not, however, the concern here.

Becky is the interpreter. She does not have to endorse, support, accept, or agree with the instruction she hears. She does have to interpret it, however. Professional interpreters must find within themselves the ability to separate their own church and state. Becky must remove her religious biases and background from the classroom, even a classroom that is full of religious bias. She must be professionally aloof and work to interpret the content as well as the spirit of the content with the same skill that she would use to interpret any other academic material.

Becky will likely need support in coming to this decision, however. Having a mentor or friend who could offer that support is important. This returns us to the recommendations of Linda Siple (1991) and the functions of a mentor. These functions include acceptance, confirmation, protection, coaching, and counseling. Becky's growth as an interpreter in WRE class may come about if she is able to turn to someone who offers her the acceptance, confirmation, protection, coaching, and counseling she needs in this difficult situation.

Departure Points for Discussion

1. Shouldn't Becky tell the WRE teacher that she is Jewish and opposed to her using school time to instruct the students in Christianity?

2. Even if she accepts that she, as an interpreter, should separate her own religious beliefs from her interpreting role, shouldn't she let someone know that she is offended by the situation?
3. Shouldn't she tell the students that she does not agree with the WRE lessons?

The Case of the Locker Room

Maryanne was a new interpreter in the middle school. Her assignments included sixth-grade English, math, physical education, and social studies. She also had lunchroom duty and assisted the language arts teachers with grading, photocopying, and other preparations. Maryanne enjoyed the interpreting role with each of the four different teachers and classes she had. The two boys she interpreted for were good students, a little backwards at times, but nice kids who wanted to fit in this new middle school.

Several weeks into the school year, one of the boys asked Maryanne to ask the physical education teacher, Coach Smith, what he had talked about to the boys in the locker room the day before. Coach Smith, as Maryanne interpreted the question from the boys, said that he was just telling everyone to remember to take their dirty gym suits home that weekend, that some of them were smelling really bad. Maryanne went on to ask if Coach Smith needed an interpreter in the locker room. Coach Smith laughed and told her that she might get embarrassed down there. Maryanne laughed in response but added that she would be willing to work something out if the boys were missing important information. Coach Smith assured her that if he needed to tell them anything, he would remember to say it up in the gym while she was available to interpret.

Several weeks later, one of the boys said that something funny had happened in the locker room but they did not know what it was, that everybody had laughed and Coach Smith had teased some of the boys but they didn't hear what was going on. They asked Maryanne if she would find out what was so funny. Maryanne again approached Coach Smith and interpreted for the boys that they were curious about what had happened that caused everyone to laugh. Coach Smith said something about one of the students always singing in the shower and how he had called him "Elvis." Again, Maryanne suggested that maybe the boys needed an interpreter in the locker room. Coach Smith again discouraged her participation.

Maryanne went home that afternoon thinking that the boys should have a male interpreter for physical education and in the locker room and family-life education class and for all the other "male" things that they were being exposed to. She wondered if her role as a female interpreter presented barriers for them rather than removed barriers. She wondered if the school would be willing to hire someone just for physical education, or if bringing up the situation might jeopardize her own position within the school. What should she do?

Suggested Best Practice   Maryanne's concerns are legitimate and should be reported to the supervisor or administrator responsible for the deaf students' program. The male-interpreter-for-male-students and female-interpreter-for-female-students issue is one that is likely to emerge for the first time in the preadolescent or adolescent age group. School administrators who are able to match interpreters to students by gender are probably among the fortunate few, however.

Maryanne's concerns, outside of telling the responsible administrator, have already led her to a responsible action. By continuing to interpret to Coach Smith the boys' questions about conversations that occur in the locker room, she, but more importantly, the boys, are educating the teacher about the role of the interpreter and the nature of communication exchanges. The more casual exchanges that occur in the locker room may not be fundamental to the activities of the class, but they are part and parcel of the overall communication the students experience as part of the class. Supervision that is provided by the teacher in the locker room includes communication, and the deaf boys are not able to access this communication.

If the boys and Maryanne are successful in their continued pursuit of access to the teacher's communication as it occurs in the locker room, they will probably see a change in Coach Smith's pattern. He may learn to indicate to the boys that he will share with them what was exchanged on their return to the gym and Maryanne. He may learn to use a blackboard or clipboard to write topics that will be interpreted later when Maryanne is available. He may learn enough signs himself to signal the nature of the communication exchanges that occur in the locker room, again to trigger a promise that they will be shared, although delayed, through the interpreter. He may also learn enough about his own communication style to realize that a change needs to occur—either by reducing the communication that occurs in the locker room when an interpreter is not available or by encouraging the school to hire an interpreter who could be in the locker room. Maryanne's reporting of the situation to her supervisor and her encouragement of the boys to continue to seek access to locker room exchanges are both good practices in this situation.

Departure Points for Discussion

1. What if Maryanne offered to enter the locker room at a certain point in the class period?
2. What if the administration failed to renew her contract the next year because of what might be interpreted as a gender issue?
3. Shouldn't the boys be expected to assume some responsibility in this situation?
4. Shouldn't Coach Smith own some of the responsibility?

The Case of Cheating

Dan was a new fifth-grade student in the school system. He had moved to the community from another state and his IEP called for an educational interpreter in his full inclusion placement. Stephanie enjoyed her first few weeks interpreting for Dan. He was very attentive and very interactive in the class. He was physically attractive to the girls, physically competitive with the boys, and charming with his teacher. He had a low tolerance for making errors, though, and appeared somewhat compulsive about making As on all his assignments. He frequently watched the other students and tried to outpace them. On one assignment, Stephanie thought his watching led to cheating. It appeared he changed an answer on the test. A few days later, she saw it again. He was cheating. What should she do?

Suggested Best Practice   Coming to a consensus on the interpreter's role when cheating occurs is always difficult. Some interpreters, when discussing this case, are quick to recommend telling the teacher. Others are just as quick to recommend letting the teacher discover it on her own. Both sides can effectively argue their interpretation of the Code of Ethics. Similarly, teachers (general education, special education, and teachers of the deaf) are likely to have different opinions on the appropriate protocol for this case. So are administrators; so are instructors in interpreter training programs (Warren-Norman, 2002). There simply is no one-size-fits-all answer here. (The same is true for hearing students who cheat. Single-sanctioned responses are always controversial.)

Of interest here is yet another point. Many deaf students like Dan are accustomed to watching their peers. This watching is sometimes applauded as a compensatory skill. When the watching leads to cheating and the observant interpreter catches it, it's punishable as an offensive skill. Interpreters who have hard-and-fast rules regarding cheating are wise to reflect on their logic and their values. Seeing both sides of the coin is likely to put us in the gray zone where we can appear wishy-washy, indecisive. At the same time, it may be easier to see others' points of view from that gray zone.

Departure Questions for Discussion

1. Couldn't Stephanie alert the teacher that Dan might be inclined to cheat because of his visual monitoring, and then hope that will lead the teacher to catch him?
2. What if Stephanie just told Dan that she saw him cheating, and that if she sees it again, she will have to report it? Wouldn't that discourage him from doing it again?
3. Isn't it better to stop cheating now in the fifth grade than to let it go on to higher grades?

The Case of Mocking

Liz was the interpreter for Anna Leigh, a fourth grader who had been mainstreamed since preschool days. Anna Leigh was a very capable student who handled the academic and social demands of the classroom and school environment well. Mrs. Wall, the fourth-grade teacher, had a routine in the opening activities that involved "show and read." Mrs. Wall invited students who chose to participate to read a favorite poem or short story to the class at the opening of each school day. The students had to make the book or resource available to the rest of the class throughout the day, and students could do no more than one reading per week. The fourth graders loved to choose Shel Silverstein poems; the silliest ones seemed to be used most. Generally, two or three students would volunteer to show and read each day. Anna Leigh volunteered as frequently as the others and more than many. Anna Leigh loved to read and she was forever seeking something funny to bring in for show and read.

Liz's role during the show and read was to sit and observe, to offer either oral interpreting, cued speech interpreting, or sign language interpreting as Anna Leigh indicated she needed it. When Anna Leigh was the reader, Liz also sat and observed. Occasionally, she would advise Anna Leigh on how to say a particular word; otherwise, Anna Leigh was on her own.

Early in the school year, Liz overheard a couple of the boys in the back of the room mocking, or imitating, the way Anna Leigh read. Liz ignored it the first time, but on the second occasion, she looked directly at Mrs. Wall to see if Mrs. Wall had heard the boys. Mrs. Wall's facial expression showed that she clearly had heard the boys; so had most of the other students in the classroom. Anna Leigh showed no awareness of the teasing; she continued to read the poem as gaily as she had begun it.

Because Liz did not interpret during the show-and-read activities, she wondered whether bringing the boys' behavior to Anna Leigh's attention was appropriate. Later in the morning, when all the students went to gym, Mrs. Wall approached Liz and asked her if she had overheard the boys imitating Anna Leigh's speech. Liz responded that she had and that she had wondered if she should have signaled their behavior to Anna Leigh—that, as her interpreter, she probably had a role to draw Anna Leigh's attention to distracting sounds as they occurred. She admitted she was unsure of her role in this situation and that the last thing she wanted to do was to inform Anna Leigh that she was being made fun of. Mrs. Wall responded that she was glad Liz had not brought the boys' cruelty to Anna Leigh's attention, and that she would need to think about a strategy to handle this, that she hoped to find an indirect strategy rather than a direct approach. Mrs. Wall also asked Liz if she would think about the situation, that perhaps the two of them together could come up with a strategy. What should Liz do?

Suggested Best Practice   Fourth graders (and students in other grades, too) can be insensitive in their mocking and teasing. Teachers generally are accustomed to squelching cruel teasing when it occurs. Some teachers even have policies that address teasing and mocking. Liz's confusion about her role in this situation is understandable. All variables considered, Mrs. Wall probably has the right attitude—an indirect approach is probably more advisable than a direct approach, and making Anna Leigh aware of the teasing may be unnecessary and hurtful.

Liz has two decisions to make: (1) whether she was right in ignoring the boys' teasing and not informing Anna Leigh; and (2) whether she should "think about the situation," as Mrs. Wall has suggested, and help her develop a strategy for handling it.

One approach, which might be helpful in this situation, one that could come from either Liz or from Mrs. Wall, would involve establishing a policy about "judging" the effectiveness of each of the reader's presentations. Part of the teasing that occurred may have stemmed from the intelligibility of Anna Leigh's spoken delivery. In fact, when reading out loud to a group, most students speak at a more rapid rate, which also reduces speech intelligibility, than when they communicate in discourse. Selecting a table of students, or two or three students within the classroom (one at the front, one in the middle, and one in the back) to act as judges of the students' presentations could focus everyone's attention to presentation style. If the judges found that the speech was difficult to understand, they could merely raise their hand to alert the student to speak slower or louder or more clearly. Changing judges each day would also enable all students to have a turn giving feedback to the readers. This strategy, although intended to redirect listeners who might be inclined to mock or tease, would be equally helpful to all students in the class and to all readers. This should improve the show-and-read activity for everyone.

Departure Points for Discussion

1. Shouldn't Anna Leigh's parents be informed of the incident? Don't they have a right to protect their daughter from insensitive teasing?
2. Shouldn't the boys be punished?
3. Wouldn't this incident be perfect for a role-play?

Summary

This chapter has provided information about and for educational interpreters who service elementary- and middle-school students. Interpreters play an important role in facilitating communication with this age group, communication that enhances relationships that frequently define a student's social competence. Interpreters benefit from understanding the types of relationships that occur in this age group and learning to represent the communication styles of different communication partners. The challenges presented in textbook instruction and instruction that is not bound by textbooks require interpreters to develop expertise in vocabulary, in syntax, and in discourse strategies. Sign language interpreters who hone their skills in both ASL interpreting and English transliterating are most likely to achieve this needed expertise. Interpreting tests, interpreting for students who present with mixed communication profiles, and working with students as they learn to become consumers of interpreter services are all discussed as critical areas in interpreting for elementary- and middle-school students. Other difficult interpreting situations are discussed with suggested best practices.

REFERENCES

Akamatsu, C. T. (1998). Thinking with and without language: What is necessary and sufficient for school-based learning? In A. Weisel (Ed.), *Issues unresolved: New perspectives on language and deaf education* (pp. 27–40). Washington, DC: Gallaudet University Press.

Barefoot, S. M., Bochner, J. H., Johnson, B. A., & vom Eigen, B. A. (1993). Rating deaf speakers' comprehensibility: An exploratory investigation. *American Journal of Speech-Language Pathology: A Journal of Clinical Practice, 2,* 31–35.

Beaver, D. L., Hayes, P. L., & Luetke-Stahlman, B. (1995). In-service trends: General education teachers working with educational interpreters. *American Annals of the Deaf, 140,* 38–46.

Bienvenu, M. J., & Colonomos, B. (1985–1988). *An introduction to American deaf culture: Rules of social interaction* (video). Silver Spring, MD: Sign Media.

Bloom, P. (2000). *How children learn the meanings of words.* Cambridge, MA: M.I.T. Press.

Boothroyd, A. (1998). The perception of speech by children with hearing loss. In A. Weisel (Ed.), *Issues unresolved: New perspectives on language and deaf education* (pp. 103–116). Washington, DC: Gallaudet University Press.

Brice, A. (1994). Spanish or English for language-impaired Hispanic children? In D. N. Ripich & N. A. Creaghead (Eds.), *School discourse problems,* 2nd ed. (pp. 133–153). San Diego: Singular Publishing.

Caccamise, F., & Lang, H. (2000). *Signs for science and mathematics: A resource book for teachers and students, 2nd ed.* Rochester, NY: National Technical Institute for the Deaf.

Carney, A. E., & Moeller, M. P. (1998). Treatment efficacy: Hearing loss in children. *Journal of Speech, Language, and Hearing Research, 41,* 561–584.

Cartwright, B. (1999). *Encounters with reality: 1001 interpreter scenarios.* Silver Spring, MD: RID Press.

Cazden, C. B. (1988). *Classroom discourse: The language of teaching and learning.* Portsmouth, NH: Heinemann Educational Books.

Cokely, D., Baker-Shenk, C., Isham, W., & Colonomos, B. (1992). *Interpreters on interpreting: Interpretation models and process* (video). Burtonsville, MD: Sign Media.

Daimco, J. S. (1991). Descriptive assessment of communicative ability in limited English proficient students. In E. V. Hamayan & J. S. Daimco (Eds.), *Limiting bias in the assessment of bilingual students* (pp. 157–217). Austin, TX: Pro-Ed.

ETS Committee for People with Disabilities. (1994). *Recommendations and guidelines for the use of interpreters in ETS test administrations with deaf and hard of hearing candidates.* Princeton, NJ: Educational Testing Service.

Gallagher, T. M. (1993). Language skill and the development of social competence in school-age children. *Language, Speech, and Hearing Services in Schools, 24,* 199–205.

Kayser, H. (1989). Speech and language assessment of Spanish-English speaking children. *Language, Speech, and Hearing Services in Schools, 20,* 226–244.

Kelly, J. (2001). *Transliterating: Show me the English!* Alexandria, VA: RID Press.

King, C. M., & Quigley, S. P. (1985). *Reading and deafness.* San Diego: College-Hill Press.

Luckner, J., & Humphries, S. (1990). Helping students appreciate humor. *Perspectives in Education and Deafness, 8,* 2–4.

Marschark, M., Lang, H. G., & Albertini, J. A. (2002). *Educating deaf students: From research to practice.* New York: Oxford University Press.

Merritt, D. D., & Culatta, B. (1998). *Language intervention in the classroom: School-age children series.* San Diego: Singular Publishing Group.

Miller, G. A., & Gildea, P. M. (1987). How children learn words. *Scientific American, 257,* 94–99.

Nippold, M. A. (1998). *Later language development: The school-age and adolescent years, 2nd Ed.* Austin, TX: Pro-Ed.

Nussbaum, J. (1992). Communicator style and teacher influence. In V. P. Richmond & J. C. McCroskey (Eds.), *Power in the classroom: Communication, control, and concern* (pp. 145–158). Hillsdale, NJ: Lawrence Erlbaum Associates.

Padden, C., & Ramsey, C. (2000). American Sign Language and reading ability in deaf children. In C. Chamberlain, J. P. Morford, & R. I. Mayberry (Eds.), *Language acquisition by eye* (pp. 165–189). Mahwah, NJ: Lawrence Erlbaum Associates, Publishers.

Schloss, P. J., & Smith, M. A. (1990). *Teaching social skills to hearing-impaired students.* Washington, DC: Alexander Graham Bell Association for the Deaf.

Seal, B. C. (2000). Working with educational interpreters. *Language, Speech, and Hearing Services in Schools, 31,* 15–25.

Shepherd, G. D., & Ragan, W. B. (1992). *Modern elementary curriculum, 7th Ed.* Fort Worth, TX: Harcourt Brace Jovanovich College Publishers.

(1988). Sign materials for technical/specialized vocabulary. *RID Views, 5,* 5.

Siple, L. A. (1991). The functions of mentoring. *RID Views, 8,* 28–29.

————. (1998). The use of addition in sign language transliteration. In A. Weisel (Ed.), *Issues unresolved: New perspectives on language and deaf education* (pp. 65–75). Washington, DC: Gallaudet University Press.

Sofinski, B. A., Yesbeck, N. A., Gerhold, S. C., & Bach-Hansen, M. C. (2001). Features of voice-to-sign transliteration by educational interpreters. *Journal of Interpretation,* 47–59.

Stevenson, C., & Carr, J. F. (1993). Goals for integrated studies. In C. Stevenson & J. F. Carr (Eds.), *Integrated studies in the middle grades: "Dancing through walls"* (pp. 7–25). New York: Teachers College Press.

Stewart, D. A., Schein, J. D., & Cartwright, B. E. (1998). *Sign language interpreting: Exploring its art and science.* Boston: Allyn & Bacon.

Swisher, M. V. (1991). Visual reception of sign language in young deaf chilren: Is peripheral vision functional for receiving linguistic information? In D. S. Martin (Ed.), *Advances in cognition, education, and deafness.* Washington, DC: Gallaudet University Press.

Tattershall, S. S. (1994). Upping the ante: Increasing demands for literacy and discourse skills in adolescence. In D. N. Ripich & N. A. Creaghead (Eds.), *School discourse problems (2nd ed.)* (pp. 63–89). San Diego: Singular Publishing Group.

Warren-Norman, H. (2002, August). *Parameters for interpreter services in public school settings.* Paper presented at the National Educational Interpreters Conference, San Antonio, TX.

Winston, E. (1989). Transliteration: What's the message? In C. Lucas (Ed.), *The sociolinguistics of the deaf community,* (pp. 147–164). San Diego: Academic Press.

5 Best Practices in Interpreting in High School and Vocational Settings

Interpreters in high school and vocational settings encounter many experiences that are unique to adolescence. The questions and answers discussed in this chapter should provide readers with greater insight into these unique experiences and the roles interpreters play in these experiences.

Question 1: What is expected of interpreters in secondary educational settings?

The operative word for interpreters in secondary settings is *flexibility*. Flexibility is necessary for at least two important reasons. First, the *heterogeneity* of students with hearing loss enrolled in secondary settings continues to match the heterogeneity of students without hearing loss. Tom Kluwin, Donald Moores, and Martha Gonter Gaustad (1992), in their book *Toward Effective Public School Programs for Deaf Students,* provided characteristics of the variety of students who are currently mainstreamed, included, and otherwise educated in public school programs today:

1. *Social skills and communication.* Some secondary students have high levels of participation with hearing students; others have little participation with hearing students, but high levels of participation with other deaf and hard-of-hearing students. Some students prefer oral communication, some prefer American Sign Language (ASL), others prefer simultaneous communication (Stinson & Whitmire, 1992).

2. *Motivation, self-concept, and achievement.* Some secondary students identify themselves as highly motivated and likely to succeed, while others identify themselves as less motivated with "no sense of control over their own situations" (Kluwin, 1992, p. 178). Some students come from homes where parental support enhances the student's achievement potential (e.g., the

parents value and check homework, provide deafness technology and use captions on TV) while other students come from homes where parental involvement with their child and their child's education is minimal, possibly even a deterrent to the student's achievement potential (Kluwin & Gaustad, 1992).

3. *Extracurricular involvement.* Some students who are deaf and hard-of-hearing engage in structured activities such as clubs and sports, both inside and outside the school, and others do not participate in extracurricular activities. Those students who participate in structured activities during and beyond the school day are more likely to perceive themselves and to be perceived by others as socially competent than students who resist participating or fail to join in extracurricular activities (Stewart & Stinson, 1992).

In essence, there is *no prototype for a deaf or hard-of-hearing student* at any educational level, including the high school level. Consequently, there is no single role that an educational interpreter can play in meeting the variety of interpreting needs of the variety of deaf and hard-of-hearing students in the secondary educational setting.

A second reason for educational interpreters to demonstrate flexibility at the secondary level stems from the fact that educational programs across the country are tremendously varied (and necessarily so) in their approaches to educating secondary students. The teaching styles, classroom environments, curriculum offerings, extracurricular opportunities, technological support, geographical and sociological environments, and the philosophical and pedagogical underpinnings of an educational program represent the larger society of our country. Because today's society is pluralistic, the schools that represent the society are likewise pluralistic.

Ordinary high schools across the United States today are experiencing some pretty extraordinary changes. Their relatively homogenous teaching staff is responsible for a widely heterogenous generation of learners. Traditional curriculum offerings are undergoing tremendous social and political reform. Technology is increasingly more invasive. Student outcomes have never been so scrutinized. In many ways, secondary schools today have never been so vulnerable. Educational interpreters who walk into any secondary school setting can be overwhelmed.

Imagine an interpreter who interprets for inner-city students in New York moving to a site in rural Alaska, or an interpreter from a traditional lecture-style classroom in a middle school transferring to an interactive web-based class in high school. An interpreter who interprets a tenth-grade algebra class cannot expect "sameness" when walking into the vocational school's auto mechanics class. Interpreters at the secondary level must possess a spirit of flexibility. The interpreter who demonstrates flexibility because of multiple skills, inclusive attitudes, and pluralistic knowledge is truly a valuable asset to a school program; *this interpreter is the prototype that we would all aspire to be.*

One of the many variables that sets the secondary student apart from the middle-school student involves experience, particularly experience with language, learning, and communicating. Terms like *metacognitive, metalinguistic* and *metacommunication* have been popular in language learning literature for several years. These terms relate to the ability to think about one's thinking; to talk about one's language or communication; and to demonstrate a consciousness of one's thinking, language, and communication skills. As adolescents move to higher cognitive levels, they become more introspective about their thinking, learning, and communication. Their social dialogues show this development: *Tell me what you're thinking; Why did you say that? What do you mean by that? I should have said . . .; I didn't know.* Their comprehension of abstract idioms, similes, and metaphors advances; and their use of ambiguity and sarcasm increases (Nippold, 1998). Their slang even shows metalinguistic processes: *geek, hook up, dude, my bad, whatever.* Metacognitive verbs (e.g., *agree, conclude, assume*) are increasingly common in their classroom discussions (p. 27). Their phrases show increased sensitivity to discourse cohesion: *actually, we didn't; as I was saying; back to your story.* Because interpreters play such an intimate role in reading or attempting to read a student's thinking, learning, and communication, and in representing the communication of the social and academic environment, secondary education interpreters may indirectly play a critical role in the development of a student's metalinguistic knowledge. Think about the following exchange that occurred in a senior English class:

TEACHER: The first syllogism. Doug, wanna try the first one?

DOUG: All fruit contains vitamin C. Some vegetables contain vitamin C. So some vegetables are fruit. That's valid.

TEACHER: That's valid. All right. Go through all the rules and prove that it's valid.

DOUG: The rules?

TEACHER: Yes.

DOUG: I think it's valid.

TEACHER: I know, but you have to prove that it's valid.

DOUG: I just think it's valid.

TEACHER: I know, but that doesn't work. Six rules, right? What are the three terms?

DOUG: Three terms? All fruit, vitamins, and vegetables.

TEACHER: Right, those are the three terms. Now, do you have any negatives?

DOUG: Oh, fallacy. Four terms.

TEACHER: You have four?

DOUG: No, I don't have four.

TEACHER: No, you don't have four. There's no fallacy. The second premise has vitamin C—which is a B term, so you have only three. Are there any negatives?

DOUG: No.

TEACHER: No, so you don't have to test for the negative. Now look at the major term. What is the major term?

DOUG: All fruit.

TEACHER: Fruit.

DOUG: And some vegetables is the minor term.

TEACHER: OK, vegetables is a minor term and fruit is the major term in the conclusion. Distributed in the conclusion?

DOUG: Undistributed.

TEACHER: That is correct. Is vegetables undistributed?

DOUG: Not distributed.

TEACHER: Undistributed.

DOUG: Undistributed.

TEACHER: So those are OK. Check. So look at the middle term. What is the middle term?

DOUG: Contains vitamin C.

TEACHER: Correct. Is that distributed at least once?

DOUG: No.

TEACHER: So what's the fallacy?

DOUG: No, it is distributed.

TEACHER: In which one—the major or minor premise?

DOUG: I don't understand undistributed.

TEACHER: All right, where's my eraser.

Metalinguistic knowledge presents itself to interpreters with much variability. In borrowing from Bloom's (1956) taxonomy of thinking levels, students demonstrate thinking across a range of levels:

1. At the *knowledge* level, a student demonstrates basic recall or recognition of material. The student in this example responds with basic recognition or basic knowledge when he attempts to defend his syllogism with the phrase, "It's valid; I just think it's valid." The teacher recognizes that Doug is responding at a low level and she demands that he demonstrate his comprehension at a higher level, "I know, but that doesn't work."

2. At the *comprehension* level, a student interprets or explains knowledge, generally in a descriptive way. The student in this dialogue demonstrated comprehension when he responded to the teacher's question, "What are the three terms?" His comprehension of *terms* as they apply to syllogisms led to the correct answer and opened the door for even higher levels of processing.

3. At the *application* level, a student demonstrates use of knowledge. By providing the correct question, "Are there any negatives?" the teacher prompts Doug to apply another of the six rules that determine the validity of a syllogism. His comprehension of the meaning of negatives allows him to apply the negative rule accurately.

4. At the *analysis* level, the student breaks knowledge into its component parts, showing relationships between the parts, and building from a whole to its parts. In this example, Doug analyzes his earlier response to the comprehension of *three terms* with a change in response, "Oh, fallacy. Four terms." Again, the teacher prompts his thinking about the terms and he analyzes the number of terms again.

5. At the *synthesis* level, a student works from parts to whole, showing the relationships between parts that build to the whole. In this example, Doug must analyze the meaning of *a major premise* and *a minor premise* and determine the relationship that these two parts have to a syllogism as a whole. His ability to synthesize this material is compromised by a problem in his comprehension of the terms *distributed* and *undistributed*. Even though we see him move across several thinking levels in this interaction with his teacher, and even though it appears that he has a good handle on syllogisms, his response at the end of the thinking exercise reveals the ultimate level in Bloom's taxonomy.

6. At this *evaluation* level, students are able to make judgments about their learning and the knowledge possessed by others. This judgment goes beyond "hard" and "easy," reaching into areas of interest and disinterest. Students determine when they evaluate their thinking that they either will (a) think more about this knowledge or (b) abandon their thinking for some new or more interesting body of knowledge. When Doug responds that he does not understand distributed and undistributed, he indicates to his teacher that he needs more information in order to think more about his new knowledge. He describes to his teacher that his own evaluation of his knowledge points to a weakness. He succeeded in communicating with her a metacognitive, and in this case, metalinguistic, message. And, in this case Doug communicated all of these thinking skills in a classroom of 20 peers, directly communicating with his teacher, with his hearing-impairment specialist, and an interpreter looking on. Eureka!

If we accept that deaf and hard-of-hearing students are just like hearing students, then some deaf and hard-of-hearing students demonstrate higher thinking levels in their educational programs, while other students struggle to analyze, synthesize, and evaluate their learning (Ennis, 1987). Most secondary students demonstrate a variety of thinking levels throughout the variety of subjects or learning experiences in which they may be involved. An educational interpreter who works at the secondary level attempts to determine early on in the interpreting relationship with each student where that student's thinking skills tend to cluster or predominate. If the student's cognitive functioning clusters around the basic recall and comprehension levels, the interpreter will need to adjust his or her interpreting when a teacher or a body of knowledge demands higher thinking. Whether the interpreter is able to "up the cognitive ante" is yet to be researched.

In Doug's case, the teacher was able to up the cognitive ante without the intervention of the interpreter. Educational interpreters are required to match the source language and target language to the best of their linguistic ability, imposing their own higher thinking skills on the material being studied and the persons involved in the interaction or exchange, then applying the linguistic match that best suits the student's cognitive level. Most interpreters do this intuitively; that is, they come to their roles as interpreters with ample experiences in analyzing, synthesizing, and evaluating linguistic information to determine the applicability of a linguistic match. (Research on interpreters' cognitive skills appears in Chapter 7.)

In addition, successful educational interpreters are able to analyze metalinguistically what worked and what did not work in the interpreting process; that is, skilled and qualified educational interpreters are engaged in the "constant process in which a range of components influencing the participants and the sL message must be assessed and in which the effect of any influencing component must be accurately and appropriately accounted for in the tL message" (Cokely, 1992, p. 19). Educational interpreters, then, are engaged in their own higher-order thinking skills as they assess the thinking and communication skills of the students with whom they work and the linguistic medium with which they are working.

In "Issues in Interpreter Education," Janice Kanda and Betty Colonomos (1990) reported that the interpreter engages in several processes in rendering equivalent messages and conveying form. These higher-functioning processes involve perception, memory, semantic chunking, lexical retrieval, message analysis, visualization and imagery, and composition (p. 182). Engaging in these processes of interpreting at secondary and higher levels is extremely fatiguing, such that interpreters may find their cognitive stamina challenged as frequently as or more often than their physical stamina. For this reason, I propose that interpreters at the secondary level need to find ways to "gear down," to go on "cruise control," to concentrate their engagement at lower cognitive levels in order to perform maximally when higher cognitive thinking is required. An interpreter who develops familiarity with routines in the teaching style is able to gear down his or her cognitive processing by moving into a lower-level *recall* when the routine presents itself for interpreting. The following illustration may serve to make the point.

> Mrs. Garber's first-period government class begins with a cafeteria count each morning. The cafeteria count is a two-minute procedure that involves reading the daily menu for Line A, Line B, and Line C. Line A is always a different menu, although the difference usually involves the same 8 or 10 entrees that are recycled throughout the school term. Line B is always the burgers/fries/pizza/hot dogs menu, fast food that smells like fast food and dominates the majority of the cafeteria business. Line C is always a soup/salad/fruit/vegetable bar that changes only according to seasonal availability of vegetables and fruits.

By the second week of the school term, the interpreter in Mrs. Garber's class is able to go to *basic recall* in interpreting the menu as it is read to the class each day. The vocabulary does not change; the syntax does not change; the demands of the sL are fixed so that the interpreter moves them to the tL in a rather fixed or rote fashion, much like a driver sets his cruise control on an open highway, which is less cognitively demanding than a congested highway.

The cognitive load for the interpreter in the "News Update" part of government class is heavy:

> Following the cafeteria count and menu reading comes the 15 to 20 minutes of "News Update." This learning experience requires the students to listen to Mrs. Garber as she reads a headline from a daily paper, reads selected sentences that accompany the headline, and then asks students to make comments about the article. Students are given participation grades for their responsiveness to the items. Students who do not routinely volunteer comments are asked particular questions, which are sometimes embarrassing.

The interpreter needs to be fully engaged with the material. Preparation prior to the reading and an additional copy of the material for particularly difficult vocabulary are both necessary to this engagement. Listening carefully for phrases and sentences that may be revisited during the interpreting requires message analysis, semantic chunking, and evaluative processing: "Will she come back to this later? How will she connect this item to the one yet to come?"

This interpreting exercise is in stark contrast to the cognitive demands of the same interpreter as she interprets the menu. This interpreter, if successful, has learned to think about her interpreting and to be flexible in handling these contrasting demands. Her knowledge of the teacher's style, the classroom routine, the teaching material, her preparation for the process of interpreting, her cognitive analyses during the process, and her ability to switch gears during the process are all part of the flexibility that is required to be successful. The interpreter in the secondary setting must be flexible in working with students who present with a wide variety of language, communication, and cognitive skills; with teachers who demand a wide variety of language, communication, and thinking skills over a wide variety of content; and with herself in capitalizing on experiences with language, communication, and thinking to represent the most accurate linguistic match between source and target languages.

Question 2: How does curriculum differentiation affect the interpreter?

Curriculum differentiation is a controversial topic in contemporary education practices (e.g., Pool & Page, 1995). Most secondary schools in the United States differentiate their program of studies to *track* college-bound students into college-preparatory courses and work-bound students into a vocational curriculum. Many schools have a third track—a general education track that is intended to bridge the disparity between the other two curriculum tracks and enable students to move between the tracks (Camarena, 1990). In addition, some schools acknowledge a fourth track that may or may not be intrinsically involved with the other three, a special education track for students with disabilities or special needs.

Tracking decisions for high school students typically are made at the end of the elementary- or middle-school years, at a point to facilitate scheduling. Tracking decisions are based on four criteria: (1) teachers' recommendations from the previous grade, (2) grades earned by the student in the previous grades—generally in the seventh and eighth grades, (3) performance on achievement tests, and (4) personal and parental requests (Camarena, 1990). The first criterion, the teachers' recommendations, contributes more to tracking decisions than the second, the student's grades; and these first two play a more prominent role in tracking decisions than the third and fourth criteria. A hierarchy exists, then, in the perceived importance of and impact on decisions administrators make about a student's high school curriculum track (p. 166). The validity of this hierarchy is not without question. As a colleague at a technical education program indicated, bright students who want to be chemical engineers or architects are usually discouraged from pursuing technical courses because technical courses are not perceived to be cognitively equivalent to traditional college-bound courses. Indeed, one of the controversies surrounding curriculum differentiation is that social differentiation, or separating students by ability levels, is viewed by many educators and noneducators as discriminatory. (Pool & Page, 1995). Research has revealed that students tracked in the work-bound curriculum are more likely to be "disproportionately poor, male, and minority" (Page, 1990, p. 17). Others who advocate curriculum differentiation see tracking as a necessary procedure to meet individual needs. The compromise, the general or standard, or core curriculum with its free electives may satisfy some heterogenous balance in some schools and for some students. That is, all students, college-bound or work-bound on entering high school, are required to have so many credits of mathematics, English, and sciences, in addition to so many credits of electives that are not necessarily bound to a particular track (e.g., physical education).

For educational interpreters, the critical point in discussing curriculum differentiation or tracking, of course, involves the assigned load and how it impacts the interpreter's performance. An interpreter who serves a work-bound student may find his or her consumer math course is heavy in worksheets, not lectures; and the interpreter who serves a college-prep student may find the English literature class is heavy in oral readings, not worksheets. Interpreters are also likely to find the discourse patterns of the two classrooms completely different. Reba Page (1990), in *Curriculum Differentiation,* explained that teachers who work with lower-track students may feel a need to talk less in all their classrooms. Because these teachers may anticipate trouble from students who are not interested in academics or assume that students do not have the critical thinking skills or the communication skills to participate in classroom discussions, they discourage discourse and prescribe, instead, lots of seatwork, which often becomes a "deadening routine" (p. 22).

Interpreters in these classes also may find themselves in such a deadening routine, unsure of what to do in the down time. Imagine this scenario:

John enters consumer math class, takes his assigned seat, and makes eye contact with his interpreter who is seated about six feet to the right of the teacher's desk.

John takes out the packet of tax forms he is working on for Mr. Davis. The W-2 forms are to be completed by the end of the week and Mr. Davis is available to work with the students when they hit a snafu or problem. John started on his forms yesterday and has only four more to do today. The interpreter watched him in yesterday's class and asked, on those occasions when he looked toward her, if he wanted her to interpret, if he needed to speak to Mr. Davis. John answered no all of the four or five times she asked and then told her to stop watching him, that she wasn't his mother.

The interpreter decided to bring a book to the class today—to read to help pass the time while John worked on his forms. The 53-minute class period dragged on endlessly.

To sit idle or to engage in some form of self-stimulation is a common dilemma for educational interpreters who find themselves with a lot of down time. The perceptions that are conveyed when an interpreter balances her check-book, writes a letter, reads the newspaper, prepares a grocery list, and so on, are not viewed with the same level of respect as when the interpreter reads the text-book, discusses with the teacher next week's unit on job applications, or watches tomorrow's videotape on setting up a bank account (if these activities can be done without distracting the working students). Regardless, at some point, and in some classes that have lots of down time, the interpreter may find that the best intentions and most thoughtful efforts at engaging in meaningful preparation are eventually replaced with efforts to consume the down time in any way possible, including reading the newspaper and balancing a checkbook.

In the world of best interpreting practices, educational interpreters are able to negotiate a secondary role with their teachers, students, and administrators that is professionally relevant and sustaining. In those classes with heavy seat-work and low discourse demands, the interpreter may need to negotiate excused absence time to attend a social studies class where she may hear parts of the lecture before being expected to interpret it in fifth period. The interpreter, of course, must be careful not to jeopardize her immediate need in the consumer math class in such a way that she might be pulled from it altogether, or to place herself at risk of being given assigned duties that are not within the interpreting contract. Balancing down time for preparation with time for rest must be negotiated with the administration and carefully handled with respect to the needs of students and teachers.

The curriculum of the college-prep and Advanced Placement (AP) classes may present challenges that are in polarized contrast to those in the lower-track course just described. Susan Hanson's (1990) ethnographic research of college-prep courses in two high schools showed wide variety in the following:

- *Student expectations.* Although all teachers stressed high performance from the students, the teachers varied widely in how they allocated class time and encouraged critical thinking, independent work, self-expression, and creative work. In some classes, students were expected to read broadly and spend quiet time thinking and analyzing their thoughts. In other classes, students were

given 10 or 15 minutes of free time in which they could begin the next assignment, get a head start on homework, get individual help from the teacher, or
simply chat quietly with their peers.

- *Communication.* Two types of general communication were observed throughout
  the classes: lecture and discussion. In some classes, students were encouraged to
  pay attention as the teacher lectured, and, in other classes, students were
  encouraged to develop their personal opinions and express their ideas. Humor
  was used liberally by some teachers, even as a vehicle for keeping the class
  under control. Some teachers were strict in specific guidelines for communicating and others were lenient, encouraging student creativity of expression.

- *Curriculum.* Many differences were found in the knowledge offered to students,
  with some courses bound to particular textbooks that influenced the nature of
  the topics, and with other courses centered around student selections for learning (e.g., the students were asked to select a time period in American literature
  from which readings would be assigned and chosen). Some teachers spent considerable class time discussing and working through homework assignments
  and other teachers made no homework assignments at all.

In spite of the variability interpreters may encounter in student expectations,
communication patterns, and curriculum demands of college-track courses, a fundamental principle exists: These students, *including students who are deaf and hard-of-
hearing,* are expected to have more cognitive ability than students not enrolled in
the same courses, and greater intellectual ability generally means more difficult
content with more difficult discourse. Imagine the following scenario:

> Mr. Powell's tenth-grade AP social studies class has just begun a unit on the judicial
> system. The discussion today centers around this reading that Mr. Powell places on
> the overhead:
>
> Substantive due process has to do with the content of the law, as opposed to
> the way a law is administered. If a law is found to be unreasonable, it is ruled as
> violating substantive due process. Here are some examples of laws that the
> Supreme Court has found to be unreasonable and consequently to violate substan-
> tive due process: a law that limits dwellings to single families, thus preventing
> grandparents from living with their grandchildren; a school board regulation that
> prevents a female teacher from returning to work before three months after the
> birth of her child; a law that requires all children to attend public schools and,
> hence, that does not permit them to attend non-public schools.
>
> After reading the passage, Mr. Powell asks these questions, almost without
> pause: "So what's substantive due process? What's unreasonable about a law that
> prevents grandparents from living with their grandchildren? And why should the
> Supreme Court concern itself with the business of a city or locality that determines
> the number and location of single- and multiple-family dwellings?

As if the literal content of the passage that is read to the class is not challenging enough, the interpreter in this classroom must work rapidly to interpret the
teacher's rapid-fire questions and just as rapidly to interpret the students'
responses that, even if they do occur one at a time (and they rarely do), are likely

to hit the air like ignited fireworks. Intense! In fact, in some college-prep courses, the question–answer dialogue that occurs between teacher and students constitutes the entire class period. The *Socratic method of inquiry*—directing students to reason through illuminating questions—is *the* teaching method. Teachers who use this method may ask hundreds of questions throughout a class period, following each response with another provocative question.

The types of questions teachers ask of students has received a great deal of attention at all grade levels over the past several years, but "categorizing teacher questions for their cognitive value is surprisingly hard to do" (Cazden, 1988, p. 100). Although all teachers use procedural questions (e.g., "Did everyone remember to bring in the homework assignments this morning?"), most teachers ask factual questions (e.g., "What's the answer to number 7?"), and many teachers use punishing and intimidating questions (e.g., "Mark, why don't you know the answer to this?"). Teachers who use questions that require complex cognitive work are more likely to be found in upper-track classes than in lower-track classes. Also, their questions take on many different types. (Re-read the dialogue that occurred between Doug and his teacher in the advanced placement (AP) English class. Look carefully at how Doug's teacher guided him with factual questions to the final question: "What's the fallacy of this syllogism?" (Also, examine the questions the teacher uses in the upcoming driver education class.)

Bruce Frazee and Rose Rudnitski (1995), reported that several question types exist: questions that introduce a topic; questions that encourage discussion; questions that redirect, expand, extend, clarify, justify, explain; and questions that close discussion (pp. 146–148). Cazden (1988), in her earlier discussion of questioning techniques, explained that variation in question type is critically linked to the sequencing of questions and to the wait time after a question is asked. Questions that have high cognitive load, when followed by a lengthened wait time (typical wait time is one- to one-and-a-half seconds), result in more high cognitive responses from more students (Shepherd & Ragan, 1992). Implications for the interpreter are probably obvious: Working with the classroom teacher to encourage an increase in wait time following a question not only results in better answers, but it also results in better interpreting.

Interpreting in fast-paced, cognitively demanding classes can be invigorating for educational interpreters; it also can be debilitating. Interpreters who learn to match the pace of the discourse and the reciprocity of question–answer often love the challenge educational interpreting offers. The adrenalin rush these interpreters experience is compromised only by the fatigue they also can experience during, but most likely, *after* the class ends. The physical drain from interpreting an intense discourse may make it difficult to keep up in the next class, or, in some cases, make it impossible to interpret for the rest of the day.

Interpreters who find themselves in fast-paced classes are at a higher risk for musculoskeletal disorders (e.g., tendonitis, carpal tunnel syndrome) that result from repetitive motion injury (RMI) than interpreters who are assigned to classes with a slower pace. Interpreters who experience recurrent and increasing pain in their upper limbs and hands must inform their administrators of their symptoms and seek ways to reduce the physical demands of the job. (Susan Smith, Tyler Kress, and William Hart, 2000, reported females to be at a significantly higher risk for problems than males.) Early contact with the administration is critical, particularly because school administrators may be unfamiliar with RMI and its consequences. Because the consequences can include loss of time in the classroom, medical costs that may be connected to worker's compensation or school insurance claims, and, most seriously, the loss of highly skilled interpreters (Stedt, 1990; Wisowaty, 1996), administrators are often appreciative of interpreters' efforts to educate them regarding RMI. These administrators are also likely to be willing to work with the interpreter and the teachers to find ways to reduce the physical demands of the assignment. Team interpreting, as discussed in Chapter 2, is increasingly more common in intense secondary and postsecondary settings.

In order not to give the impression that all lower-track classes function at the pace of a tortoise or that all higher-track classes function at the pace of a hare, two more vignettes are in order:

Driver Education Class:

This tenth grade driver education class contains about 30 students, more males than females, all at the eager age to drive. Students are seated in conventional rows with the teacher on a stool in front, and the interpreter stands about six feet from the teacher and another six feet from the deaf student. He is seated on an end row, about midway from the front where he can see about 90% of the students, as well as his teacher and interpreter. This lesson is on tailgating:

TEACHER: If you slow down, that's telling them what?

[Several students respond simultaneously. The interpreter points to two and starts to interpret the loudest student, but pauses, turning his head back to the teacher, and resumes interpreting for the teacher who keeps talking.]

TEACHER: That you're willing for them to pass. All right, but let's say you slow down and they still don't pass.

[At least two students respond simultaneously. The interpreter points to both but quickly turns his head back to the teacher as she continues to talk.]

TEACHER: No, you don't want to tap your brakes at this point. What else should you do?

[Several students answer but no one is acknowledged and the teacher starts talking again before they are finished. Again the interpreter looks to the students and then redirects his gaze back to the teacher as he interprets.]

TEACHER: If you're traveling in the center of the lane and you have a car tailgating you, and you move . . .

STUDENT: . . . off the road.

[A student finishes her sentence. The interpreter points to the student and successfully interprets the student's statement.]

TEACHER: Why would you do that? No, you don't move off the road now. You move to the right. Why?

[The interpreter successfully interprets but does not add question markers to the WHY. Several students answer simultaneously, the interpreter attempts to point to each one, and starts to interpret the most audible answer when he pauses, redirects his gaze back to the teacher and interprets.]

TEACHER: Then maybe he's not passing 'cause he can't see.

[A student says something. The interpreter looks at him but turns immediately back to the teacher.]

TEACHER: No, he's still not passing, so what do you do?

SEVERAL STUDENTS respond, *[some louder than others]*. Now you pull off the road . . . *[several others interrupt]*: Tap your brakes. *[The interpreter points to four or five students and interprets: TAP BRAKES.]*

Without acknowledging any student, the teacher and interpreter, whose gaze is back to her, continue.

TEACHER: Tapping doesn't mean slamming them. It means a gentle light touch to get his attention, to let him know that you're not going to go faster than you already are, and . . .

STUDENT: *[interrupting] The interpreter points and tries to take in what the student is saying but the teacher continues.]*

TEACHER: OK, what if you've done all these things and he's still on your tail and you're getting more and more upset. Why?

STUDENTS: *[At least three different voices answer simultaneously and the interpreter points to each, but just as he starts to interpret one of the responses, the teacher continues.]*

TEACHER: 'Cause you're spending more time with your eyes on the rearview mirror than on the road.

[A student is talking at the same time and the interpreter looks back and forth between the student and the teacher but continues interpreting the teacher.]

TEACHER: No, you can't get in the other lane. Now you get off to the side of the road. All right *[two-second pause]*. Now get out your workbooks.

At least 20 students moan and the interpreter points to several and signs: NOOOO (*interpreted on both hands with directionality showing multiple voices*), NOT THE WORKBOOKS.

Not only was this a challenging lesson for the interpreter because of the fast pace (all this occurred in just under two minutes), but it was also particularly frustrating because the teacher never acknowledged the students' responses. Even though she asked questions, she never permitted answers to be fully heard. She interrupted the students as they answered, and the students, in turn, interrupted her and each other. The interpreter's inability to interpret the simultaneous voices was clearly shown, however, in his rapidly moving eye gaze, head turns, and pointing.

Surprisingly, the dynamics in this class were quite positive, and the deaf student appeared to be totally alert to the quickness of it all. The interpreter, who managed a spirited and highly accurate (if somewhat incomplete) interpretation, said it was a typical class.

English Class:
The eleventh-grade English literature class is heterogenous or mixed (i.e., it contains some students who are bound for college, some bound for work, and some who are in the general education track). The English teacher enjoys the mixture and has welcomed the deaf student and her interpreter. The first-period class goes something like this—on the overhead is a Shakespearian sonnet:

> **Sonnet 18**
> Shall I compare thee to a summer's day?
> Thou art more lovely and more temperate.
> Rough winds do shake the darling buds of May,
> And summer's lease hath all too short a date.
> Sometime too hot the eye of heaven shines,
> And often is his gold complexion dimmed.
> And every fair from fair sometime declines,
> By chance or nature's changing course untrimmed.
> But thy eternal summer shall not fade,
> Nor lose possession of that fair thou owest,
> Nor shall Death brag thou wander'st in his shade
> When in eternal lines to time thou grow'st.
> So long as men can breathe, or eyes can see,
> So long lives this, and this gives life to thee.

Mrs. Roland begins class by asking the students if anyone has read any of Shakespeare's sonnets. No one responds. She then tells the class of 16- and 17-year olds that the sonnets are usually discussed for their universal themes of time, death, beauty, moral integrity, and love. She then asks the class to read Sonnet 18, which is presented on the overhead, and think about which theme—time, death, beauty, integrity, love—Shakespeare intended.

The students proceed to read to themselves, looking at the screen in front of the room. After three or four minutes, Mrs. Roland reads the first two lines: *"Shall I compare thee to a summer's day? Thou art more lovely and more temperate."* She then asks, "So what's the theme? How many think he's talking about beauty?" Four or five hands go up, including the deaf student's. She calls on the deaf student, "Why do you think he's talking about beauty, Jonathon?" "Because 'lovely,'" Jonathon responds for himself. "Well, Jonathon thinks the theme is beauty because Shakespeare used the word *lovely*. Maybe. Let's read on and see if anyone disagrees: *"Rough winds do shake the darling buds of May, And summer's lease hath all too short a date."*

"Is beauty addressed here?" A hand goes up and another student says, "I think he's talking about time. He's talking about the seasons and that means time." Mrs. Roland responds, "OK, now Ginger says that Shakespeare's theme in this sonnet is time. Jonathon says it's beauty and Ginger says it's time. Let's read on and see if we can find one that we all agree on."

The dialogue continues, with Mrs. Roland reading lines and asking the students questions, which they answer in a rather pensive and subdued manner. The discourse is moderately paced, no rush, lots of pause time. The interpreter finger-spells comfortably as she transliterates verbatim the words of the sonnet. She leaves the 50-minute class feeling good about her performance and about the learning she facilitated.

Question 3: What is different about interpreting in vocational and laboratory settings?

The topic of curriculum differentiation would not be complete without addressing the vocational setting, but the expansiveness of issues involved in interpreting in vocational and technical education settings deserves to be treated as a separate area. As Diane Elliott, Pamela Luttrull, and Sharon deFur (1997) described, an increasing number of students with disabilities are participating in vocational education where the demands of general education transfer to vocational education.[1] The communication or teaching style of teachers in technical and vocational tracks is every bit as challenging to the educational interpreter as the fast-paced demands of the social studies class, the deadening-pace demands of the consumer math class, or the moderate pace of the literature class that were just described. The critical difference in most vocational-technical classes, however, is that "teaching by showing" (Kemp & Cochran, 1994, p. 46) defines the instructional style.

The same pedagogical principle is common to laboratory settings, such as those found in biology, chemistry, geology, and physics, where students with special needs have traditionally been underserved. Frequently, advisors and counselors have either counseled deaf students away from laboratory sciences or simply failed to offer them as part of the students' options. Many counselors, teachers, and parents have assumed deaf students to be at increased risk for accidents, but these assumptions are not valid (Minor, Nieman, Swanson, & Woods, 2001). Preventive measures are critical for all students, and required safety orientations on protective eye and skin wear, and procedures for responding to a spill, leak, fume, or other accidents, are often videotaped for mandatory viewing and periodic review. These measures are equally as applicable to deaf students as they are to hearing students, but may require certain accessibility accommodations, including visual alarm systems, unobstructed views, and interpreters (pp. 71–72).

Deaf students also may not be offered, or may not choose a curriculum with laboratory sciences, because of the shortage of interpreters knowledgeable of and comfortable with the language:

---

[1]If Virginia is representative of the other 49 states, half of all secondary-aged students with disabilities participate in some form of vocational education (deFur, Getzel, & Kregel, 1995).

The language of chemistry is . . . full of Latin and mathematics and acronyms, passive voice and questions and obscure pronouns. It's not so much a conversant language as it is a language of two or three topic turns. It's a language bound by visual activity. It's a dynamic language, in which the simplest phrase can be so difficult to interpret for semantic accuracy (Seal, 2001, p. 10).

The challenges of interpreting in science laboratories can be extremely gratifying, however, and deserve increased visibility in ITPs and practicum experiences. In fact, the National Science Foundation, in its efforts to increase deaf science majors in postsecondary programs, has provided funding for training educational interpreters who work with high school and college students in summer research programs (Seal, Wynne, & MacDonald, 2002).

Interpreters in vocational classes may be scheduled for part of their day or for a full day over an extended period, depending largely on the nature of the training and the needs of the student(s). Most large school systems have a vocational or technical department or division that is an integral component to the secondary curriculum. This department is usually located within a wing of the school building or in a building that is adjacent to the main building. Others, especially smaller school systems, may share a centralized vocational or technical school with other high schools in the school district. In addition, many states have regional vocational centers funded by the Department of Rehabilitative Services (DRS) that accept students who are at least 15½ years old for vocational evaluations and prevocational and vocational training programs, and 14 years old for transitional programs. Programs at DRS centers may have their own staff interpreters or they may expect local schools to provide interpreters for the students they send to the center.

Common to all of these vocational-technical–laboratory settings are certain pedagogical principles: Students learn best by *doing* and teachers teach best by *showing.* The role of the interpreter is to provide communication access to the doing and the showing. Herein lies the challenge. The nature of the doing and showing varies widely across the range of courses and training programs offered in these settings. Science education generally spans four or five courses. Vocational education can span hundreds of fields, but commonly includes education in agriculture and business, marketing and distribution, health, business and office, trade and industry, and occupational home economics (Gajar, Goodman, & McAfee, 1993). Some programs include technology as a seventh vocational area, although each of the other areas relies heavily on technology in the training.

The scope of courses within the vocational fields is virtually unlimited. An interpreter may find himself or herself interpreting automotive electrical systems, body work, engine repair, exhaust systems, computer programming, computer manufacturing, computer graphics, word processing, desktop publishing, telecommunications, food services, dishwashing, waiting/waitressing, clothing and textiles, sewing-machine operation, dry cleaning, shoe repair, upholstering, furniture making, furniture refinishing, painting and wallpapering, small-appliance repair, tool-and-die making, furnace repair, welding, forklift driving, farm equipment mechanics, farm equipment operations, heavy equipment operations, electronics, housekeeping, greenskeeping, gardening, landscaping, pollution control, sanitation, water treatment, forestry, cosmetology, janitorial and custodial care, kennel care, meat inspecting, meat cutting, meat packing, shipping, receiving, office machine operations, office equipment repair, lithography, electrical engineering, roofing, drywalling, floorcovering, heating and air conditioning, plumbing, carpentry, cabinetmaking, bricklaying, stonemasonry, nursing aide courses, medical records, paramedics, safety inspection, quality-control management, and/or many others (Littrell, 1991, pp. 157–188). The diversity of course content is unlimited. The vocabulary is likewise unlimited.

A look at a blueprints course should expose the challenges that occur, even in a classroom/shop setting that resembles a typical lecture setting in a typical high school:

MR. MAYS: OK, we're gonna work on blueprints today, reviewing the alphabetic lines, the different types of lines used on the drawings and their purposes. Does that scare you, Lance? *[teasingly]*

LANCE: Yea, I can handle the abbreviations, but the lines give me trouble.

[Mr. Mays then distributes a handout to each of the students, puts a transparency on the overhead and takes a pointer in hand.]

MR. MAYS: OK, all the line types are on your handout and I want to make sure you understand everything before the quiz on Thursday. The various lines represent what the draftsman is trying to get across to you. One line that is always on the print is the visible line or the outline.

[Mr. Mays points to a line on the overhead.]

MR. MAYS: What's the definition of a visible line?

[Most of the eight students respond, reading the definition from their handout.]

MR. MAYS: OK, it's used to represent the visible edges of the part being drawn *[pointing to several lines on the overhead]*. But depending on what the view looks like *[puts pointer down and goes to a board that is sectioned off like a grid, picks up a colored marker and begins to draw a box]* . . . this is the top view of a box. What if we changed the front view of the box *[drawing a second box]*, you need a line down the middle. Why do we have to add the line in the center? *[Silence]* To show where the two tops come together. What's that called? The center line. We had that just the other day. Now what if I move it to the side *[erasing one line and drawing another]*, now it's an off-center line. What if I change these two angles to a radius *[erasing the line and drawing an arc]*. What does this mean?

JOAN: It doesn't mean anything unless you add a point.

MR. MAYS: Why is that? What is that certain point when two lines meet or cross?

JOAN: An intersection.

MR. MAYS: Anytime you have an intersection, you need a line to designate that intersection. What about when a radius and circle meet but do not cross?

LANCE: That's a tangent.

MR. MAYS: Right. Anytime you have a tangent, there isn't a visible line signified. If you have a radius, there's no visible line, so where you have a break or intersection you have to have a visible line, right? And two lines that become tangent will not have a visible line *[erases the board and goes back to the overhead]*.

MR. MAYS: The next line shown on your handout is a hidden line. A hidden line does what?

JESSE: Shows the surface.

MR. MAYS: Shows the surface, right. It represents outlines or parts of the surface that you can't see, like on the back of this surface *[pointing to a point an the overhead]* that you can't see. It's three-dimensional, well, not necessarily, but it does tell you that there's another part *[pointing to another spot on the overhead]*, a back view or some other view. Hidden lines are only used when they clarify a drawing, not if they make it more confusing. They're up to the draftsman. Now, what if it's an object line *[pointing to another point on the overhead]*? Visible lines are object lines. What about section lines? What do they represent *[pointing to another line on the overhead]*?

ROSE: Something has been left out.

MR. MAYS: Yes, see this section here *[pointing]*. The arrows show which half of the object you're supposed to look at. If we cut this part out at that point *[moving pointer across the section]*, this section is now the cross section. The only time section lines are used is with a cutting plane or a sectional view. They're normally very thin. Will the pattern change? No, just straight lines at a 45-degree angle. Does the pattern ever change? If the material is different, what changed? We have various types of material or sectional lines that signify the different materials. This one *[pointing to the overhead again]* represents lines at a 45-degree angle. What's that mean?

LANCE: Steel.

MR. MAYS: Not steel, but cast iron. *[He puts down the pointer and goes back to the board and starts drawing lines.]* Steel has two lines close together, then a larger space between them. We also have aluminum *[drawing another set of lines]* and brass *[another set of lines]* up to eight line spacings for section lines.

OK, now let's look at center lines *[returns to pointer and overhead]*. This drawing has a center line here *[points]*, one here *[points to a different place]*, and another one here *[points to another place on the overhead]*. These two have a center line that signifies the whole *[pointing at a different place]* and this center line represents the part *[pointing at another place]*. One center line can be the center line of the object itself *[moving the pointer]* and the other is the center line of any feature on the object. This line *[pointing]* has a vertical orientation for the center line of a part or feature *[moving the pointer up and down]*; same way with this one *[moving to another line with an up-and-down sweep]*. It's the center line of a feature, not a whole. Are center lines present on all drawings? Yes, they should be because every drawing has center lines.

Now let's talk about dimension lines . . .

[Mr. Mays continues for the next 15 minutes, talking about *cutting plane lines, short break lines, long break lines,* and *phantom lines.* The students attend carefully, moving their eyes from the pointer on the overhead screen to their handout to the grid on the board to Mr. Mays.]

Interpreting for this class is particularly challenging, even though the lecture resembles the type of lecturing found in traditional classrooms, even though the teacher lectures at a comfortable pace, and even though there are only eight students in the classroom whose questions and responses must be heard and understood in order to be interpreted. At least two challenges, however, should be immediately apparent: (1) the semantics or meaning of the words used, and (2) the mutual demand on the students' eyes and ears to comprehend the meaning of the words used.

A scrutinizing look at the meaning of Mr. Mays's words exposes the variations on vocabulary that can be particularly difficult for educational interpreters in vocational classes. In this class, for example, the interpreter must understand LINE, but not *just* LINE; the interpreter must be able to represent all the variations on LINE that are used. This requires comprehension, at least to the degree that meaningful differences can distinguish vocabulary that may involve only discrete changes. Transliterating technical vocabulary requires more than finding "word-meaning" or "pairing one sign with each word conveyed" (Lawrence, 1987, p. 88). It requires "message-meaning" in order to represent the intentions and context of the speaker. Conceptual accuracy is particularly challenging for interpreters who attempt to render message equivalence with technical vocabulary.

Another problem exists with the vocabulary used in vocational classes and laboratories. When teachers use diagrams, graphs, charts, tables, figures, instruments, machines, tools, and even the blackboard as part of their lecture, their word choices take on a heavier concentration of pronouns than when they lecture without visual supports. Interpreting "this line," "the line here," "another one here," "the center there," is meaningless without first establishing a referent for each "this, here, another, and there." In this lecture, Mr. Mays's pointer designated the referents. Each time he pointed to a specific line or point on a line, the students' eyes established the referent while their ears took in the verbal information about that referent.

Elizabeth Winston, in several of her writings on educational interpreting (e.g., Winston, 1995), discussed the "incompatibility" of some classrooms for interpreting. She explained that in those situations in which the "hearing student must use both the ears and eyes at the same time, the activity is not compatible with interpreting" (p. 35). In Mr. Mays's class, the deaf student's eyes are likely to be fixed on the interpreter while the hearing students' eyes are fixed on the teacher's pointer. When the deaf student moves her eyes from the interpreter to the overhead or to the board, she experiences a gap in the auditory information; when she moves her eyes from the overhead or board to the interpreter, she experiences a gap in the visual information. If the auditory or verbal information refers to the visual information, a gap in either one reduces the comprehension of the other.

The challenge to make both the auditory and visual information accessible to the student who is deaf or hard-of-hearing requires mutual efforts from both the interpreter and the teacher.

> Teachers who are conscious of how their instructional (and noninstructional) time is allocated and how they use their time to engage students in learning (Goodman, 1990) are teachers who have an upper hand on teaching. . . . Even these talented teachers may be surprised at the additional time required for a student who has a hearing loss. These teachers learn that every auditory message that accompanies a visual message (like all those found in books, on worksheets, transparencies, maps, computer screens, in video, filmstrip, and slide presentations) requires the student with a hearing loss to attend sequentially, not simultaneously (Seal, 1997, p. 265).

Several strategies for teachers to improve the accessibility of their classrooms for deaf or hard-of-hearing students have been recommended (Seal, 1997):

- Addressing the class from an established location in the lab, room, or shop
- Providing descriptive statements before, not during, demonstrations
- Pausing to facilitate a shift in attention from the teacher or interpreter to the transparency, computer monitor, chart, and so on
- Sequencing hands-on activities during the instructional phase
- Repeating student comments, questions, and answers to the whole class (p. 265)

Interpreters who support teachers in these strategies are likely to experience mutual support from the teachers. The reciprocity of this support is fundamental as interpreters attempt to employ their own strategies to make the information accessible to the students.

At least two strategies are commonly used by interpreters in technical and laboratory settings: One strategy involves proxemics and the other involves timing. The interpreter who closely shadows the teacher may enable the deaf student to track the teacher's pointings or references to visual information directly while taking in the interpreter's linguistic message indirectly in the peripheral visual field. Likewise, the interpreter who moves in close proximity with the teacher may enable the student to track the interpreter directly while taking in the teacher's pointings indirectly in the peripheral visual field. As Nancy Frishberg (1990) explained, moving along with the teacher may be helpful in allowing the "deaf student to comfortably attend visually to the signed message and the speaker, blackboard, film, etc." (p. 109).

Virginia Swisher and her colleagues (Swisher, Christie, & Miller, 1989) investigated the ability of adolescents to identify signs that were presented in the periphery. Their results (see Chapter 4 for comparative results with children) revealed that students between 15 and 18 years of age were able to identify as many as 80% of the signs presented in their peripheral visual fields. They interpreted this finding to have "implications for the presentation of visual information in the classroom, and for the positioning of educational interpreters, particularly where the teacher is performing a demonstration and talking about it at the same time" (p. 170).

Moving along with a teacher also should enable the teacher to sense the pace that the interpreter has in keeping up with the pace that the teacher has. This sense of timing is necessary for both the teacher and the interpreter in situations where sequential eye gaze is required. The unique challenges that are presented in technical classrooms, shops, labs, and other secondary settings, where showing and doing are important to the teaching and learning, are only met when the interpreter and teacher work in tandem.

The next two vocational scenarios offer an additional challenge—one experienced when the interpreter cannot be in close proximity to the instructor. In certain situations, the practicality of close shadowing of the teacher negates the possibility. Issues of space and safety require a different approach for interpreters and teachers in the following classes.

Welding Class

One of the students in Mr. Raymond's welding class approaches him with a plate he has just welded.

Mr. Raymond tells him to, "Put a clamp here *[pointing to a place on the horizontal pipe]* to hold the pipe down. The weight should keep this one from slipping *[pointing to the vertical pipe]*. Clamp it down, cut it square, and weld it."

Mr. Raymond observes as the student clamps, cuts, and picks up a welding torch. As the student slips the welding helmet over his head and starts welding, Mr. Raymond steps between me *[the observing interpreter]* and the welding torch. When the welding stops, he redirects his attention to the student and says, "Go in like this *[pointing directly into a point on the pipe]*, not like this *[pointing at an angle]*." Mr. Raymond then says to me, "I'm blocking you because the TIG welder's slow and the electric arc can burn your retina, just like looking through a magnifying glass at the sun can burn your eyes, so you don't want to look at it." I then ask, "But how can I interpret if I don't look at it." "You can't; you can't look at it."

Diesel Engine Class

Mr. Harsh leaves his perch inside the hood of a large truck and goes over to two students who are working inside a clutch that's resting on the floor. "All right, what have you turned?" The students point and mumble something as Mr. Harsh pulls a flashlight from his shirt pocket and shines it inside the clutch. He then takes "the adjusting tool" and says, "Now get in here where you can see it. See how that ring is moving *[as he demonstrates]*, that's how you need to adjust the clutch."

He looks to one of the students and says, "Now push in the clutch with this tool *[handing him a large rod]*, and you *[handing the other student the tool from his hand]* turn the ring with this tool." As the boys start to work with the tools, Mr. Harsh comments, "Notice how the bearing is fast, stuck in there, you can't move it without the tool. *[They continue to turn.]* See how much closer it is now. Now use the gauge *[handing one of them another tool]* to measure the distance between the throw-out bearing and the clutch plate."

In both classes, the teacher's interactions with the students involved doing and showing; and, in both classes, seeing what was being done and what was being shown was either dangerous or impossible. When the teacher's hands are deep within a clutch, when the teacher is perched inside the hood of a truck, when the welding torch light requires a welding helmet, the challenge is to find compensatory ways to make the information accessible. Again, the challenge belongs to both the teacher and the interpreter. Both Mr. Raymond and Mr. Harsh reported that their classroom instruction prior to entering the shop is an important precursor to the hands-on instruction that goes on in the shop. They also reported that they rely heavily on videotapes that illustrate the safety precautions required in working with dangerous tools and equipment. They also indicated that the interpreter must abide by the same safety rules that everyone else abides by: wearing protective glasses and observing at safe distances from activities that pose danger.

In *Planning for Effective Technical Training*, Kemp and Cochran (1994) made several recommendations to make demonstrations visually accessible: arranging equipment and materials so everything is visible (like in a circle), suspending video cameras for those views that need to be over the shoulder, building in ample time for students to practice a skill, and building in additional time for students to discuss what they have practiced and to ask questions about what they are learning. Each of these strategies, though not intended just for deaf or hard-of-hearing students, would be particularly helpful for interpreters in challenging vocational and laboratory settings.

Another strategy that may be helpful in situations like these is the use of consecutive interpreting. Anna Witter-Merithew and Richard Dirst (1982) described the differences between simultaneous and consecutive interpreting:

> *Consecutive.* The interpreting format where the interpreter receives small amounts of information from a speaker, then pauses to represent the information into the other language. Then the process continues in this alternating until completed. This is the most appropriate format when ASL and English are used, but because it is time-consuming, it is usually reserved for one-to-one situations.
>
> *Simultaneous.* The interpreting format where the interpreter is interpreting at the same time the speaker is talking or signing. The interpreter will tag behind only a few words or a sentence. This format is the expected norm for interpreters and works well when interpreting from one form of English to another (p. 401).

Although most interpreters use simultaneous interpreting in educational settings, the feasibility of consecutive interpreting in vocational classes and other classes that involve lots of showing and doing should be explored. Several characteristics of these classes make them compatible for consecutive interpreting: small class sizes, increased opportunities for individual instruction, larger blocks of scheduled time devoted to learning, and testing (and grading) that is competency-based. Interpreters should work with their teachers and students to determine those situations that are incompatible for simultaneous interpreting and better suited for consecutive interpreting. In those situations where close proximity and timing prohibit simultaneous interpreting, consecutive interpreting should be used.

Question 4: How does technology affect interpreting?

The technical, vocational, and laboratory settings just described are filled with technology used both in the instructional (the showing) and experiential (the doing) phases of learning. Instructional technology is not unique to these settings, however. In fact, instructional technology has permeated all phases of our educational programs today. Typical high schools may have multiple computer resource labs, multiple computer terminals in their libraries, and at least one computer in each classroom. The increased use of computers in students' homes has led many schools to expect students to arrive at high school with keyboarding and navigating competencies. If anything, today's schools are more likely to focus attention on their teachers' needs in gaining computer proficiency than on their students' needs. Staff development for technology is common. Resource personnel are hired to assist teachers in their instructional use of word processing, simulations, telecommunications, and mathematical computing and modeling. Most high schools today are, or are rapidly becoming, high-tech settings.

Interpreting in high-tech settings can impose different dynamics. Interpreting a teacher's Power-Point lecture may require only a few adjustments: previewing the slides to ensure terminology, gaining familiarity with graphics and any special viewing options (e.g., animation, sound bites, video clips, and so on). Lighting can be a special consideration, especially if reduced lighting for increased visibility of the screen means decreased visibility of the interpreter. Background templates and font style and size can also be problematic if the interpreter's need for a quick view of the screen is compromised (Lightfoot, 2002). Interpreters accustomed to working with multimedia presentations typically attempt to position themselves for maximum viewing (both for the students and for themselves). Migrating away from the speaker to the screen, or finding a middle ground to hear and see both the speaker and the screen is not uncommon. Some interpreters work with mirrors for increased access to a screen positioned behind them. This area of interpreting with multimedia is also fertile for research, particularly in determining the effects of divided attention, in both interpreters and students, on interpreter performance and student learning. Are they enhanced or diminished?

Interpreting in high-tech classrooms, vocational shops, and laboratories where the students are engaged *with* the technology raises other access concerns. Proximity to the activity may be impossible, as in the welding and diesel engine class; or access may depend on the interpreter's agility in moving, as explained in this chemistry laboratory:

> Faucets and fixtures reach out from waist-high sinks. Pipettes and purifiers rest ominously on and around cabinets. Goggles, gloves and gadgets occupy the hands while heads are engaged in measuring, condensing, diluting, timing, plotting, graphing, and sometimes, dumping and starting over when just one small step has been miscalculated. The activity level is all-consuming; yet, there are long lulls as

some mixture liquifies, and then there are frantic sprints as the solutions from one beaker are transferred to another (Seal, 2001, p. 10).

When the focus of attention involves changing activities, interpreters have to find the best place to sit or stand, and the best path in which to move from one activity to another. This may be particularly difficult when long lulls are followed by quick sprints; interpreter vigilance is often challenged in these settings.

When the student is at a computer monitor, the nature of the discourse is heavily influenced by changes on the screen. Online searches, online communication (both synchronous and asynchronous), and links from one site to another, may place the interpreter in a role similar to that discussed in Chapter 3 (the role of the interpreter during free play) and in Chapter 4 (the role of the interpreter in instructional groups). The interpreter may simply need to be available, within eye- or earshot. In these cases, responding to a student's bid to interpret will occur when the student needs to communicate with the teacher or peers with whom the student might be working (see Stewart and Kluwin, 2001, for grouping students in technology assignments). This interpreter will likely rove with the teacher in approaching the student's terminal, and provide interactive interpreting as needed. Interpreters who are distanced from the screen's changing activities may find a problem when they begin to interpret. Their background knowledge may be insufficient for immediate interpretation. The deaf student who points to the computer screen with nothing more than a lost look leaves the interpreter with nothing more than a lost look. My experience is that teachers are often more comfortable with these looks than interpreters, and sometimes the fix requires the student and teacher to catch the interpreter up to the problem. Then, sometimes, the teacher's hand on the mouse simply clicks away the problem.

Secondary educational interpreters are increasingly placed in classrooms where they interpret *alongside* technology. The use of Computer Assisted Real-time Translation (CART) and computer-aided speech-to-print transcription (C-Print captioning) are increasingly more common in secondary and postsecondary settings, in some cases because of increased enrollments of students with cochlear implants. Interpreters who work alongside recorders often enjoy the visual access to low-frequency vocabulary and spelling. These interpreters also develop an attitude of flexibility in maintaining vigilance when students' eyes linger on the transcription.

An attitude of flexibility in accepting changes *in* technology and changes in our interpreting *because of* technology is critically important today. Communication technology in our daily lives is rapidly changing (Hallett, 2002). Two-way pagers, faxes, e-mail, video interpreting, and Internet Protocol (IP) relay are accelerating changes in our communication patterns in ways unprecedented in the history of the world (Bowe, 2002; Nelson, 2002). The influence of this technology on our interpreting is largely uncharted, yet we suspect it is, or soon will be, pervasive. E-mail etiquette or *netiquette* (Norton & Sprague, 2001) calls for certain behaviors in our electronic communication—like conciseness. We are cautioned not to type more than a screen, or, when our message necessarily exceeds a screen, to include the word *long* in the subject line (p. 145). We are advised to use subject lines or topicalization to reduce ambiguity in our messages. We are advised not to open messages from unknown sources, not to *flame* or *spam* (p. 148). These behaviors will likely influence our interpreting in two ways: Most obviously, new signs will emerge for commonly used "tech speak." More subtly, consumer expectations for quick access and reduced ambiguity will continue to raise expectations for quick access and reduced ambiguity in our educational interpreting.

Question 5: What about interpreting in transition programs for secondary students?

Another consideration in secondary educational interpreting involves transition. Transition services are defined in the 1997 Amendment to IDEA as coordinated activities for students, designed with an outcome-oriented process that promotes movement from school to postschool activities, including postsecondary education, vocational training, integrated employment, continuing education, and independent living or community participation (Stewart & Kluwin, 2001). IEPs must reflect transition planning, including the anticipation of interpreting as a related service. The impact of transition programs on an educational interpreter is that the interpreter, like the student, may be moved from the school or vocational center to an employment or community site.

At the site, the interpreter's role involves facilitating the student's orientation to the school's expectations (he or she is still a student), to the employer's expectations (he or she is also an employee), and to the job responsibilities (he or she is learning to work). Interpreting orientation meetings and conferences that focus on general expectations, such as attendance and punctuality, safety practices and regulations, and personal appearance and initiative, are likely to occur at the onset of the transition program. Interpreting specifics about the student's job responsibilities and performance criteria also are likely to occur at the onset of the program. Then, at some point mutually agreed on by the school transition personnel, the employment site personnel, and the student, the interpreter's role may end or be rescheduled. If the interpreter is rescheduled, the change most likely will involve interpreting in an as-needed capacity. *As needed* may involve a new schedule (e.g., the interpreter reports to the work site to interpret the weekly conference involving the student and the supervisors from the school and employment site). *As needed* also may mean that the interpreter will be contacted when the student masters a certain job skill and is ready to move to a higher skill level or to a new job. *As needed* can also take on a negative connotation—the interpreter will be called when and if problems occur at the work site.

In the successful transition program, the interpreter may be viewed from this perspective: *less is more*. That is, the less the student is perceived to need an interpreter, and the less the employer perceives that he or she needs an interpreter, the more successful the transition program. If independence at a job is the hallmark of a successful transition program, then independence in communication, as determined by the absence of an interpreter, may also represent success. The impact of this thinking—that less interpreting means more success—on the true success of the transition program is worth contemplating for at least three reasons: (1) If the interpreter is truly a facilitator, then he or she is in a position to guide those involved (including the student and his or her immediate supervisor) in certain communication tips that might reduce any negative impact because of the interpreter's absence; (2) if the student's learning is enhanced by engaging in communication with individuals at the employment site, then the absence of the interpreter may lead to failure, not success; and, finally, (3) if the educational interpreter in a transition program is to facilitate himself or herself out of a job, then it is important to work with the school system and/or the employment agency in determining how the as-needed interpreting role is to be handled.

With regard to the third point first: Negotiating what it means to be available, or on call, to interpret as needed is important. The school system or employment agency may not want to pay interpreters when they are not providing direct services. At the same time, if being available prevents the interpreter from accepting other paying assignments, some type of financial guarantees or compensatory arrangement needs to be made. Furthermore, if the interpreter truly facilitates herself or himself out of a job and accepts other assignments, her or his availability to the transition program has been nullified. The lack of access to the original interpreter may be detrimental to the student's success and/or to the employer's willingness to take future students who work with interpreters. One of the recommended strategies for transitional settings involves the use of pagers, which allow the interpreter to be on call without having to totally abandon other assignments.

With regard to the first and second points about an interpreter's presence or absence, the student's independence in communicating at the job site is a highly individual matter that involves much more than working with an interpreter. The school's communication skills specialist, speech-language pathologist, teacher of the deaf or hearing-impaired, and social worker may all need to be involved in assisting the student with pragmatic communication skills that are considered important for communicating with others at the job site. Instructing individuals at the site in basic signs, which can reinforce the quality of work or provide directions to the student during work, may require a brief inservice with follow-up tutorials. Instructing individuals at the job site on attention-getting devices and the appropriate use of touch in securing attention may eliminate some awkwardness for both the deaf and hearing parties. Instructing the deaf student to request an interpreter when she or he perceives a need to communicate important thoughts or questions to others at the job site may also reduce the interpreter's presence on a routine basis. In each of these cases, the interpreter's role in assisting other members of the communication team in observing, monitoring, and providing meaningful intervention at the job site may be a far more important indicator of a successful transition program than relying on the employer's and student's assurance that the interpreter is not needed.

Question 6: How does scheduling affect secondary-level interpreters?

Although scheduling can be a critical variable in the success of the interpreter at the elementary- and middle-school levels, it holds a very prominent place in the variables that contribute to or prevent success for the interpreter at the secondary level. As indicated, the curriculum demands at the secondary level require flexibility on the part of the interpreter. Even experienced interpreters who are masters at flexibility need special consideration in scheduling. A schedule that affords *optimum interpreting performance* for optimum communication access is most likely to afford optimum student learning.

Student schedules are usually arranged in the summer, prior to school's opening in the fall. Changes in the schedule may be possible during the first week of the school term or even throughout the first grading period, but changes after that are rare. Traditionally, student scheduling is done en masse, without particular attention to an individual student's needs. In the world of best practices, however, administrators who schedule students and their interpreters are aware of the physical and cognitive demands that interpreting involves and include either the interpreter or a knowledgeable supervisor in the original scheduling that focuses on the student as an individual.

Because newly matriculating interpreters may not know the teaching styles of the teachers or classes that are being considered, feedback on the pace of particular classes and teachers from previous interpreters is important in order to create the best possible schedule for the next year. Whenever possible, videotaped segments of interpreters at work can serve as a valuable resource for administrators and members of a student's IEP team when the time for scheduling arrives.

A *traditional* high school schedule involves six or seven periods, ranging anywhere from 47- to 53-minutes long. All periods are divided equally; all periods meet every day, five days a week. Monday's schedule is identical to Tuesday's schedule and Wednesday's schedule, and so on. An example of a traditional high school schedule that covers seven periods or courses can look like this:

1st period:	AP World Studies
2nd period:	Ninth-grade Health and Physical Education (PE)
3rd period:	AP Science
4th period:	Foundations of Technology
5th period:	Algebra I
6th period:	Spanish I
7th period:	English

This particular schedule may be ideal for the interpreter. The first-period class, assuming it is like Mr. Powell's social studies class, can be a high-demand class, but it is followed by PE, a low-demand class, one in which the discourse possibilities are low. The third-period class is likely to be heavy in lecture and demonstrations, and the technology class that follows is likely to involve lots of showing and doing. If the interpreter has a restful lunch break before the fifth, sixth, and seventh periods, he or she may be in top form to handle the heavy homework discourse (reading from the book and checking the homework that corresponds to the reading) during the first 20 minutes of Algebra, followed by 15 minutes of the teacher's instruction on new material (using the blackboard), followed by 15 minutes of graphing calculator work (computer time). If Spanish (sixth period) involves lecturing in Spanish and if English (last period) involves lots of oral reading, the interpreter will likely need to team with a second interpreter.

Several changes in the traditional high school schedule have come about in recent years in an effort to improve sensitivity to learning styles, curriculum demands, and the human biological clock. The *block* schedule is probably the most widely accepted break from the traditional high school schedule. The block schedule involves longer blocks of time devoted to courses, with fewer classes scheduled each day, and with alternating schedules occurring on an even–odd day basis. In a six-course schedule, the student meets three classes one day and three the next day. In a seven-course schedule, the student meets four classes a day, with one class scheduled at some point in the school day for the traditional 47, 50, or 53 minutes. On the odd days (starting with a Monday as the first odd day), Student A goes to her first-, third-, fifth-, and seventh-period classes, or, with the schedule just described, to World Studies, Science, Algebra, and English. On the even days (starting with Tuesday as the first even day), the student goes to second-, fourth-, fifth-, and sixth-period classes, or to PE, Technology, Algebra, and Spanish I. In this schedule, Algebra, the fifth-period course, meets daily for 50 minutes; all others meet every other day for 75 minutes. A 25-minute lunch period is scheduled at the same time each day, just before Algebra.

Comparing the impact of this course sequence to the same sequence in a traditional schedule probably leaves us thinking that the odd days are too fast-paced and that the even days have too much down time. In week 1, the interpreter has three days of intense interpreting; in week 2, there are only two days of intense interpreting. This type of schedule alternation may not be ideal for interpreting. On the other hand, interpreters who have made the switch from traditional scheduling to block scheduling generally report that their early fears that they could not maintain for 75 minutes were soon relieved. Apparently, in many block classes, teachers increase their lecture time only slightly, but increase their seatwork, or down time, considerably. My colleagues who interpret in block schedules report that they prefer the longer periods because they have more down time in intense classes, and less course preparation.

The impact of scheduling on the educational interpreter is often outside the interpreter's control. The educational interpreter who advocates for input in the original scheduling, or for changes in a difficult schedule, realizes how important scheduling is to the goal of optimum performance. Interpreters who move from school to school benefit in knowing each school's scheduling system at the onset. These itinerant interpreters sometimes find that their driving time is their only rest time, that lunch time occurs in the car, and that traffic and parking become additional concerns to the day's schedule. These concerns are best handled at the opening of the school year, when negotiations and orientations are more likely to result in accommodation. Finally, interpreters who are aware of how they perform under different scheduling conditions should experiment with their personal accommodations (e.g., adjusting sleeping and eating schedules) when scheduling challenges their best performance.

Question 7: What other curriculum issues present extraordinary challenges to educational interpreters in secondary settings?

The interplay between course content, teacher style, and student dynamics make every learning situation in any secondary setting a potentially volatile situation. Recognizing this volatility is particularly important. What could be an easy interpreting situation in one school or with one grade level or one group of students could become an impossible situation in another school or with another group of students at another grade level. The flexibility that was mentioned at the beginning of this chapter should be stressed again as a major theme for interpreters working with adolescents. With that introduction, however, there still exist certain courses that, by their very nature, present challenges that differ from other courses. In this section, I will discuss three of these: family life instruction, driver education, and foreign language classes.

Family life instruction has been an integral part of secondary education for several years, although it may exist under curriculum names such as "Sexuality Education," "Body Systems," and so on. State and federal mandates have responded to the crises in teen pregnancies, AIDS and other sexually transmitted diseases, and drugs and substance abuse among adolescents with increased efforts to educate students about their bodies.

Interpreting in classes that focus on sexuality issues can be difficult for many interpreters and students. Teachers who are comfortable with the content frequently know the areas of increased sensitivity and work carefully to present the material in ways that minimize embarrassment. Imagine the lectures and activities that could accompany this tenth-grade sexuality curriculum (courtesy of Harrisonburg City School's Family Life Education Curriculum Director):

Unit 1: The Media's Portrayal of Sexuality
Unit 2: Sexual Violence
Unit 3: Family Values
Unit 4: Decision Making
Unit 5: Sexually Transmitted Diseases and HIV/AIDS
Unit 6: Attraction and Intimacy
Unit 7: Sexual Coercion
Unit 8: Birth Control and Parenting

Topics covered in Unit 7 include: incest, sexual harassment, child abuse, rape (date rape, marital rape, sodomy), obscene phone calls, exhibitionism, and voyeurism. Topics covered in Unit 8 include: abstinence and outercourse, oral contraceptives, injectable contraceptives and implants, the diaphragm, the vaginal sponge, the cervical cap, spermicidals, the condom (male and female), body temperature method, calendar method, and withdrawal method. In many school systems, sensitive topics like some of these are taught in single-sex classes, not in co-ed classes. The implication for the interpreter who may be of a different sex from the students and teacher of the class can be unsettling. Making arrangements for same-sex interpreters should begin early enough in the school term to ensure that the alternate interpreter will be available and prepared for the sensitive material.

Even in same-sex classes, with same-sex interpreters, issues surrounding interpretation can be delicate. I recall one interpreter friend who borrowed a videotape of human sexuality signs from the local university's library, only to reject a large number of the signs in favor of fingerspelling. As she explained, some of the more graphic signs would have lured a select group of girls to watch with the intent of using them in solicitous ways. The young girl for whom she was interpreting would have been seriously embarrassed if the other girls were to have used her language in such an exploitative way. Other interpreters have indicated they use sexual signs, regardless of their graphic appearance, just like teachers use words that have duplicitous connotations. These interpreters argue that their role is not to censor.

Interpreters in sex education classes have also reported surprise when approached by a student with questions or a desire to talk more about information presented in the classroom. One interpreter indicated she felt comfortable answering her student's questions about intercourse, knowing that she probably had no one else with whom to have these conversations. Indeed, communicating about sexuality is awkward for most students and their parents, and deaf adolescents who have hearing parents may find it particularly difficult to have detailed conversations about sexual topics with their parents. Antonio Maxon and Diane Brackett (1992) reported that most hearing adolescents gain their sexual knowledge, at least half of it, from their peers, between the ages of 12 and 13. Interpreters who are asked to elaborate on classroom discussions or sexual information not learned earlier from peers may find themselves at an ethical crossroad. Judgments on best practices will vary, with a not-my-place attitude for some, and a part-of-my-cross-cultural-role attitude for others. Many interpreters will find a middle-of-the-road stance, responding to some questions and agreeing to interpret for other questions, which they feel should be directed elsewhere.

Interpreting in foreign language classes creates interesting challenges to secondary interpreters, too. The first question generally asked is, How? Interpreters who don't speak Spanish, who don't read French, who don't know Japanese cannot be expected to interpret what they don't understand. A second question that is generally asked is, Why? Why would a deaf student want to take German? Isn't English enough of a challenge for spoken languages? My experiences have revealed many secondary students who are deaf who choose to study foreign languages (just as increasing numbers of hearing students choose to study ASL as a foreign language). The following interview with a deaf eleventh grader should make an impression on any doubters:

INTERVIEWER: What languages are you taking now (this year)?

STUDENT: *[responding in spoken English that is supported with cued speech]* I'm in ASL I right now, but I'm not very good at it. I know how to sign Exact English, not American Sign Language. And I have three years of Spanish.

INTERVIEWER: Why do you prefer cued speech in the classroom?

STUDENT: Because you can get a lot of information from it and you feel more comfortable knowing what is going on in class. And it helps to improve your English. You can talk to other hearing people without feeling awkward, And you can write in complete English and people will understand what you write and what you say.

INTERVIEWER: Do you mind answering this next question in sign language so we can see some of your signing skills?

STUDENT: Sure *[in sign language]*.

INTERVIEWER: Do you speak other languages?

STUDENT: *[still signing]* Yes, I speak Spanish, level III, and I speak some Indian languages, but not very well.

INTERVIEWER: Do you plan to take other languages?

STUDENT: *[still signing]* Yes, I really want to learn more about my native languages, like Tamil and Hindi. And I would like to learn more about French but I think it would be hard for me because the voicings and the wordings are so different.

At least two possibilities exist for interpreting foreign languages. One involves using cued speech, fingerspelling, or orally transliterating what the teacher says when she or he instructs in the foreign language. This possibility may be more promising at the introductory level than at advanced levels. At the introductory level, the interpreter is like all other students in that the interpreter must learn the material from the introductory point, and in learning the material, the interpreter learns to code the material into its transliterated equal. The second possibility involves interpreters who know both the foreign language and the student's language. These interpreters are likely to sign the foreign language in ASL or an English-based sign code while mouthing the foreign language. Interpreters who master this feat are usually in high demand in school programs that have large numbers of deaf or hard-of-hearing students. These interpreters should be encouraged to make their techniques and strategies available to a larger audience of interpreters.

Cheryl Davis (2000) offered several guidelines for teachers, students, interpreters, and service coordinators in college programs where deaf and hard-of-hearing students may need or request foreign language classes. Her recommendations are equally relevant at the secondary level where the focus on different cultures is increasingly prominent. Central to her recommendations is an attitude of acceptance toward language learning. This attitude was particularly relevant to those interpreters who attended the 2002 World Symposium for Sign Language Interpreters (Burch, 2002). Their awareness that sign language interpreters work in hundreds of countries with hundreds of deaf cultures across the globe is not likely to impact secondary foreign language programs, however, without appropriate sharing.

Another foreign language, ASL, has entered the secondary curriculum in recent years (Wilcox, 1992), and many progressive school systems hire deaf teachers who instruct the language in ASL. Interpreters also may be hired to provide voice-to-sign interpreting for the deaf teacher and sign-to-voice interpreting for the hearing students, sometimes for just the opening weeks of the school year, and sometimes as classroom assistants (interpreter-aide) or team- or co-teachers (interpreter-teacher) for the entire year. The hyphenated roles interpreters play in these classrooms can be just as awkward as the hyphenated roles interpreters are sometimes expected to play with hearing teachers. (See Stewart and Kluwin, 2001, for concerns common to team teaching and for issues of diversity in the classroom.) Careful attention must be given to the expectations of the teacher and his or her supervisor, the interpreter and his or her supervisor, and the students (and frequently their parents). Inservice meetings, collaborative decision making, and ongoing communication about what works and what needs changing is important to this interpreting assignment, too.

Some ASL teachers may want the interpreter to provide sign-to-voice interpreting when they offer announcements, assignments, and information *about* the lesson, but they do not want the interpreter to provide sign-to-voice interpreting *during* the lesson. These same teachers may want voice-to-sign interpreting when the students are talking about announcements, assignments, and information relative to their participation in the class, but no interpreting during students' participation in the actual lesson. Wide variation is also likely among deaf teachers in their use of spoken language, speechreading, and writing, as well as in their teaching skills. This same variability was mentioned by David Martin and Richard Lytle (2000) in their article on "Deaf Teacher Candidates in Hearing Classrooms." The program they described, the benefits of having deaf teachers in hearing schools, and the critical role the interpreters play in these intern experiences, merits reading.

ASL classes may also be mixed, with deaf and hearing students, including international deaf and hearing students who come to the classroom with very different cultural, linguistic, and educational backgrounds. Multiple interpreters may be needed to serve multiple roles with these students. Flexibility is again the key to success for interpreters who work in foreign language classes.

One final look at curriculum involves driver education, not necessarily the classroom material, discussed previously, but the behind-the-wheel instruction that many schools provide their sophomores or juniors. Behind-the-wheel instruction can be challenging enough to teachers who communicate casually and confidently with adolescents. Adding an interpreter in the backseat presents a whole new experience for the teacher. If we let ourselves relax, the newness of this situation for everyone can be amusing: a student's first experience behind the wheel, an interpreter's first experience in the backseat, and a teacher's first experience with a deaf student behind the wheel and an interpreter in the backseat. (This may be more amusing to those of us who have sons and daughters who are just learning to drive. We seek humor in a lot of these new experiences to avoid nervous breakdowns.) My interpreting colleagues, who have experienced behind-the-wheel instruction, have shared with me the need to do the following:

1. Teach the teacher these fundamental signs: RIGHT, LEFT, SLOW DOWN, STOP.
2. Work with the teacher on the importance of instructing *before* the engine is started, not after the car is moving.
3. Find a position in the backseat that enables a quick move into the rearview mirror's visual field for emergency interpreting.
4. Learn to extend the arms between the two front seats.

Again, for many students and many interpreters, these strategies work.

Question 8: What is the interpreter's role regarding consumerism in the educational program?

The question of *consumerism* was raised in Chapter 4, but appears again in this chapter to focus on the older, more mature student. By the time the student enters high school, especially if that student has experienced educational interpreters in middle- or elementary-school grades, he or she should demonstrate certain behaviors that, when nurtured appropriately by the interpreter, will lead to increased sophistication as a consumer. Anna Witter-Merithew and Richard Dirst (1982) discussed these behaviors and offered five responsibilities that represent increased independence in the secondary student's use of interpreters:

1. Informing the interpreter or teacher when there is a misunderstanding or when comprehension is challenged
2. Being prepared for class by reviewing new and difficult vocabulary
3. Engaging in problem solving as it is needed
4. Demonstrating a spirit of cooperativeness with the interpreter and teacher
5. Assisting the interpreter with copies of materials that are necessary in the interpreter's comprehension of the content to be interpreted (p. 403)

Witter-Merithew and Dirst also addressed the interpreter's responsibility in nurturing these consumer behaviors in the student. They indicated that the interpreter who maintains integrity and intent in the interpreted communication, remains impartial, even in the face of conflict, and honors confidentiality by protecting the privacy of all communication partners, and indirectly teaches the student how to use the interpreter appropriately. This interpreter also nurtures the hearing teachers and students as consumers when he or she demonstrates these apparently simple, yet deceptively complex, professional skills. I would add yet one more area to this topic of increasing maturation in consumerism for the secondary student, the area of evaluation.

Although all students should be encouraged to take on increasing responsibility in evaluating the interpreting situation and their role in it (refer to Chapter 2), older students should be encouraged (perhaps even taught) to evaluate their interpreter in a systematic manner. Figure 5.1 provides a sample evaluation instrument for secondary students to use in their annual or semi-annual assessment of their interpreter. Supervisors or responsible administrators should ensure that the students have been trained to use the instrument appropriately and to understand the importance of the assessment process. Encouraging use of this instrument is probably best illustrated with the following story:

> I ran into them at the mall. I hadn't seen Laura in five or six years. This attractive 17-year-old stood there with her mom, showing vague recollections of me as I reminded her of our years together when she came to the university. She was in our preschool from ages 3 to 5, then in our summer program until she was 10 or 11. I had also visited her elementary classes many times in supervising practicum students.
>
> Laura's classmates had transferred to the deaf school between third and fifth grades, but Laura continued to succeed in her local school with support from her teacher, who also did some interpreting for her. Then, after fourth grade, this teacher left and, according to Laura's mom, instead of hiring another teacher, they hired four different interpreters over the next six years. The one who stayed longest (eighth through tenth grades) was a sweet woman, but Laura just couldn't understand her. (At this point, Laura excused herself to go try on jeans.) Laura's mom went on to explain that Laura started getting headaches around age 13, at the onset of her menses. Doctor after doctor, hospital after hospital, test after test—all showed nothing. Laura was prescribed a variety of drugs; none seemed to eliminate the headaches. She missed 43 days during her sophomore year; she begged not to go to school. She also failed that year.
>
> I asked Laura's mom if she felt there was a connection between the headaches and Laura's interpreter. She said she didn't think so at first, particularly with onset of her periods. But, this year there had been a complete turn-around. For some reason, the interpreter hadn't come back. Laura's new interpreter turned out to be a good signer and Laura understood her. This new interpreter told Laura that the previous interpreter had been in the schools for three years but she had never even registered to take the interpreting test, so the school had to let her go. Laura's mom also said that Laura's headaches had stopped and she's doing really well in school. Her grades have climbed and she has two junior classes with her best friend. The administration told her if she goes to summer school, she might even graduate with her class next year.
>
> Laura's mom also shared that now that she looks back on the last few years and all that they had to go through, she wished she had said something about the interpreter. But, at the time, she was afraid of not having an interpreter at all. As it turns out, that woman really wasn't an interpreter at all.

FIGURE 5.1   A Student's Instrument for Evaluating the Interpreter

Interpreting Skills

1. I understand my interpreter's signs:

   _____ all the time   _____ most of the time   _____ sometimes   _____ not at all

   Comment: _____

2. I understand my interpreter's spoken language/oral interpreting/cued speech transliterating:

   _____ all the time   _____ most of the time   _____ sometimes   _____ not at all

   Comment: _____

3. I understand my interpreter's fingerspelling:

   _____ all the time   _____ most of the time   _____ sometimes   _____ not at all

   Comment: _____

4. My interpreter understands my sign language:

   _____ all the time   _____ most of the time   _____ sometimes   _____ not at all

   Comment: _____

5. My interpreter understands my speech:

   _____ all the time   _____ most of the time   _____ sometimes   _____ not at all

   Comment: _____

6. My interpreter understands my fingerspelling:

   _____ all the time   _____ most of the time   _____ sometimes   _____ not at all

   Comment: _____

7. My interpreter understands what he or she is interpreting:

   _____ all the time   _____ most of the time   _____ sometimes   _____ not at all

   Comment: _____

8. I understand what my interpreter is interpreting:

   _____ all the time   _____ most of the time   _____ sometimes   _____ not at all

   Comment: _____

9. My interpreter uses appropriate (check all that apply):

   _____ facial expressions   _____ processing (lag) time
   _____ body language   _____ professional behaviors
   _____ gestures   _____ communication skills
   _____ signaling devices   _____ personal appearance

   Comment: _____

10. My interpreter is:

    _____ always on time for class   _____ frequently on time
    _____ sometimes late   _____ always late

    Comment: _____

(continued)

FIGURE 5.1   **continued**

11. I wish my interpreter could improve:

_____

_____

12. I wish I could improve:

_____

_____

Question 9: What are the best practices for these difficult situations?

The following cases, like those presented in the previous chapters, are intended to challenge our thinking, especially ethical thinking, not necessarily to set a precedent to which we become rigidly fixed, but to expose the myriad of issues that ethical dilemmas can present to educational interpreters.

The Case of the Knife

Jolene was the interpreter for a Gourmet Cooking class, an eleventh-grade course that had a deaf student enrolled. The deaf student, Marcos, used sign language to communicate. The class had 13 students—eight boys and five girls. Marcos attended regularly and enjoyed the course, especially the different menus they were learning to make. They had previously studied Spanish cuisine, French cuisine, and were currently studying Japanese cuisine and learning to use the knives to chop, slice, butterfly, julienne, and so on. Mrs. Gonzalez had instructed the students in the importance and care of using sharp knives.

On Monday, when the students entered the kitchen, Mrs. Gonzalez announced that a large knife had been missing since Friday afternoon. She explained that she noticed the knife was gone before she left Friday, and had pinned the theft, or misplacement, to that class. She announced that if the knife was returned by Tuesday's class, there would be no discussion or punitive actions taken, but that if the knife was not returned by Tuesday's class, the entire class would be sent to the principal for punishment. She also explained that anyone who knew anything about the missing knife should come forward and share it with her confidentially.

Jolene became nervous as she interpreted. She had seen Eduardo near the knives Friday before they left, and she thought he was acting suspicious during Mrs. Gonazalez's comments. What should Jolene do?

Suggested Best Practice   We can view this case as an ethical case in which the interpreter's values determine the rightness of "informing," or, we can view this case as simply a case of honoring school policy. School personnel are obligated by contract to abide by the system's policies in matters of safety and violence. Although all interpreters may agree to the school's policies by virtue of signing a contract, the reality of this case is that some inter-

preters are reluctant to speak up about their suspicions. These interpreters may have difficulty negotiating within themselves the rightness of their actions. Some hide behind the
RID Code of Ethics, others hide behind a principle called "mind your own business." Where
issues of human safety are concerned, however, interpreters who possess critical information are expected to come forward with that information.

In their book *Deaf Students in Local Public High Schools: Backgrounds, Experiences, and
Outcomes,* Tom Kluwin and Michael Stinson (1993) addressed the topic of *complaints* among
high school students who are deaf. In comparing the typical complaints made by deaf students in the ninth, tenth, eleventh, and twelfth grades, they reveal a trend that involves
violence. "The focus of the ninth-grade comments were to a large extent about being bul-
lied or confrontations with hearing students. By twelfth grade, [their] concern was over
guns and drugs" (p. 141). Kluwin and Stinson interpreted these "concerns for personal
safety" as a move from "big-kids-bother-me" to "drugs and guns [are] in the schools"
(p. 141). While this information may not surprise interpreters in urban areas, it can come
as a surprise to interpreters in rural areas. Increasingly, though, safety issues that once were
owned by cities are becoming reality in all communities. Many schools have security
guards who patrol the halls, who periodically examine lockers, who arrest students who
conceal weapons. The interpreter who is naive to his or her responsibility where these precautions and other issues of safety are concerned owes it to himself or herself and consumers to become more knowledgeable and cooperative in preventive strategies.

Departure Questions for Discussion

1. Shouldn't she wait until Tuesday and see if the student comes forward?
2. What if Jolene puts herself in danger by informing on Eduardo?
3. What if she puts Marcos in danger?
4. What if she's wrong?

The Case of Driver Education

Mr. Farnsworth adapted well to Beth and her sign language interpreter, Karen. The 15-
hour behind-the-wheel class was scheduled from 1:45 to 3:00, for two weeks. By the third
day, he was signing comfortably to Beth, she was driving with increasing confidence, and
he was chatting comfortably with Karen. Karen's responsiveness to his talk was guarded.
She felt awkward talking in the car while Beth was driving. She didn't like it when Beth
looked at her through the rearview mirror and saw her mouth moving. She found herself
explaining what she and Mr. Farnsworth were talking about.

On the fourth day, Beth joked to Karen that she was going to get a new interpreter if
she and Mr. Farnsworth didn't stop talking so much and distracting her. Karen took her
comment more seriously than Beth probably intended it, though, and told Mr. Farnsworth
their talking might distract Beth; he responded that he would try to monitor it. That day's
75 minutes was awful. Karen noticed that Beth was looking in the rearview mirror more,
not less, frequently, and Karen felt that the silence between her and Mr. Farnsworth was
very uncomfortable. What should she do?

Suggested Best Practice   Karen's options include doing nothing and working with herself to deal with the silence, bringing something to read to pass the time, and/or to engage
Mr. Farnsworth *and Beth* in short segments of chit-chat that simulate the real world of

driving without distracting either from the process of teaching and learning to drive. Karen might also take advantage of the opportunity to direct the conversation to issues of cultural differences between deaf drivers and passengers and hearing drivers and passengers. In acting as a cross-cultural mediator, Karen might share strategies that involve lights for night driving, preferential seating for interpreting between passengers and driver, and so on. She might also suggest that a deaf driver be invited to demonstrate some of these strategies for both Beth and Mr. Farnsworth to learn. The involvement of deaf adults in this instruction should be welcomed by all parties.

Departure Questions for Discussion

1. But it's not Karen's place to teach the driver's education teacher how deaf individuals communicate when they drive, and it's not her place to invite deaf role models to come into the car. Shouldn't someone else do that?
2. What's wrong with Karen and Mr. Farnsworth talking? Beth has no right to ask them to stop.
3. Shouldn't Beth learn to adapt to the hearing people in the car? Won't their talking be a reality in her day-to-day driving?

The Case of the Student Teacher

Mr. Harris is the student teacher in the ninth-grade English class under Mrs. Meggel's supervision. Cory's grades in Mrs. Meggel's class include a B the first six weeks, a C the second and third six weeks. The portfolios due each Friday constituted a large part of the grade. Creative writing topics were given each Monday, drafts were worked on in class, help with editing was generous during class time, and the revisions were expected to be near perfect when the portfolio was submitted each Friday.

Ray is the interpreter in this class. He and Cory have a good relationship. They frequently chat during the down times when the teacher permits students to talk with each other. Cory prefers to chat with Ray, and Ray participates willingly unless the discussion involves editing. The students must present their work to at least two people during the week for editing feedback. Ray interprets for Cory during the editing blocks.

Mr. Harris maintains the same procedures Mrs. Meggel uses, but his grading of Cory's portfolio is much more critical than Mrs. Meggel's. At the midterm point, Cory's portfolio had an F. Mr. Harris gave Cory the midterm grade to take home to his parents; their signature was required on the report.

Cory was really upset during the class, commenting to Ray that he hated Mr. Harris, that Mr. Harris was too strict, and that he wanted Mrs. Meggel back. Ray was also upset, knowing that Mr. Harris was operating by a different standard than Mrs. Meggel. He wanted to advise Cory to go talk to Mrs. Meggel, but he suspected that Mrs. Meggel had to approve the grades before they could be distributed; Ray also knew that offering advice was not within his role. What should Ray do?

Suggested Best Practice   Ray's choices in this situation are rather clear—to listen and sympathize, to listen and advise, or not to listen at all. Because of the relationship he and Cory have, refusing to listen to Cory would probably be more harmful than helpful. Ray could listen sympathetically and inform Cory that he would make himself available to interpret if Cory wanted to set up an appointment with Mrs. Meggel and/or Mr. Harris.

That type of listening could be viewed as suggestive, however, and might just add to Cory's confusion. Probably the best of all choices would be to listen and sympathize, to be available for Cory's venting, to offer emotional support and understanding, but to refrain from making suggestions that, even indirectly, could constitute advising.

In her chapter "Inclusion in the Secondary School," Judy Montgomery (1997) discussed some of the issues involved in grading special needs students:

> Grades take on new meaning in high school. They are no longer merely a number or letter for parents to ascertain progress compared to the rest of the class. In high school, grades determine if a student is eligible for athletics, assembly programs, schoolwide honors, extra-curricular activities, college acceptance, scholarships, and eventually job interviews, and letters of recommendation. There is clearly a feeling that grades suddenly MATTER! There is little time left to earn them, and each year brings the student closer to the point after which low grades can no longer be lifted by a critical number of corresponding high grades. Should students with disabilities be held to the same standards for grades? The answer is, sometimes (p. 189).

The issue in this case appears to involve two sets of standards, Mrs. Meggel's standards, which have resulted in passing grades for Cory, and Mr. Harris's standards, which result in failing grades. The ownership of this issue, regardless of the relationship Ray has with Cory, rests with the teachers and the student, not with the interpreter.

Departure Questions for Discussion

1. If this student teacher is to remain all semester, Cory could end up failing the course. How can the interpreter stand by and let that happen?
2. What if Cory asked Ray to interpret a meeting with Mrs. Meggel? Could Ray then make a recommendation that he also include Mr. Harris?
3. What if Cory's parents call him to find out what's going on? What should he tell them?
4. What if Mrs. Meggel asks Ray what he thinks has happened to Cory's work this six weeks?

The Case of the Work Transition Assignment

Mary Jane, a community interpreter, had agreed to work for the school system this fall, interpreting every afternoon from 1:00 to 3:00 at a local day-care center, where the deaf student, Juanita, a 17-year-old in the work transition program at the high school, would be working. Details about the assignment were given at the first orientation meeting at the day-care center where Mary Jane was asked to interpret.

At that meeting, different expectations for the student, her school supervisor, and the day-care mentor were explained. Mrs. Hedrick, the day-care center's director and Juanita's mentor, had questions about the pass-fail grading, and about Juanita's communication skills with young children. Juanita responded with Mary Jane's interpreting that she had lots of experience with babies, including her sister's newborn and 2-year-old, and that the interpreter would be her link to what the children and caretakers were saying. Necessary paper work was signed, and the school supervisor left, wishing everyone good luck.

During the next 45 minutes, Mrs. Hedrick assigned Juanita to the 2-year-old room where the five children were waking from their naps. Mrs. Hedrick directed her to attend to Caleb first, then Miguel. Mrs. Hedrick then proceeded to the other toddlers, chatting cheerfully as she talked with each child, offering lots of verbal interaction, playful singing, and using a mothering kind of voice. Juanita carefully watched Mary Jane as she interpreted Mrs. Hedrick's communication. Juanita appeared to enjoy Mrs. Hedrick's modeling and used some playful facial expressions when she interacted in ASL with Caleb. He was easy. Miguel, on the other hand, was afraid of Juanita and cried the entire time she tried to change him. Mrs. Hedrick had to take over.

When 3:00 o'clock arrived, Mrs. Hedrick walked to the door with Juanita and Mary Jane and told them that she would give it the week, but that she didn't think this arrangement was going to work. She said she had not expected the interpreter to be interpreting for her; she thought the interpreter would just be interpreting for Juanita. She also added that she knew Juanita couldn't talk to the children, but she didn't realize that she would be signing to them. She added that she hadn't cleared it with the parents for her to be using sign language with their babies.

Juanita looked devastated and turned to Mary Jane with a *helping* expression. What should Mary Jane do?

Suggested Best Practice   This assignment appears to have been made without all the necessary preliminary work, particularly in orienting Mrs. Hedrick to the communication differences Juanita would bring to the site, and to the role the interpreter, Mary Jane, would have at the site. Mary Jane also realized that in interpreting the orientation, she had not explained her role, something she frequently did when she interpreted for hearing persons who had not previously worked with an interpreter. The circumstances also were different in another way: Mary Jane's interpreting Mrs. Hedrick's interactions with the babies had not been anticipated by her, either, but Mary Jane assumed this was part of the mentoring that Juanita was to have. Mary Jane suggested that Mrs. Hedrick try to reach the supervisor at school before she and Juanita left and set up a meeting as soon as possible to go over these concerns.

Departure Questions for Discussion

1. Why should Mary Jane make this suggestion? Shouldn't Juanita do the communicating?
2. Wouldn't an interview and/or observation weeks earlier have eliminated these misunderstandings?
3. Should Mary Jane agree not to interpret what other caretakers are saying to the babies, just language directed to Juanita?
4. Why wouldn't parents want their children exposed to sign language? If the parents are aware that the school participates in the school-to-work transition program, how can they reject any participant from that program because of his or her language difference?
5. Shouldn't Juanita be advised that a future job in a day-care center is not likely for a deaf person, or is it?

The Case of the Grandmother

Robert's grandmother called Ginger, Robert's interpreter, the night before school started to tell her about Robert's trouble during the summer. It seems that Robert got involved with that kid, Jim, who lives in the trailer park, and the two of them stole some money out of the cash box at the local pool. They were arrested and had to go to court. Robert got 40 hours of community service; Jim got 80 hours. The judge told Robert to stay away from Jim, that if he goes near him again, his grandmother's supposed to call the sheriff.

Ginger listened with many interruptions—"It sounds like you had a hard summer, Mrs. Belmont, but I don't think this is information that Robert would want me to know." Mrs. Belmont insisted Robert knew she was calling Ginger, because she had told him when they had an interpreter at the courthouse that she was going to tell Ginger to keep an eye on him when school started. "He listens to you, Ginger, and he won't listen to none of us around here." Ginger reminded Mrs. Belmont that Robert just found it easier to talk to her because she understood his sign language. She also reminded Mrs. Belmont that, as his school interpreter, she really didn't have any right to give Robert warnings or reprimands, that she just focused on his academic work. Mrs. Belmont continued to insist, though, that Ginger needed to keep him away from Jim and she knew Ginger could do it; the whole family had faith in her to keep him out of trouble.

Ginger hung up wondering what she should do now.

Suggested Best Practice   Ginger is in a position many small-town and rural-area interpreters find themselves in. She may be one of a few people, perhaps even the only person, who can truly communicate with Robert. Plus, Robert might be one of a few, perhaps the only deaf student, in the whole school and community. Robert's grandmother may have done the best she can to raise him, but she always defers to the professionals when things get out of hand.

Amy Wilson Tripp (1994), in her article "Turning Students into Grownups: Values and Decision-Making," reminded us that deaf adolescents experience not only the normal conflicts that arise during the teenage years, "including a drive toward independence, physical and emotional growth, and peer pressures," but that these conflicts are "further magnified by the inherent problems of communication" (p. 12). The interpreter's knowledge of this fact probably sets her up as being the problem-solver, a role she neither wants nor welcomes, but a role that she is sometimes forced into because of the logistics of her small-town surroundings. Right or wrong, Robert's grandmother will probably continue to ask Ginger to play a role in his maturation. Ginger's responsiveness, right or wrong, could make a critical difference in his maturation. In this case, Roberts's grandmother expects Ginger to monitor Robert's interactions with Jim. Ginger can passively listen to Mrs. Belmont's requests and can even alert Robert that his grandmother expects her to watch him, and hope that the situation goes no farther.

Departure Questions for Discussion

1. Ginger has no business even talking to Mrs. Belmont about Robert. Shouldn't she tell her not to call back?
2. Shouldn't Ginger turn this problem over to her supervisor or principal or the guidance counselor, and let them handle it?
3. What if Robert tells her he doesn't want her to watch who he hangs out with at school?
4. What if Robert asks Ginger not to talk to his grandmother when she calls?

The Case of the Vocational Test

Craig had just completed the training program in precision machinery and registered to enter the Student Apprenticeship Program, which would place him in a skilled trade job. All of the local companies that participated in the Student Apprenticeship Program required a passing grade on an entry examination, the Bennett Mechanical Comprehension Test. Craig registered to take the test and asked Mr. Marshall at the technical school if he would arrange to have an interpreter there on the test day. Mr. Marshall agreed and an interpreter who had worked with Craig before showed up to interpret for him.

The proctor of the test discussed the interpreter's role before distributing the test booklets, and responded that the Spanish interpreters were permitted only to interpret the directions at the beginning of the test and the time announcements during the test. Because literacy was an important part of the entry examination, Craig would be expected to read and respond to the test items on his own. The proctor also reported to Craig, through the interpreter, that the questions on the test were simple, with pictures that helped most individuals to understand them.

The test began; Craig's interpreter interpreted the instructions and found a seat about 10 feet from Craig. The interpreter looked at Craig several times during the onset of the test to determine if Craig was proceeding as expected. At first, when Craig signed NOT UNDERSTAND WORDS, the interpreter remained detached (Craig's just talking to himself, he thought). Then Craig looked directly at the interpreter and signed the same thing. The interpreter asked, "Do you want me to interpret for you?" Craig answered no.

Throughout the test, Craig showed flustered behavior, to the point that the proctor approached the interpreter and asked what was wrong. The interpreter stopped to think before he responded—Should I tell him he's having trouble reading the test or should I offer to interpret for him so he can ask Craig himself? What should the interpreter do?

Suggested Best Practice   The interpreter's role in the test had already been spelled out. He was not to interpret the text of the test. Furthermore, Craig had already told him not to voice his signs, that he was just talking to himself.

In this case, offering to interpret for Craig kept the ownership of control in Craig's hands, not the interpreter's. This lesson is hard for some interpreters and for some consumers to learn. In an effort to be "used," interpreters sometimes tend to assert their availability, leaving the consumers with the notion that the interpreter makes decisions about what and when to interpret. In this case, in spite of Craig's obvious frustration and the interpreter's desire to minimize his frustration, remaining detached but available for Craig and the proctor is probably the best choice.

Departure Questions for Discussion

1. But isn't the interpreter's role to equalize the communication situation? Doesn't that mean the interpreter needs to assess the situation and take action?
2. What if Craig asked the interpreter to interpret the test items? Should the interpreter refuse or approach the proctor for permission?
3. What if the proctor asked Craig to be quiet and stop distracting other students?

Summary

This chapter has presented several topics that are relevant to educational interpreters in high school and vocational settings. The focus on cognitive development, especially as it applies to learning, thinking, and responding, and, as it applies to interpreters who engage in critical thinking during the process of interpreting, was presented as important to the success of educational interpreters. Issues of curriculum differentiation—particularly the college-preparatory track, the general education track, and the vocational track—were explored. Interpreting in technical and laboratory settings was discussed for their particular challenges, namely, interpreting when instruction and learning are bound to showing and doing, and the challenges that are brought about because of safety and limited visual access. Different types of schedules common to high schools were discussed with regard to their impact on an interpreter's performance, as were unique curriculum challenges commonly found in human sexuality, driver education, and foreign language classes. Issues of consumerism completed the didactic information, and finally, several ethical cases were presented for discussion.

REFERENCES

Bloom, B. (1956). *Taxonomy of educational objectives: Handbook I. Cognitive domain*. New York: David McKay.

Bowe, F. G. (2002). Relay online. *NADmag, 2,* 19.

Burch, D. D. (2002). World symposium draws interpreters from around the globe. *RID Views, 19,* 1, 12.

Camarena, M. (1990). Following the right track: A comparison of tracking practices in public and catholic schools. In R. Page & L. Valli (Eds.), *Curriculum differentiation: Interpretive studies in U.S. secondary schools* (pp. 159–182). Albany, NY: State University of New York Press.

Cazden, C. (1988). *Classroom discourse: The language of teaching and learning*. Portsmouth, NH: Heinemann Educational Books.

Cokley, D. (1992). *Interpretation: A sociolinguistic model*. Burtonsville, MD: Linstok Press.

Davis, C. D. (2000). *Foreign language instruction: Tips for accommodating hard-of-hearing and deaf students*. Monmouth, OR: Western Oregon University.

deFur, S. H., Getzel, L., & Kregel, J. (1995). Transition services outcomes: Virginia's Project UNITE. Unpublished manuscript. Richmond, VA.

Elliott, D. C., Luttrull, P., & deFur, S. H. (1997). Vocational education: Options to meet the varying needs of students. In L. Power deFur & F. Orelove (Eds.), *Inclusive education for students with disabilities: A practical guide to meeting the least restrictive environment requirements* (pp. 195–214). Gaithersburg, MD: Aspen Publishers.

Ennis, R. H. (1987). A taxonomy of critical thinking dispositions and abilities. In J. B. Baron & R. J. Sternberg (Eds.), *Teaching thinking skills: Theory and practice* (pp. 9–26). New York: W. H. Freeman.

Frazee, B. M., & Rudnitski, R. A. (1995). *Integrated teaching methods: Theory, classroom applications, and field-based connections*. Albany, NY: Delmar Publications.

Frishberg, N. (1990). *Interpreting: An introduction* (rev. ed.). Silver Spring, MD: RID Publications.

Gajar, A., Goodman, L., & McAfee, J. (1993). *Secondary schools and beyond: Transition of individuals with mild disabilities*. New York: Macmillan Publishing Company.

Hallett, T. L. (2002). The impact of technology on teaching, clinical practice, and research. *The ASHA Leader, 7,* 4–7, 13.

Hanson, S. (1990). The college-preparatory curriculum across schools: Access to similar learning opportunities? In R. Page & L. Valli (Eds.), *Curriculum differentiation: Interpretive studies in U.S. secondary schools* (pp. 67–89). Albany, NY: State University of New York Press.

Kanda, J., & Colonomos, B. (1990). Issues in interpreter education. In C. Baker-Shenk (Ed.), *A model curriculum for American Sign Language and teachers of interpreting* (pp. 175–192). Silver Spring, MD: RID Publications.

Kemp, J. E., & Cochran, G. W. (1994). *Planning for effective technical training: A guide for instructors and trainers.* Englewood Cliffs, NJ: Educational Technology Publications.

Kluwin, T. N. (1992). Considering the efficacy of mainstreaming from the classroom perspective. In T. N. Kluwin, D. F. Moores, & M. G. Gaustad (Eds.), *Toward effective public school programs for deaf students: Context, process, and outcomes* (pp. 175–193). New York: Teachers College Press.

Kluwin, T. N., & Gaustad, M. G. (1992). How family factors influence school achievement. In T. N. Kluwin, D. F. Moores, & M. G. Gaustad (Eds.), *Toward effective public school programs for deaf students: Context, process, and outcomes* (pp. 66–82). New York: Teachers College Press.

Kluwin, T. N., & Stinson, M. S. (1993). *Deaf students in local public high schools: Backgrounds, experiences, and outcomes.* Springfield, IL: Charles C. Thomas Publisher.

Lawrence, R. W. (1987). Specialized preparation in educational interpreting. *Journal of Interpretation, 4,* 87–90.

Lightfoot, M. H. (2002). Interpreting in technology settings and the impact of technology on the field of interpreting. *RID Views, 19,* 8–9.

Littrell, J. J. (1991). *From school to work.* South Holland, IL: The Goodheart-Willcox Company.

Martin, D. S., & Lytle, R. R. (2000). Deaf teacher candidates in hearing classrooms: A unique teacher preparation program. *American Annals of the Deaf, 145,* 15–21.

Maxon, A. B., & Brackett, D. (1992). *The hearing impaired child: Infancy through high-school years.* Boston: Andover Medical Publishers.

Minor, D. L., Nieman, R., Swanson, A. B., & Woods, M. (Eds.). (2001). *Teaching chemistry to students with disabilities: A manual for high schools, colleges, and graduate programs, 4th Ed.* American Chemical Society.

Montgomery, J. K. (1997). Inclusion in the secondary school. In L. Power deFur & F. Orelove (Eds.), *Inclusive education for students with disabilities: A practical guide to meeting the least restrictive environment requirements* (pp. 181–194). Gaithersberg, MD: Aspen Publishers.

Nelson, J. (2002). The state of the wireless industry. *NADmag, 2,* 20–21.

Nippold, M. A. (1998). *Later language development: The school-age and adolescent years, 2nd Ed.* Austin, TX: Pro-Ed.

Norton, P., & Sprague, D. (2001). *Technology for teaching.* Boston: Allyn & Bacon.

Page, R. (1990). A "relevant" lesson: Defining the lower-track student. In R. Page & L. Valli (Eds.), *Curriculum differentiation: Interpretive studies in U.S. secondary schools* (pp. 17–43). Albany, NY: State University of New York Press.

Pool, H., & Page, J. A. (1995). *Beyond tracking: Finding success in inclusive schools.* Bloomington, IN: Phi Delta Kappa Educational Foundation.

Seal, B. C. (1997). Educating students who are deaf or hard-of-hearing. In L. Power deFur & F. Orelove (Eds.), *Inclusive education: A practical guide to meeting the least restrictive environment requirements* (pp. 259–272). Gaithersburg, MD: Aspen Publishers.

———. (2001). Interpreting in the chemistry laboratory. *RID VIEWS, 18,* 10–12.

Seal, B. C., Wynne, D., & MacDonald, G. (2002). Deaf students, teachers, and interpreters in the chemistry lab. *Journal of Chemical Education, 79,* 239–243.

Shepherd, G. D., & Ragan, W. B. (1992). *Modern elementary curriculum, 7th ed.* Fort Worth, TX: Harcourt Brace Jovanovich College Publishers.

Smith, S. M., Kress, T. A., & Hart, W. M. (2000). Hand/wrist disorders among sign language communicators. *American Annals of the Deaf, 145,* 22–25.

Stedt, J. D. (1990). Carpal tunnel syndrome: The risk to educational interpreters. *American Annals of the Deaf, 134,* 223–227.

Stewart, D. A., & Kluwin, T. N. (2001). *Teaching deaf and hard of hearing students.* Boston: Allyn & Bacon.

Stewart, D. A., & Stinson, M. S. (1992). The role of sport and extracurricular activities in shaping socialization patterns. In T. N. Kluwin, D. F. Moores, & M. G. Gaustad (Eds.), *Toward effective public school programs for deaf students: Context, process, and outcomes* (pp. 129–148). New York: Teachers College Press.

Stinson, M. S., & Whitmire, K. (1992). Students' views of their social relationships. In T. N. Kluwin, D. F. Moores, & M. G. Gaustad (Eds.), *Toward effective public school programs for deaf students: Context, process, and outcomes* (pp. 149–174). New York: Teachers College Press.

Swisher, M. V., Christie, K., & Miller, S. L. (1989). The reception of signs in peripheral vision by deaf persons. *Sign Language Studies, 63,* 99–125.

Tripp, A. W. (1994). Turning students into grownups: Values and decision-making. *Lessons for today: Diversity, responsibility, maturity: A folio of articles from Perspectives in Education and Deafness* (pp. 12–16). Washington, DC: Pre-College Programs.

Wilcox, S. (1992). *Academic acceptance of American Sign Language.* Burtonsville, MD: Linstok Press.

Winston, E. (1995). An interpreted education: Inclusion or exclusion? *RID Views, 12,* 11, 35–36.

Wisowaty, S. (1996). Repetitive motion injury (RMI) impacts the workplace. *RID Views, 13,* 20–23.

Witter-Merithew, A., & Dirst, R. (1982). Preparation and use of educational interpreters. In D. G. Sims, G. G. Walter, & R. L. Whitehead (Eds.), *Deafness and communication: Assessment and training* (pp. 395–406). Baltimore: Williams & Wilkins.

6 Best Practices in Interpreting in Higher Education Settings

Interpreting in higher education settings provides exciting opportunities for professional growth. Interpreters in these settings encounter students of different ages, different educational backgrounds, and different expectations as consumers of their educational interpreting services.

Question 1: What can educational interpreters expect in higher education settings?

The curriculum differentiation that characterizes secondary education programs continues into postsecondary educational programs, with two distinct tracks: academic and vocational. Academic programs "encompass four-year college or university settings and graduate degree institutions" while vocational programs "include two-year community college programs, trade and business schools" (Gajar, Goodman, & McAfee, 1993, p. 236). This distinction is somewhat arbitrary because community college programs frequently award an Associate of Arts (AA) degree to students who complete a two-year program, and they transfer credits to other institutions, which grant four-year degrees. Likewise, most higher education institutions are vocationally oriented, offering degrees that lead to professional occupations. The two-track system is widely accepted, however, and enables different entrance and exiting criteria that further distinguish the programs and the students who enroll in them.

Gary Sanderson, Linda Siple, and Bea Lyons (1999) reported in *Interpreting for Postsecondary Deaf Students* more than 20,000 deaf and severely hard-of-hearing students attending approximately 2,000 two- and four-year colleges and universities in the United States. Approximately 10,000, or about half of these students, use interpreters in their classes and various campus activities. This figure represents a sizeable increase over the previous 13 years when 11,000 deaf and hard-of-hearing students were reported in about 100 higher education programs

(Rawlings & King, 1986, p. 233). All evidence points to continued increases in enrollments of deaf and hard-of-hearing students in postsecondary programs in the early years of the twenty-first century.

Several possible reasons are offered to explain today's increased enrollment. One involves increased incidence in the number of deaf and hard-of-hearing students in K–12 programs (see Chapter 1). There simply are more students—deaf, hard-of-hearing, and hearing—going to college. Another reason centers around the influence of IDEA, the Rehabilitation Act of 1973, and ADA. Some scholars who advocate mainstreaming and inclusion point to higher standards, increased academic rigor, and better curriculum opportunities for deaf students because of these laws. Consequently, deaf students who were mainstreamed in K–12 are more likely to go on to college than students who graduate from special schools (see Marschark, Lang, & Albertini, 2002, for discussion). Increased enrollments of deaf students in postsecondary programs may result from increased support services—notetaking, tutoring, alternative testing, captioning and transcription services, and interpreting services—provided by colleges. Some scholars also point to the increased use of ASL and English in total communication and bilingual-bicultural programs in K–12 programs, and improvements in cochlear implant and amplification technology over the past two decades. Consequently, many deaf students who graduate from high school today are more sophisticated in their communication than previous generations, when fewer deaf students were likely to go to college.

Most likely, each of these reasons is valid in explaining some of the increased enrollments, and none of the reasons is independently valid in explaining all of the increase. Clearly, the point of discussion for educational interpreters is simply this: More deaf students are enrolled in postsecondary programs across the United States, and more educational interpreters are employed in these higher education settings than ever before.

David Stewart and Tom Kluwin (2001) discussed transition to college and postsecondary life. They detailed the phases—*before* the IEP meeting, *during* the IEP meeting, and *following* the IEP meeting—in which a student's reflection on his or her communication skills is fundamental to the successful transition plan. They also stressed the individuality of transition: "Critical to the process of transition is the ubiquitous fact that deaf students do not think and act alike no matter how similar they might be with respect to academic levels, communication style, family environment, degree of hearing loss, and other biodemographic characteristics" (p. 230). Among deaf students entering college today are those who are primarily oral; those who are primarily ASL users; those who use sign supported speech, cued speech, and speechreading to communicate; those who use tactile signing (increased incidence of deaf-blind students has also been reported in higher education); and those who prefer to access their classroom communication with advanced technology.

CART and C-Print were mentioned in Chapter 5 for their increased use in secondary programs. Higher education programs essentially have provided training ground for their use. *Emerging* technologies are common to college settings, too, most likely because of the high premium placed on research. Colleges are often the birthplace for new developments in technology where they can be field-tested and then disseminated to the wider public. Viable Realtime Transcription (VRT), or online transcription, recently made its debut on my college campus, with mixed reviews at this point. The iCommunicator™ (speech-to-text transcription) made its debut the previous year, again with mixed reviews. At this point (and with only anecdotal evidence to support these claims), it appears that at least two critical factors are involved in college students' acceptance of new communication technologies. One factor is accuracy; students who doubt the accuracy of their transcript are quick to abandon it. The point at which errors are intolerable has not been scientifically determined. Some students report they must have confidence that at least 90 to 95% of what they are reading is accurate. Others have indicated they don't mind errors in transcribing if they can figure them out. Some students might figure out the following error, others may not. The professor said, "What we need in deaf education is a little more money." The transcript read, *"What we need in deaf education is a little Mormon."*

The second critical feature that appears to weigh on communication technology's use is individual preference. Literacy levels are certainly critical factors, but personalities may also be the basis of a student's choice for an educational interpreter instead of, or in addition to, transcription. As one student reported, she loved the transcript provided by the VRT, but she felt like a voyeur in the class. She did not have access to the humor, to speaker identification, to the dynamics of the interactions. This student, like many in higher education classrooms, prefers an interpreter.

Student acceptance of their postsecondary interpreters may also be dependent on accuracy level and on individual personalities (see discussion of interpreters' personalities in Chapter 7). The current generation constitutes the largest generation of students who could have been mainstreamed, integrated, or included for the duration of their formal educational years. With their backgrounds of integrated experiences, we may assume that these college students are well acclimated to educational interpreters. Their cumulative experiences, along with their continued communication development across the late teens and early 20s, are likely to result in specific negotiations in requesting and working with interpreters. A return to the work of Marilyn Nippold (1998) is appropriate to this discussion.

Language and communication development were once thought to end with the critical learning years, around age 5. Indeed, these first five or six years are important and impact language development during later childhood, teenage, and early adult years. Truly, language learning occurs across the lifespan. One of the enticements for many interpreters in higher education settings is language learning—new vocabulary, new concepts, new information, new ways of looking at and using old knowledge and old language. Educational interpreters, as a whole, are highly verbal, and their own thirst for language learning is often satisfied in higher education settings.

Back to the student. Developmentally, students who enter college in their late teens or early 20s arrive with ongoing communication maturation. Part of this maturation involves continued growth in their conversation and narration skills. They stay on topic longer, shift more gracefully from one topic to another, and tell better stories than their younger peers (Nippold, 1998, p. 178). Another part of their maturation involves growth in persuasion and negotiation skills. They learn to influence the thinking of others, change their minds after being influenced by the thinking of others, and resolve interpersonal conflicts with others through language (p. 189). All of these communication skills—conversation, narration, persuasion, negotiation—involve discourse, the ability to exchange with a communication partner. Discourse skills are complicated (see Cynthia Roy's book, *Interpreting as a Discourse Process*, 2000), and this discussion focuses on only two of the skills expected to be developing in college students (and frequently tested in Public Speaking 101): persuasion and negotiation.

Deaf students who successfully make the transition from high school to college are likely to have followed the same developmental course that hearing students have followed, with multiple experiences in their childhood and adolescent years with bargaining, arguing, even nagging and whining, to achieve an end. Nippold's examination of this course concludes that the development of persuasion and negotiation are incomplete at age 17 and further growth occurs during early adulthood. This growth is highly contingent upon experiences in taking on the perspective of others. (Think back to Chapter 3 and the development of theory of mind.) Students who have multiple communication experiences show improvement in "perspective-taking, verbal reasoning, cooperation and collaboration with others, and concern for group welfare" (p. 201). Their increased use of metacognitive phrases: *I know what you are thinking, Before you say 'no';* and their increased use of sentence cohesives (subordinating and coordinating conjunctions): *consequently, rather, furthermore, on the other hand* (pp. 168–169) are offered as evidence that this development continues to mature in college. The extent to which this maturation occurs because of multiple communication experiences through childhood and adolescence, the degree to which these skills are tapped or primed in the college classrooms, and the interplay between the two, have not been teased out. In fact, Nippold suggested more research in these discourse skills because wide variability in negotiation and persuasion is evidenced in late adolescence and young adulthood. Furthermore, she suggested that this variability may be related to literacy levels (past correlations), and that improvement over the young adult years may relate to later vocational and social success (future correlations).

The impact of this development on educational interpreters is probably apparent. Interpreters working with postsecondary students generally expect them to negotiate their own access needs, to persuade their university and college representatives in decisions involving communication accommodations (refer to the case of the changing technologies in Chapter 2). Interpreters at this level also expect students to negotiate with them how best to meet their communication needs. Proximity decisions, sign choices, preferences for fingerspelling, mouthing or offering oral shadow, transliterating and interpreting, frequently need to be negotiated between the student and interpreter. Increased requests for oral interpreters or transliterators (e.g., Grisham, 1997, p. 9) have also led to increased training opportunities in oral transliterating in recent years, particularly for cochlear implant students who are increasingly more common on the college scene (Flexer, Wray, & Leavitt, 1990; Troiano, 2000).

Student independence in working with their sign language and oral language interpreters, in selecting and rejecting supportive technologies, in negotiating with their college administrators, and in communicating with their classmates and faculty is highly variable. Some newly matriculated college students come to their developmental changes quite easily. Others require lots of support (Porter, Camerlengo, DePuye, & Sommer, 1999). At least two characteristics stand out in profiling today's college students who are deaf and hard-of-hearing: **diversity** and **individualism**. These two characteristics serve as the theme for this chapter.

Question 2: What can the interpreter expect regarding curriculum?

The curriculum in most colleges recognizes the metamorphosis that occurs from adolescence to adulthood and attempts to provide a combination of general, or liberal, education courses with major and minor courses. General education courses are designed to improve the changing student's knowledge of self, culture, and the world. Major courses are designed to satisfy the student's need for a degree that leads to a job, profession, career, or entry into a higher degree program.

The curriculum of many colleges and universities is constantly in a state of change. Never before has society demanded from higher education a more radical transformation that is associated with "excellence, accountability, and achievement" (Smith, Wolf, & Levitan, 1994, p. 1). This demand is revolutionizing the way we look at teaching and learning. From a teacher's perspective, Wilbert McKeachie (1991) wrote:

> In addition to thinking less about covering all the facts and more about teaching conceptual structures, we need to think about how our students learn the material. When we make assignments, we need to be explicit about why we are making the assignment and why it's important for students to do it—write a paper, read a textbook, work on a team project, or whatever learning methods are assigned (p. 8).

McKeachie also described college students according to five groups or types:

1. The "A" student who is highly motivated and has good strategies for learning
2. The student with poor grades who has low motivation with poor strategies for learning
3. The student who has good learning strategies but low interest in the course and earns average grades
4. The student who has good learning strategies, values the course and wants to do well, but has low self-confidence; this student feels he or she just can't do well and earns only average grades

5. The student who is interested in the course, is highly motivated but has poor learning strategies, is anxious about tests and grades, and earns only average grades (adapted from McKeachie, 1991, p. 9)

Interpreters in higher education programs will probably encounter each of these five types of students, who are even more diverse by virtue of their age, economic status, ethnic origin, language, culture, and sexual orientation. Interpreters will service these students in courses taught by faculty who are increasingly more likely to be Mexican American, Asian American, African American, Native American, and non-American (Hirano-Nakanishi, 1994). The courses will range from World Civilization to Principles of Economics to Public Speaking to Abnormal Psychology to African Dance to Web Technology to . . . well—there is no limit to what might be taught in the name of higher education. Diversity is the benchmark of the modern curriculum and those who participate in it.

Given this information, how is an interpreter expected to represent the diversity he or she will encounter? One answer comes from research on the retention of verbal information. Fatema Olia's (1991) research on *mental imagery* involved 72 deaf undergraduates (ages 18 to 25) divided into two groups. One group received instruction and encouragement on the formulation of mental images when they were presented with verbal information. The other group received training in relaxation techniques and were encouraged to use those techniques when they were presented with verbal information (verbal refers to both sign and spoken languages). Both groups watched three videotaped short stories in signed English. Students in the experimental group were encouraged, at 15-second pause intervals, to form mental pictures throughout their viewing. The control-group students were told to practice their relaxation techniques at the same 15-second intervals. Students who were encouraged to use mental imagery retained significantly more verbal information from the stories than those who were encouraged to relax. Olia's conclusions were that deaf students should be taught and encouraged to generate mental images as they receive verbal information, especially lecture information in the college classroom.

Olia's results have important applications for educational interpreters. Interpreters are experts in mental imagery. In voice-to-sign interpreting, for example, an educational interpreter's reception of auditory and visual information is cognitively processed, or *churned,* until it can be seen. Then, once the interpreter sees it (in her or his head), she or he reproduces it into an image that is presented, hopefully with timed precision, to the student consumer. In sign-to-voice interpreting, the interpreter receives visual and/or auditory information, cognitively churns it and reformats it into an auditory signal that, hopefully with timed precision, enables the consumer (student or teacher) to receive it and form a meaningful mental image of the message. In oral interpreting and in cued speech transliterating, the educational interpreter receives a visual and/or auditory message, cognitively churns it and reproduces another visual message that is presented in a way that enables the consumer to receive it and process it with meaningful mental images.

Thinking is all about mental imagery. Interpreting is all about thinking; therefore, interpreting is all about mental imagery. This next classroom vignette should serve to illustrate:

TEACHER: OK, tonight we're going to start with a brief mini-lesson on efficiency in reading. We are going to look at two study methods. We are going to make a very deliberate effort to remember the methods. You will discuss this information in your group, you will write about it, and I hope you will transfer it to your course work.

The first method we're going to learn about is called ARC: Anticipation, Realization, and Contemplation. *[She writes it on the board.]*

Anticipation means to think, to become aware of, to predict. What other words come to mind? Anticipation. *[silence]* That something's happening? *[continued silence]* Come on, now, we all want to get out of here tonight. Anticipate! *[silence]* Well, did you anticipate the verdict yesterday at the trial? Did you deal with the information in advance? Did you think about it? *[lots of YES responses]* Well, that's what you need to do when you read, develop the strategy of anticipation.

A lot of students say to me, "Hey, I don't remember what I read. I can read all the paragraphs but then I don't remember what I read." I caution you that this is where the breakdown occurs *[pointing to Anticipation on the board]*, that you aren't thinking about what it is you are going to read. Sometimes you actually feel like you have a limited amount of knowledge, so, maybe to learn about that topic, you have to brainstorm when you anticipate. You have to think about it and make the topic personal to your learning. When it becomes personal, then you will remember it.

So, you might say, "Oh, I don't know much about brainstorming. I don't want to do that. It takes too long. It messes up my paper, with words going in all kinds of directions." Then, I say, "OK, you don't have to brainstorm. How about just making a list of questions?" Ask yourself what you might learn, or ask yourself what you want to know about this topic? Maybe you can look at the bold subheadings and turn them into your questions.

That's how I read new information. I take the subheadings and turn them into questions. I make myself focus by taking each subheading and turning it into a question, then answering that question while I'm reading, not after, but while I'm reading a particular section. Then, I check off that section as something I'm comfortable with, because I can answer my own questions about what I just read. Now, that's setting the stage for the next part of the ARC process. Realization.

Realization is the actual reading, the nuts and bolts of reading. Now, as you read, you set up a legend, a key, or something to keep you on task. For example, you can make a checklist of everything you read that you already know. Or, maybe you put a dash for something you think contradicts what you thought you knew. "I don't know about this, but I guess it's new information." And maybe your symbol for something new is a dash. What would the question mark symbolize? What do you think a question mark means during this reading stage? *[pause]* What do you think, Kristan?

KRISTAN: Something that raises a question in your mind.

TEACHER: Exactly, or something you don't understand or need a new level of understanding for. What about a plus? What could you use a plus for? Something that you already know maybe, but are adding new knowledge to. The system itself is not so important. It doesn't have to match my system. But whatever it is, it needs to work for you. Maybe you like asterisks for exciting information. Whatever system you use is fine, but I recommend you use it regularly, every time you read. Once you put it into practice, you build a new habit.

Students say to me, "Well, I underline," or "I highlight." That's fine. But, have you ever picked up a book that had every line in it underlined? Or three different highlight colors? It's not helpful at all. I refrain from highlighting or underlining. Instead, I prefer to write myself margin notes. In the margins, I make comments, often restating what the author said in MY words, not in the author's words (that's just memorizing) but in my own words. That facilitates my reading.

Now, the third stage is Contemplation. When you think about ARC and you think about an arc and how it joins or makes a relationship, you'll understand what *Contemplation* is. In this stage, you actually think about the Anticipation you had at the beginning of your reading. It merges or meshes with the Realization. Contemplation is an important stage, a stage of reflection. "Did the information that I read meet my expectations or not?" This is the stage where you confirm or reject your anticipations. *[pause]*

Now, before I go to the next method, Do you have any questions about the ARC method?

As you read these paragraphs, you formed mental images of the auditory and visual messages the professor of this reading course was offering to her 18 community-college students. Quite possibly, your mental images were visual. That is, you could visualize (in your own head) the letters A–R–C as she wrote them on the board. You could visualize someone looking at subtitles in preparation to recasting them into questions. Perhaps you envisioned yourself with a book, writing notes in the margin, or looking at a page of a book covered in several highlight colors.

The interpreter in this class, as I captured her imagery on videotape, saw these same images in her head and then portrayed them in the visual field of the deaf student for whom she was interpreting. She "set up" the A–R–C in space, referring to each letter by point or by looking at its appointed station each time it was mentioned. She drew a visual arc between the A and the R and between the R and the C, and then she connected all three letters with a larger sweeping arc. She wrote in the margins. She showed confusion when she looked at the page full of highlighting. And she did all this fluently, smoothly, effortlessly, and with apparent success, as the deaf student's affirmative head nods indicated his ability to "see" the verbal information as she interpreted it.

Just weeks after observing in this college classroom, I was asked to substitute interpret at a local university for a deaf student in a math logic class. The regular interpreter described in as much detail as she could the *image* of this class. I will portray it here, and then give you a sample of the verbal information the professor presented.

Dr. C. greeted the Math Logic class with his grade book, checking the assigned seats for absences, and entering some kind of notation as his eyes moved from seat to seat. He did not greet the students as he looked at them. In fact, he didn't really appear to look AT them. The students, mostly male (only two or three females), were all about the sophomore or junior level.

As the regular interpreter had explained, I could expect five or six students to sleep at some point in this 8:00 MWF class. Another five or six of the enrolled 20 would be absent.

Dr. C. moved to one of the two blackboards and began talking, writing as he talked. This is what he said:

If you want to prove G from R to R, defined by G of X is equal to G of X minus X, show that F plus G is equal to F of X. An associative operation doesn't have to be communicative. F of X is not necessarily the same as G of F.

Does there exist a function G from R to R or little O to little O having the property that F of little O equals F of X? *[brief pause, no responses]* This time you have to check the other side. The technique of proof requires that you must find the value of a function.

If you want F of little O of X to be equal to F of little O of X, then little O must be X. Right? *[brief pause, no response]* Yes, it's pretty obvious.

Suppose you discovered that this collection of numbers (we'll call it Set R), that this set is a ring and suppose it's a ring that has all the properties of a ring and as in this case, it's a ring with identity. You can now think of this new Set R as consisting of Z and then extending the set Z by one number by tacking on the square root of 2. What will you get if X squared equals 2 and is not solvable in Z, but it is solvable in R? *[brief pause, no responses]* Then we have found the smallest structure that allows us to solve a problem.

Well, did you see it? Was it obvious? Did you have a mental image of Function G, of Little O, of Set R, of the ring? The professor did, and I sensed that the student for whom I was interpreting was visualizing something as his eyes moved intently from me to the board, and as he jotted notes and mathematic equations and shook his head affirmatively at various points. At the end of class (I thought the 50 minutes would never end!), I asked if he truly comprehended what I was interpreting, and he answered, "MOST OF IT."

I was asked to substitute a second time that semester, just before midterm. The language was just as *un-IMAGIN-able* to me the second time as it had been the first time, and even though I had the audiotape to use for preparation, I was no better able to "see" the information presented by the professor. The student's attentiveness this time was different. He slouched in his seat; he did not take notes. He told me after class that he was dropping the course. I was a little shaken at the news, fearful that my inability to visualize the material had blown his learning opportunity. He assured me that he had a strong C and could probably do better if he worked at it. He also shared that he just couldn't tolerate the teacher's style and wanted to take the course from someone else.

I talked to the regular interpreter at the first possible chance. She explained that she had a pretty good grasp of the material and was actually visualizing it herself and for the student. It wasn't the interpreting, she said. It wasn't even the material or the course. It was the individual teacher and the individual student in that individual situation. The dynamic did not work.

We might say this student is like one of those five types McKeachie described: He had the necessary learning strategies, even valued the course material, but was not motivated by the teacher to perform to his ability. We might also say that this teacher was caught up in thinking about the facts, not in thinking about how the students were learning the material.

One more classroom scenario is appropriate to represent the diversity interpreters can encounter in higher education:

> The political science class professor, Dr. K., announced to Tuesday's class that her graduate assistant would cover her class on Thursday while she attended a national conference. She also announced that the videotape the G.A. would show them would serve as the focal point for the following Tuesday's discussion on the political history of Nigeria.
>
> As the interpreter, I was glad to have heard that a videotape was being presented. I approached Dr. K. after class and asked if I could borrow the tape overnight to prepare for Thursday's class. Dr. K. explained that the tape was on reserve under her name, only to be checked out by her G.A., but she would call the library and make arrangements for me to take it overnight. Dr. K. also warned that the tape was somewhat hard to follow, because of the different dialects used, and that she was glad I would have a chance to preview it. She said she would also e-mail the student for whom I was interpreting and make arrangements for him to take it over the weekend, in case he wanted to view it again before next Tuesday's discussion.
>
> I spent about two hours that night, previewing the tape, rewinding and fast forwarding to grasp the unfamiliar dialects used. I used my laptop to record orthographically and phonetically the different spellings of names: Dagogo Princewell, Bugma, Amenebo, Kalaberic, Kuma, Isaac Erokosima, Princess Alexandria, Halhasheho Shegari. I ended up with a three-page record of the videotape—the proper names, the sequence of events, and salient points of the narrative. I made an extra copy to give to the student.
>
> After Thursday's class, the student complimented me on how I had mouthed the dialect: "I could make out the different tones in your face and on your mouth." He also appreciated the written supplement and thought he could use it as he watched the tape again that weekend.
>
> Dr. K. returned to Tuesday's class and engaged the students in the various phases of Nigeria's political history. She discussed the assassinations, the military coups, the differences between the chiefs chosen by family clans and the British ministers chosen by Parliament. The student I interpreted for answered a question about the symbolism of the canon ball and the yam. I thought later about how he

explained it, representing in space much like I had visualized it the week before. He had retained the images. He had processed the verbal information that accompanied them. And, more important, he had retrieved it when he needed it for the class discussion five days later.

The interpreter in this political science class was motivated by the professor and by the student. The student in this class was motivated by his professor and by the interpreter. The professor was not fixed just on the facts but on how the student was learning the material. The professor's responsiveness to the videotape situation showed that she, too, was motivated by the student and by the interpreter. The dynamic worked.

Question 3: What happens when the interpreter cannot visualize the information, when there is a breakdown, or a miscue, or an error?

"If you accept the propositions that (1) humans make mistakes, and (2) that interpreters are human, then there is no question that interpreters make mistakes" (Mintz, 1993, p. 1). Excellent interpreters misread fingerspelled words, misrepresent a negative statement as a positive statement, misunderstand the intent of a speaker, miss whole sections of a presentation. Interpreters make errors; some are inconsequential, some are embarrassing, some are humorous. When learning is at stake, interpreter mistakes can be serious.

Dennis Cokely (1992) devoted considerable time and study to researching interpreter miscues: incidences in which the equivalence between the target language (tL) and source language (sL) is not achieved. His findings, "that miscues do occur and certain types of miscues may occur despite preparation and conscious effort on the part of the interpreter to avoid them" (p. 160), are partially responsible for the move away from solo interpreting to team interpreting. Indeed, two heads can be better than one when it comes to representing the verbal information of a challenging classroom or educational setting.

The terms interpreter *miscues* and interpreter *errors* should be clarified. The differences between miscues and mistakes is subjective. Cokely referred to any deviation between the sL and the tL as an interpreter miscue. He discussed the fact that some miscues are more serious (unacceptable) than others (acceptable). He did not, however, refer to an interpreter's deviations as mistakes. In spite of his work, most interpreters today, in educational and other settings, refer to their miscues as mistakes or errors. In explaining Cokely's research, I will use his terminology; but in my day-to-day work, I refer to interpreter miscues as interpreter errors.

A third term, *communication breakdown*, should also be introduced in this discussion. A communication breakdown is an interruption in the exchange of information between a "speaker" and a "listener" that necessitates a repair in order for communication turns to continue (Roth & Spekman, 1984). As experienced communicators, we all know that breakdowns are part of everyday communication. How often do you tell your husband or wife or children or parents or students or teachers something that they swear you never told them? American Sign Language (ASL), spoken English, all languages in fact, have negatives, probably because of communication breakdowns—"You DIDN'T tell me that," or "That's NOT what I meant!" (see also Tannen, 1986).

As interpreters, we facilitate communication turns. In the educational setting, the teacher or professor is usually turn dominant. When the professor fails to communicate the intent of his or her verbal message, a breakdown occurs. Several factors impact on communication breakdowns: the intelligibility of the communicator, the completeness of the message, the complexity of the message, the relevance of the message, the appropriateness of the information, the presence or absence of mutual attention or visual regard, the presence or absence of mutual desire to communicate, cultural differences, social differences, and gender differences (Roth & Spekman, 1984). A professor who is unintelligible; who uses incomplete sentences; who lectures above the heads of the students; who talks about irrelevant information; who uses inappropriate language in his or her communication; who has little interest in communicating with the students; and/or whose cultural, social, or gender orientations toward communicating are different from the students' is likely to generate breakdowns for the interpreter and for the students. Similarly, an interpreter who cannot comprehend the complexity of the message, or a student who demonstrates an absence of mutual attention can generate communication breakdowns.

Generally, during the interpretation process, the facial expressions and non-verbal communication (e.g., those affirmative head nods) offered by the student enable the interpreter to sense that the verbal information is being received, that the communication turn (even if dominated by the teacher) is being maintained. Sometimes, a frown, an eyebrow change, or head tilt can represent to the working interpreter that a breakdown has occurred. When this happens, the interpreter may continue interpreting, but with an anticipating posture that signals a preparation for the student's next action: a raised hand to ask for a clarification, or a direct question to the interpreter for a repair, or a notation to ask about "such and such" at a later point. Or, the interpreter may initiate the repair process at the point where he or she anticipates the breakdown occurred: with a "WHAT?" and a questioned look to the student, with a repetition of the interpreted message, or with a question to the student to see if he or she wants to interrupt the professor.

When the breakdown belongs to the interpreter (e.g., "I DIDN'T CATCH THAT," or "SORRY, I MISSED WHAT HE SAID"), the process for repair also varies. In my experiences, college students often become the source of the information missed, offering the correct spelling of the word, or relying on their previous experiences with the material to "cloze" off what was missed. In the math logic class, for example, the student provided signs to replace my fingerspelling of RING and SET. In other situations, however, the student may not be able to repair the interpreter's breakdown. The alternatives, then, vary, with some interpreters comfortable interrupting the professor to ask for a repetition or clarification ("Could the interpreter hear that again, please?"). Some interpreters wait out the miscue in anticipation that they will be able to catch it and repair it later as more of the message unfolds. Some interpreters, after disclosing to the student directly "I missed that" or indirectly (a change in facial expression and head orientation), expect the student to take action. The individuality of the interpreter, student, classroom situation, and the communication breakdown itself is so unique that each breakdown an interpreter experiences may potentially be handled differently.

This individuality does not suggest that there are no guidelines for handling communication breakdowns. In fact, Cokely's (1992) findings offer us several important guidelines to reduce miscues. A return to his research is appropriate in explaining them. Cokely analyzed the interpretations of six highly qualified and skilled interpreters who "had extensive experience interpreting at conventions, conferences, and interpreting lectures and speeches" (p. 36). His analyses revealed a high number of miscues by each of the interpreters, ranging from a low of 20 miscues in 5 minutes of interpreting to a high of 139 miscues in 8 minutes of interpreting. Cokely further analyzed the miscue types according to five categories: (1) omissions, (2) additions, (3) substitutions, (4) intrusions, and (5) anomalies. The range in error type varied across the six interpreters, but they tended to omit information more often than they added or substituted or offered intrusions and anomalies[1] in their interpretations.

Cokely also analyzed the interpreters' miscues according to their lag time, revealing that those interpreters who had the shortest lag times averaged miscues in 38% of their sentences while those who had the longest lag times averaged miscues in 12% of their sentences (p. 120). He also compared the miscues of the interpreters according to their native languages. The three interpreters who were native ASL users had the same frequency of miscues as those who were native English users.

Several guidelines for handling miscues or errors come from Cokely's (1992) research:

1. Interpreters should have external monitoring (as can occur with team interpreting) when the consequences of miscues are serious.
2. Interpreters must have appropriate levels of competence in both the tL and sL in order to reduce miscues.
3. Interpreters must maintain enough lag time to reduce the frequency of miscues.
4. Interpreters who can cognitively process the sL before, not during, the time that they are delivering the tL will have fewer miscues (consecutive interpreting results in fewer miscues than simultaneous interpreting).

---

[1]Cokely defined anomalies as "meaningless or confused" interpretations that could not be accounted for by the other types (p. 88). He defined intrusions as "literal" substitutions that occurred when the interpreter abandoned the tL and transliterated the sL (pp. 87–88).

5. Interpreters who request more pauses, not slower speaking rates, from the speakers of the sL can reduce the frequency of miscues.
6. Interpreters must work with their consumers to determine the strategies that will be used when breakdowns or miscues are observed.
7. Interpreters and consumers must be aware that when miscues result because of misperceptions, they can go undetected by both the interpreter and the consumer. Determining *checks* to ensure reliable interpreting (e.g., as in comparing the student's comprehension of the interpreted message with the notetaker's comprehension of the teacher's lecture) should be explored in those cases where solo interpreting is used.
8. Finally, recognizing our own vulnerability in making interpretation errors should provide us with an incentive to work toward improving them. Self-evaluations (see Chapter 2) should be an ongoing part of this effort.

In the classroom scene that follows, several examples of Cokely's points are observed. Pay particular attention to the professor's sensitivity to the interpretation process, and the success the interpreter has in avoiding errors. Note, too, the pauses that occur at the end of each utterance and the professor's eye gaze that made for a favorable learning experience for the three deaf undergraduates, and a favorable interpreting experience for the interpreter.

DR. M: In this protein *[pause, pointing to a chemical structure on the board]* we have all these amino acids linked together *[pause, raised eyebrows directed to deaf students in front]*. Now in myoglobin, there's a lot more than this. *[pause]*
   I forget the actual number. *[hearing student in back says something]*

DR. M: Deedee says it's 126. We'll go with that; that sounds reasonable. *[pause]*
OK. You have your amino acids linked together, about 126 of them, and then you have a carboxyl group. *[pause]*
   That's *[pause, looking at the interpreter]* c-a-r-b-o-x-y-l.
   That's what we call the primary structure.

[The interpreter steps toward Dr. M. and says and signs, PRIMARY AS IN FIRST OR PRIMARY AS IN MOST IMPORTANT?]

DR. M: Primary as in first.
   This group might be 1 through 35. *[writing the numbers 1–35 by the circled group]* And this group will be 45 through 90. *[writes the numbers on the board]*
   And this group will be 100 to 126. *[adds the numbers on the board]*
   This group will start curling up around each other. *[gesturing with her arms how they fold up]*
   And here's a gap, and maybe these guys don't do much, just hang out. *[pointing to the space between 35 and 45]*
   But this next group starts to form another type of structure. *[pointing to the 45 to 90 group]*
   And then these don't do much either. *[pointing to the 100 to 126 group]*
   So when we think about secondary structures, we think about the local interactions. *[pause]*

We think about the protein folding up on itself. *[pause]*

And the final product, the three-dimensional structure, then looks like these rounded globs under a microscope. *[pause]*

Maybe even rectangular globs. *[pause]*

But they're the same amino acids, just now referred to as elements in their secondary structure. *[pause]*

So in the end, the final form might look like this. *[She draws another structure.]*

Here's the 45 to 90 group, and here's the 100 to 126 group. *[pointing to the respective groups on the board]*

Now, in your textbook, myoglobin looks like this. *[She draws a circle.]*

It's a circular structure called an alpha helix. *[looks to the interpreter and spells h-e-l-i-x]*

That's what we're interested in.

Question 4: What about interpreting in graduate school?

Nontraditional students—individuals who are married, who are divorced, who have children, who have careers, who have degrees, who have debts that may require part-time attendance, who attend college to participate in the academic life, not in the social life—constitute a growing number of students enrolled in today's college programs. These students frequently enroll in graduate programs, sometimes as "special status" students who take a one-time-only course, sometimes as part-time graduate students who may matriculate at a different pace than the traditional student, and sometimes as full-time graduate students. These individuals, when they are deaf or hard-of-hearing, may require interpreters. The uniqueness of their individual situations defies general discussion. In fact, in preparing to represent the nontraditional student at a graduate level, I interviewed three individuals whose interviews speak to both the diversity and individuality of educational interpreting in higher education.

Steve Nover, director of the Center for ASL/English Bilingual Education and Research at the New Mexico School for the Deaf and author of several articles on inclusion, bilingualism, and literacy education, was a doctoral candidate at the University of Arizona when interviewed. His responses about educational interpreters provide a provocative look at some of the theoretical issues for interpreters in research degrees. Bonnie Poitras Tucker, a professor of law at Arizona State University and author of several books and articles on cochlear implants, deafness, and disability law, returned to college after a divorce, earned her law degree, practiced law for a few years, and then returned to the classroom to teach. Bonnie's use of oral interpreters in her classes provides a stimulating look at some of the interpreting issues for oral deaf adults. Donna Panko, a friend who now directs the disability services program at the University of Vermont, was interpreting for a doctoral candidate at the University of Virginia at the time of her interview. Donna's insights are similarly provocative and stimulating.

The questions asked Steve, Bonnie, and Donna were alike in content, sequence, and intent. Their answers reveal similarities and differences. I offer them with gratitude.

Interview with Steve Nover on His Use of Interpreters

SEAL: My first question involves you, your status as a doctoral candidate, and your use of interpreters. You're a doctoral student, right? In your last semester?

NOVER: Yes, actually, I'm writing my dissertation proposal right now. I have been a student, part-time, in Language, Reading, and Culture. My classwork finished last spring and I hope to finish my dissertation by December.

SEAL: How has your use of interpreters impacted your schedule? For example, when you were taking classes, would you determine what you wanted to take, then notify the university to secure interpreters for you, or would you contact interpreters to see if they were available before you would register for particular courses?

NOVER: No, I would go through the U of A and tell them who I wanted. But, you realize, I have a special status because I am a Ph.D. student. Some of the undergraduates are not always as happy with the interpreter services they receive.

SEAL: Do you have a preference?

NOVER: No, it really depends on the individual interpreter. For the past five years, I've been lucky to have one person who's on the faculty and also interprets. And I've had several other Master's degree interpreters who know the field of linguistics. I prefer an interpreter who has a background in linguistics.

SEAL: Do you require your interpreters to be familiar with the fields you are studying?

NOVER: That's definitely important. I sent you a paper on full inclusion, and the research for that paper really helped me to start looking at interpreting. My meta-awareness of the interpreting process increased. I would prefer NOT to use interpreters; I would prefer to get the language directly, or even from notes from other students, then I could see the kind of language used by the professor. With an interpreter, I don't get that kind of direct input.

SEAL: Do you prefer for your interpreters to use ASL or English?

NOVER: I don't think it really matters. I like both. What I personally prefer is something like the CART services.

SEAL: CART? court reporting? Do you have access to that technology, in addition to your interpreters?

NOVER: CART stands for Computer-Assisted Reporting Technology. No, I don't have that. Some of the students here have it, but because I use interpreters, I wouldn't be allowed to have it too. But, I'm all done anyway. Now, when I attend a conference, I prefer reading the CART notes to watching the interpreter.

SEAL: I see. Do you expect your interpreters to study the material or to read it before a class?

NOVER: Well, again, I prefer the interpreter to have a background. I have had interpreters who didn't know the subject matter, and basically they just threw out signs and fingerspelled words to me, with no cohesion. I expect background in the material.

SEAL: Do you prefer to use the same interpreter all the time or do you prefer a variety in your interpreters?

NOVER: I prefer consistency, someone who knows my thinking, my language, my communication style, and so on. If you have different interpreters, it's hard.

SEAL: What about interrupting? Do you prefer for the interpreter, if he or she misses something—perhaps a word, or a phrase, or a concept—do you prefer for the interpreter to interrupt the professor and ask for a repetition, or do you prefer for the interpreter to tell you, "Oh, I missed that," and let you handle it?

NOVER: Well, I may not always know, so if the interpreter misses something, I think it's the interpreter's responsibility to interrupt the teacher and ask for a repetition. But, if I don't understand something, if I missed it, then I will interrupt the professor and ask for a repetition.

SEAL: Did I ask you any questions that you wish I hadn't asked, or that you'd like to reconsider your answers on? Or, is there anything I didn't ask you that you wish I had asked—regarding using interpreters in a Ph.D. program?

NOVER: I think the best possible situation is to have an interpreter who has a Ph.D. in the field that I'm studying, to have the training, the background, and the knowledge in what I'm studying.

Interview with Bonnie Poitras Tucker on Her Use of Oral Interpreters

SEAL: What's your position at Arizona State University?

TUCKER: I'm a professor of law in the Law School.

SEAL: Have you used oral interpreters the entire time you've been teaching?

TUCKER: Yes.

SEAL: And how does that work for you?

TUCKER: It works just like it's working for us now. My interpreter is mouthing what you say at the same time you're saying it, and I lipread her.

SEAL: So when you lecture to your classes, your oral interpreter sits in front of you?

TUCKER: She sits in front of the class, wherever that might be. And she mouths what the students say. Half the time, I can lipread the students without an interpreter, but half the time, I can't. It depends on how large the class is. If the class has 130 students (like one class will have in the fall), then I rely on the interpreter, but if the class is 30 to 40 people, then I rarely rely on the interpreter. I can usually lipread the students myself, unless someone mumbles.

SEAL: I understand. How do you explain to your classes on the opening day that you're using an interpreter?

TUCKER: Well, I tell them about the class, the syllabus, the exams, and so on, and I say, "I'm deaf and this lady in front is an oral interpreter," and that she mouths what they say so I can read lips . . . that she is mouthing what they say, and that when I look away from them and look at her, I'm not ignoring them. I also tell them that sometimes when they are talking, I may think they're finished because there's a pause there, and I tell them that they have to just interrupt me and say, "Hey, I'm not finished." Basically, I'm a nice person; I don't want to be rude. I just want them to understand that because I'm not looking directly at them (often I look back and forth), they shouldn't think that I'm not understanding what they say. I do this with the first-year students, and the upper classes I might do it with, but most of the upper-class students I've already had before. So, I give more details to the first-year students. But, it's no big deal. I often tell them that they won't even be aware of the interpreter. And I tell them if I don't speak loudly enough or if they don't understand me, to raise their hands and let me know. I also tell them that only one person can speak at a time, and that they have to raise their hand, that they cannot speak without raising their hands.

SEAL: So, if hands are raised, students want to speak, and you're in a large class, does your interpreter signal for you that, let's say, "A male in the back row is trying to get your attention."

TUCKER: No, I call on the students. Either they raise their hands or I just call on someone.

SEAL: But, imagine it's a really volatile discussion and the students are getting carried away. Would your interpreter let you know that there's a buzz in the room and that it's getting overwhelming to follow?

TUCKER: She just points in that direction, because she can only be one-to-two words behind the speaker, and if she takes the time to say, "Student in the back row," she's too far behind.

SEAL: OK, the next question deals with errors. Interpreters are humans and humans make mistakes. Do you have any preference for how you want your interpreters to handle mistakes?

TUCKER: If the interpreter misses something, she says (or he says, I've had both male and female interpreters), "I missed that," and just keeps on going. Then, if I want it repeated, I say, "Would you repeat that please?" But if the interpreter makes a mistake . . . well, I've never had a situation. Hold on. *[speaking to the interpreter]* Well, sometimes the interpreter may have a puzzled look because they don't know the legal terminology. And, I just tell the interpreter to mouth it as it sounds and let me figure it out, because I'm pretty good at figuring out what they're trying to say. My interpreters are people that I train to interpret.

SEAL: So, they don't hold RID credentials?

TUCKER: You're right. Except for one RID interpreter I had for two years, and he was a sign language interpreter who worked for me as an oral interpreter, and he did an exceptional job. But, my other interpreters never really know what an interpreter is.

SEAL: Do you prefer it that way, or would you prefer . . . ?

TUCKER: Yes, actually, I think I prefer it that way. I want to train them myself. Some interpreters have rigid rules I don't like. My feeling is that the interpreter is there for me and things should be done my way. I don't mean that I try to be difficult for an interpreter; that's not what I mean. But, I don't want someone who thinks they have to hear every single word and if they don't, they interrupt the student to repeat it. My interpreters are not allowed to interrupt the student at all. And, if they miss something, and like you said, everybody misses something sometime, they're human, but they tell me and I make the judgment. I go to meetings where interpreters will be there, you know, for other deaf people. And I can't believe it when an interpreter interrupts a speaker and asks a speaker to repeat. They wouldn't do that if they worked for me; I don't want that.

SEAL: That's why I asked the question about interruptions, if you ask the student or the interpreter to repeat.

TUCKER: All the interaction is between me and the students. The interpreter is just there to interpret, not to interact with the students.

Interview with Donna Panko About Interpreting in a Doctoral Program

SEAL: The first question has to do with your role as an interpreter in a doctoral program.

PANKO: I'm a freelance interpreter hired by the university on an hourly basis for the semester. I have an hourly contract. This semester I am interpreting in two classes which meet for an hour and a quarter twice a week. These classes are very different in that one is straight lecture and easily manageable by one interpreter. The other is a rapid paced combination of lecture and discussion and requires a team of interpreters. The graduate student, the consumer, also teaches one class using an interpreter. In that class, he speaks for himself and the interpreter interprets student comments. I often substitute in that class. So, two interpreters cover all of his classes, special lectures, and meetings. All the interpreters used at the university are freelance interpreters. And in addition to the interpreters, there is a CART recorder in one of the classes.

SEAL: Do you feel a need to prepare for the course before attending the class? Do you read the readings assigned or listen to audiotape lectures to be familiar with the material for the next class?

PANKO: That's a great question. The university loans the interpreters sets of books for each course. I do read in preparation for each class, if not thoroughly, at least to the extent that I am familiar with the subject matter and the names and vocabulary used. When specific technical words are introduced, I finger-spell them until the consumer and I agree on a convention to use for the terms. Occasionally, a convention will last a whole semester or even carry over into other classes. You know, signs that are adopted broadly in ASL sometimes begin as classroom conventions.

I also tend to be interested in a lot of areas. I actually feel lucky to have the opportunity to be involved in whatever subject someone happens to be registered for.

SEAL: What are some of the challenges you experience interpreting in a doctoral program, regarding content of courses?

PANKO: Challenges at the doctoral level? *[laughing]* The language is deliciously sophisticated and often obtuse. It goes from being sophisticated to being incredibly tangled, almost nonsensical. I have made lists of phrases—some of them are so incredible. And, occasionally, the discussions, even though I've read the material, and I understand the language, occasionally I don't understand what they're getting at. And sometimes, like a discussion the other day, I did understand it, but it was so totally obtuse. And the class discussed it for the whole class period, and even though everyone used different words, everybody said essentially the same thing.

SEAL: Well, what happens when you don't understand? What if, during a group discussion that is difficult to monitor, you truly don't understand what was said, maybe because you didn't hear it clearly or you misunderstood what was said? Do you interrupt the students who are talking? Do you interrupt the professor? Do you interrupt yourself to let the student know you have missed something?

PANKO: Usually, I just say, "I'm missing this. He named an author, but I missed it. It started with a G." Sometimes it comes to me later or someone says it later, and I go back and say, "The name of the author I missed was G. . . ." That's usually the way it goes, but the discussions sometimes get on a roll, and my sense is that the student prefers to control that himself. On the infrequent occasions when I have requested clarification from the professor, I have the impression that everyone in the classroom was grateful.

SEAL: You mention that the doctoral student also teaches. How does it work with the interpreter?

PANKO: He lectures, but he combines interaction with it. He asks questions of the students and the interpreter will interpret what the students say. He speaks for himself in his classes.

SEAL: So, how does it work in the class where you are teaming? Is that a more intense lecture course?

PANKO: This semester, both of my classes meet for the same length of time. And in one, the professor speaks slowly. It's very manageable for one interpreter. In the other class, the professor has lots of breakouts. The discussion is incredibly intense, even frenetic. I found that it was not manageable and I requested a teammate for that class, not only for relief but to help follow discussion, getting terminology, passing notes back and forth with information, and so on.

SEAL: So, in that class, one of you is "on" and the other feeds to the interpreter, or are both of you "on"?

PANKO: No, we alternate, about every 20 minutes, depending on what exactly the professor is doing. We have to be flexible about that. We sit next to each other, and although we generally try to rest between turns, we also listen and make notes. The "at-rest" interpreter listens for obscured words. In rapid exchanges, the at-rest interpreter may sign or fingerspell a word or phrase directly to the student, a phrase that the "on" interpreter missed, but because of the pace, didn't even have time to stop to request the phrase. A good teaming situation can work like that. It can enhance the quality of the interpreting, serve as a professional development opportunity, and generally enrich the whole experience. The ideal situation is that the team functions as a comfortable unit for the student, always working toward clear communication, both in and out of class. This ideal is a bit more elusive than you might expect, though, because of the complex group dynamics involved. There are pitfalls. Sometimes, interpreters can be competitive with each other; or they may form a dyad that excludes the consumer. Or, the team and the consumer can form a triad that separates the consumer from the rest of the class. Any of these pitfalls can seriously interfere with the interpreting.

Question 5: What obligations do educational interpreters have for their own lifelong learning?

As we entered the twenty-first century, many of us born before 1970 (and 1960, 1950, 1940) realized that the Information Age requires a new attitude about learning and our own aging. Technological developments in information science have revolutionized our access to information. We can learn something about almost anything from the Internet. A recent Google search on "educational interpreting and deaf students" yielded 13,600 hits. Imagine! The impact of the Information Age on education, including our own, can be staggering. We used to refer to education as though it were a static experience: "She was educated at . . . " "He received his training in 1992 . . . " "Her degree is in . . . " And, while we still acknowledge degree programs and licensures in terms of dates and locations, there is an ever-pressing awareness that what is learned in degree programs, what our licenses and certificates provide us, are merely opportunities to enter greater learning experiences. I see educational interpreting as an incredible learning opportunity, not just because, as Donna Panko explained, it gives us "the opportunity to be involved in whatever subject [the student] happens to be registered for," but also because it gives us the opportunity to be involved in learning. For educational interpreters, learning should be held at a premium. The congruity of having educated interpreters as educational interpreters is probably apparent, but it merits brief discussion here.

Many deaf students, the consumers, assume that their college interpreters have gone to college. This assumption—having *educated* interpreters—is probably more openly expressed in higher education settings than in elementary and secondary settings. Nover's preference for having interpreters who are also experts in his line of research is not uncommon. As revealed throughout the chapters in this book, educational interpreting requires academic problem solving; and, "presumably, the longer one is in school, the more familiar and comfortable one becomes with certain forms of academic problem solving" (Karson, Karson, & O'Dell, 1997, p. 35).

This connection between interpreting and schooling is of current interest among the professionals who certify sign language interpreters at the national level. Many are pushing for all candidates for certification to hold degrees, and not only professional degrees in interpreting, but also bachelor's, master's, and doctoral degrees. These degrees guarantee the consumer two things: a certain *intellectual* level that met competitive entrance testing, and a certain *commitment* level that sustained the degree holder through a program of studies to its completion. They also suggest, although with no guarantees, that the degree holder values education. Those who value education are more likely to continue seeking educational opportunities.

Students enrolled in interpreter training programs (ITPs) are in an exciting phase of their learning. ITPs across the country have examined their curriculum offerings and many have increased their course offerings and practicum experiences in educational interpreting (Dahl & Wilcox, 1990; Shroyer & Compton, 1994). These courses, when paired with field experiences (observations and volunteer placements) and internships (required placements) enhance an educational interpreter's readiness to work in the school setting. They do not replace the learning that hopefully will continue through life. They merely better equip the interpreter for that continued learning.

One of the most exciting continuing education opportunities available today involves web-based education. Students who are unable (and some who are able) to enroll in traditional college programs are likely to benefit from the increasing availability of online courses that strive to be pertinent, current, and convenient, with the same rigor and quality of instruction expected in on-campus courses (Aggarwal, 2000; Palloff & Pratt, 2001).

Distance education courses require frequent and sustained computer access to the World Wide Web. They are not independent studies because of required participation—often a specified number of times per week in a chat room, on a bulletin board, or through e-mail dialogue with other students and the instructor. Also, Web-based courses are not free; tuition, books, CDs, and video materials may make their costs higher than on-campus courses. Web-based courses are also not for everyone. Many students need the face-to-face interaction with their peers and instructors at a given time each week. Those who have sufficient self-discipline to participate in asynchronous learning environments (interpreters may be naturals at this) are encouraged to investigate this wonderful new learning medium. Two programs are currently advertised: the University of Colorado's Project TIEM.Online, Teaching Interpreting Educators & Mentors, and the University of Tennessee's online interpreting program (Davis & Griffin, 2002). More are likely to come.

Opportunities for continued education exist outside the Internet, too. Educational interpreters can design their own independent learning programs through RID's Certification Maintenance Program (CMP).[2] (See the Appendix for CMP information.)

Membership in RID, in the National Cued Speech Association, in state interpreter organizations, and in professional organizations of deafness-related fields (e.g., the National Association of the Deaf, or NAD; Self-Help for the Hard of Hearing, or SHHH; the American Society for Deaf Children; the Alexander Graham Bell Association for the Deaf; and so on) provides educational interpreters with access to information about workshops, courses, conferences, and access to information in journals, newsletters, electronic bulletin boards, discussion groups, listservs, and more. Each of these formal contacts and resources becomes a valuable avenue to lifelong learning.

Educational interpreters in college settings may find themselves eligible for a given number of college credits or courses each year. Some schools provide tuition support for their staff to continue their education. Interpreters should request tuition reimbursement procedures or find out about tuition-free courses available to them in higher education settings. An advisor or knowledgeable supervisor may be helpful in recommending courses that would be relevant to educational interpreting. (See Lynn Hayes's article, "If I Had It to Do Over Again . . ." in the Appendix.)

Finally, lifelong learning is also enhanced by having mentors and colleagues who, on a personal level, can nurture our growth. Having someone with whom you can discuss your anxieties when you miss chunks of the sL, having someone with whom you can pose difficult ethical questions, having someone who simply talks to you in confidence about your skills and where they need improvement, about your disappointments and your enthusiasms enables a tremendous learning advantage at all stages of our development. In addition, becoming someone who listens to a colleague about his or her anxieties, who shares views about difficult ethical questions, who permits others to ask for recommendations for improvement enables a tremendous learning advantage at all stages of our development.

Formal mentorship programs have become popular in recent years. These programs vary in design—from degree programs that educate deaf and hearing interpreters and interpreter educators in the literature and techniques of mentoring, to school-based programs in which a seasoned interpreter is simply assigned, with no instructions, as a mentor to a newly hired ITP graduate. Both of these programs, and all their variations, are covered in the following metaphor:

---

[2]As mentioned in Chapter 1, your reading of this book could constitute an independent study activity for you.

Ecologists tell us that a tree planted in a clearing of an old forest will grow more successfully than one planted in an open field. The reason, it seems, is that the roots of the forest tree are able to follow the intricate pathways created by former trees and thus embed themselves more deeply (Daloz, 2000, xiii).

Interpreters who agree to mentoring relationships (both the newly planted tree and the tree from the old forest) are expected to grow. Mentors who observe, evaluate, demonstrate, explain, show, reflect, listen, inform, discuss, support, encourage, befriend, transform, question, coach, and challenge (Clark, 1995; Zachary, 2000) commonly report improvement in their own interpreting skills and knowledge. Similarly, protégés or mentorees who experience collegial nurturing, are likely to grow faster in the roots of their mentor's support.

Encouraging mentor-protégé relationships is as important for postsecondary interpreters as it is for educational interpreters in earlier grades. People sometimes erroneously assume that college interpreters need no support. All interpreters benefit from collegial relationships that enable professional stretching. A caution is offered in encouraging carte-blanche mentorship relationships, however. We know very little about the relationships that fail, and we would be naive to think that all mentor-protégé partnerships succeed. Individual preferences and/or personality types are likely to be important variables in the sustenance of mentoring relationships. Research on mentor relationships and mentorship program outcomes in educational interpreting are both needed (see discussion of personality types in Chapter 7 and the mentoring evaluation questions in Chapter 2).

In conclusion, educational interpreters represent a variety of skill levels, a variety of educational settings, and a variety of learning experiences. We, too, are diverse. Capitalizing on college offerings, distance learning, mentorship programs, and other continuing education opportunities should be part of our learning values. Each of us should embrace the concept of lifelong learning as a privilege, and encourage lifelong learning as a corporate pursuit for all those who claim a title as distinctive as "educational" interpreter.

Question 6: What are the best practices for these difficult cases?

The following cases, like those presented in previous chapters, represent a variety of ethical issues. You are encouraged to approach each case from your own problem-solving style and to discuss your conclusions with others who may share different approaches for solving problems.

The Case of Group Work

In Dr. Fratelli's social work class, the students are required to make a formal group presentation. The topic must be of current social interest with both a *pro* argument and a *con* argument given. Bob's group is scheduled late in the term, three weeks before the semester's end. A week before the group's scheduled presentation, a female student approaches Bob and his interpreter and asks if they could talk for a few minutes after class. Bob says yes and asks his interpreter if she can stay for a few minutes.

After class, the student tells Bob that the group had met already the night before and had decided on "The Illegal Alien" for their presentation topic next Friday. She indicated that three of them had picked the pro argument and that he was to work with her and another guy for the con argument. She asked him if that sounded all right. He responded OK. She asked him if he would mind if she was their side's speaker. He responded, "Of course not." She told him she would write out their argument and bring it to him in class Wednesday for his input or approval. He said, "Fine." Then she left.

Bob's response to the interpreter was, "Hmmmmm. I wonder why they met without me? I guess no one wanted to use the relay service. Do you think I should say something to the teacher?" (The teacher had distributed to each group the members' names and phone numbers, with the relay service phone number listed next to Bob's name.) The interpreter responded, "I don't know." Bob added, "I don't want my grade to be reduced because I didn't meet with the group." The interpreter asked, "Isn't group participation part of the grade?" Bob answered, "Yes, maybe I should tell Dr. Fratelli, but I don't want to get the others in trouble. What would you do if you were me?" What should the interpreter do?

Suggested Best Practice   The interpreter may be inclined to say, "Hey, I'm not you; this is your problem, not mine." But that attitude of disengagement is counter-indicated for an interpreter who engages in the course as a member of the class. Being sensitive to Bob's question does not mean offering guidance or direction. "What would you do if you were me?" is a question that begs an opinion, perhaps as a colleague or member of the class, not necessarily as an interpreter. As such, I find it appropriate to say, "If I were a student in this situation, I'd . . . probably feel compromised and unsure of how to handle it. I think I would want to approach the professor if I felt she were approachable. I think I'd feel better about disclosing my discomfort with the events, but I might ask her not to take action, other than acknowledging what I share." I would then follow my statements with another question, "What do you plan to do?" or "Have you come up with a plan yet?" I would also offer my support in being available to interpret.

Departure Questions for Discussion

1. Wouldn't comments like these made by the interpreter be suggestive, of an advising nature?
2. What if the student rejected your answer as appropriate for you, perhaps, but inappropriate for him? Should you go on to offer other suggestions?
3. What's wrong with saying, "I don't know what I'd do" and wish him the best as he comes to a decision? Isn't that safer for all parties involved?

The Case of Interpreters Teaming with Interpreters

Robin, Linda, and Lorraine were all hired to interpret a conference on "Neurofibromatosis" at the Medical School. There were two deaf persons in the audience of 50 to 60 people. There were five speakers: a doctor who specialized in surgery, a doctor who specialized in genetics, a psychologist who spoke on the impact of the disease on development, a learning disabilities specialist who spoke on special education interventions, and one of the deaf persons who spoke on the loss of hearing and its impact on her life.

The language of the conference was very technical. Each of the interpreters had received a packet of readings well in advance, but, in spite of their preparation, they found that the topics were very challenging. They worked in pairs, with one reinforcing the other, feeding her vocabulary from the overheads and slides while the third interpreter took a break.

Robin and Linda tended to read each other well and worked well together. Lorraine was of no help to either Robin or Linda, however, when it came her turn to support. During the afternoon break, as they were gearing up for the last speaker and their turn at sign-to-voice interpreting, Lorraine explained that she didn't think she could do the sign-to-voice with the difficult vocabulary that was being used and all the fingerspelling the deaf woman used. She asked if they minded if she just sat out. Robin and Linda both agreed to do the last presentation, which was scheduled to last for an hour. And Linda said, "But I don't think you should bill for this last hour and earn the same salary that we are getting." Lorraine's response was surprising: "If I have to stay, I'm billing." Robin suggested that she leave.

At the end of the conference, the coordinator approached both Robin and Linda and offered them envelopes with their checks inside. Robin explained that she should mail Lorraine's check to her and that it should be reduced since she left early. The coordinator said, "Oh, I already gave her check to her. I saw her leaving and walked out with her. She said she wasn't feeling well. I can understand that. You all have worked so hard today. But don't worry about the money. I told her that it's too much trouble to have her return the check and have to do another voucher. There shouldn't be that much difference in the pay anyway."

Robin called Linda the next day, really upset about the chain of events. She asked Linda if she felt a call to the state interpreting agency was appropriate, that she wanted to report Lorraine for unethical conduct. Linda said she would have to think about it. What should Linda do?

Suggested Best Practice   Most interpreting referral agencies adhere to a code of ethics or conduct and expect their participating interpreters to abide by the same. Even in cases such as this one where the interpreters could have contracted independently of a referral agency, reporting infractions of ethical behavior to a state or national agency could still occur. How the agency responds to such reports may vary from state to state. Unless the agency has an ethical practices board that judicates decisions in cases involving alleged infractions, registering the report may be the end of it. That is, agencies that promote a conformity to ethical behaviors are not always equipped to execute judgments and punishments.

But another question is raised here. Should interpreters in teaming situations take action against each other? When, in this case, Lorraine, perhaps the C interpreter, could not support Robin and Linda, the A and B interpreters, should she have quit early? Or, should she have made a stronger effort to be an equal member of the team? Should the A and B interpreters have provided the C interpreter more support? Did the infraction occur because Lorraine accepted the same salary Robin and Linda accepted, or did an earlier infraction occur when each member did not work for the good of the team? Obviously, Linda's decision to join Robin in reporting Lorraine's behavior goes far deeper than the salary. In my opinion, both Robin and Linda should accept some ownership of the problem.

Brian Cerney (1996), in his article "Interpreting Working Conditions: Sharing the Vision," recommended that interpreting team members should conference prior to an assignment to "discover their areas of concern for professional growth" (p. 32). He pointed out that in these meetings, the interpreters should agree on what areas they will focus on: feeding missed information, verifying fingerspelling, monitoring text (e.g., overheads), monitoring problems, or just agreeing to "note only positive things about each other just to keep up morale" (p. 32). Recognizing and promoting the collegiality that can occur in team interpreting is important in reducing tensions such as the one created here. At the same time, we do not know why team interpreting works for some individuals in some assignments and fails for the same individuals or others in other assignments. We do not know the dynamics that tend to foster a successful situation and how they differ from those that foster an unsuccessful situation. Educational interpreters who have extensive experience in teaming should be encouraged to reflect on the variables that impact their successes and failures and document these variables for the benefit of other interpreters.

Departure Questions for Discussion

1. Shouldn't Robin and Linda just agree not to work with Lorraine in future situations and to report to the agency that hired them that they would not work for them again if Lorraine were hired?
2. Don't interpreters have an ethical obligation to report infractions to their state referral agency? Wouldn't Linda and Robin be jeopardizing their own ethical reputations by not reporting?
3. Couldn't Robin support Linda in calling to report Lorraine, but ask her to keep her name out of it?
4. What if the referral agency wants written documentation from Robin and Linda? Would they be able to send it to Lorraine for her review and rebuttal?
5. Aren't anonymous reports safer in the long run than identifiable reports of ethical misconduct?
6. What if Lorraine mailed half of the salary she earned for that hour to Robin and half to Linda? Would there still be an ethical issue?

The Case of the Sleeping Student

Carrie was the only deaf student in the Legal Aspects of Education class, a graduate course she was taking to complete her certification requirements for endorsement in supervision. Becky, her interpreter, had interpreted the course before and knew how exciting the material could be. She was disappointed after the first class meeting to find that the new professor, Dr. Miles, was very soft-spoken, hesitant, and somewhat dull in his lecture style. There was little discussion during the first two classes and the three-hour class seemed to drag on forever.

In the third week of this evening class, Becky became sensitive to the fact that Carrie was heavy-eyed again. Because both she and Carrie were in the front, just about everyone in the classroom could see them. She thought it looked bad when Carrie slept. During the break, one of the students approached Becky in the bathroom and asked her why she kept on interpreting when the deaf woman fell asleep? Becky was a little shaken by the comment but was prepared to respond when Carrie walked in. What should Becky do?

Suggested Best Practice   Students who use interpreters, especially in evening classes, and especially in classes where the activity level is slow, become heavy-eyed when their gaze cannot shift frequently enough to rest their eyes. In these cases, interpreters should work to adjust their positioning so the student's eyes have to move. Acknowledging fatigue and sleepiness in students when it occurs may help in reducing it. Being sensitive to the fatigue of other students might also relieve some of the strain. If hearing students are also sleeping, chances are the problem lies with the teaching or the temperature, not just with the deaf student and the interpreting.

The question raised here, however, involves Becky's response to the student who asked her why she continued to interpret when Carrie slept. Becky should answer as she would have had Carrie not entered the restroom. An answer that explains the role of the interpreter to provide access to the verbal information might satisfy the question without drawing additional attention to the student's role. If, as Carrie approached, Becky's response now necessitated the addition of sign language, then some explanation about the question is in order. Responding politely and directly, rather than with embarrassment or a mind-your-own-business attitude, should also reduce the sensitivity of the situation.

Departure Questions for Discussion

1. Shouldn't Becky get Carrie a cup of coffee at the break?
2. Why shouldn't Becky stop interpreting while Carrie sleeps? Isn't it hard to interpret if the recipient of the tL isn't participating?
3. Wouldn't a second interpreter improve the situation for Carrie? That is, if two interpreters were available and they each switched off every 15 or 20 minutes, wouldn't Carrie's eyes get to move more? Shouldn't Becky request a team interpreter for this long class?

The Case of the New Signing Student

Jessica received her cochlear implant at age 4, following spinal meningitis and the diagnosis of a profound hearing loss. Her educational years included public, home, and private schooling. She was oral. She was also very bright and had been accepted at several colleges. She based her final decision on the reputation of the college, both in the major she desired and the availability of support services.

Jessica's declared major, deaf education, also had a wonderful reputation and she was welcomed into the introductory class with an override from the professor. She also enrolled in the Sign Language I class during the fall term and pre-registered for Sign II in the spring. She was very happy in her new college!

During the closing weeks of the fall semester, Jessica made an appointment with the disability offices director and requested a sign language interpreter for her spring courses. As she explained, her need to develop fluency in sign language was critical to her career, and the introductory course had made it apparent to her that progress was limited without ongoing exposure and use. The director was hesitant at first but agreed that an interpreter might be appropriate, at least on a trial basis. She advised Jessica to select a course and agreed to schedule an interpreter.

The course Jessica picked was U.S. History from 1860. The nationally certified interpreter was informed of the nature of her assignment to this class well in advance, and she agreed to give it her best. She was surprised that Jessica did not use sign language but appreciated her eagerness to learn.

During the third week of the spring semester, the interpreter told Jessica that her signing skills were obviously growing. Jessica responded that she was enjoying the opportunity she had to learn from her, but that the history course was proving to be more difficult than she expected. She also admitted that she had trouble focusing on the language of the course with her attention on the language of signs. She said she planned to drop it. She asked the interpreter if she would be willing to interpret in her Sign II class, indicating that the teacher talked about half the time and signed the other half. She thought she would get more out of it if the talking were interpreted. The interpreter's first response was, "No way, that would be too awkward." Jessica's insistence left her baffled. Furthermore, Jessica asked the interpreter if she would go with her to the disability services office to make the change. The interpreter responded that she would think about it. What should she do?

Suggested Best Practice   The interpreter's role has certainly been stretched here, and even if she enjoys the new experience, going to the office with Jessica could suggest that she is agreeing to the change. Denying Jessica's request is reasonable, but in a way that removes her from the decision making.

I suspect the disability services office will also deny Jessica's request to move the interpreting services to the Sign II class. Jessica's goal in having an interpreter is to enhance her sign language learning, not equalize communication access. The disability services officer may have erred in agreeing to an interpreter in the first place, Indeed, it appears here that the interpreter's presence actually prevented Jessica's learning in the history course. Other possibilities (study groups, volunteer work in the deaf community, observing interpreters in other approved settings) are logical alternatives for Jessica's learning.

Departure Questions for Discussion

1. What if the interpreter really wants to do it, just for the experience? Should she volunteer to continue?
2. Should the sign language instructor be involved in the decision making?
3. Should Jessica be applauded for her creative thinking? After all, her goal is to be a teacher of deaf students.

The Case of the Final Semester Presentations

Patrick knew on the first day of the semester that the final presentation week would require additional interpreters—40 students required to give three- to five-minute presentations on a topic in case law. He notified the interpreter coordinator early on, again at midterm, and again as the semester drew to its end. Each time, the coordinator shared that all the interpreters were over-scheduled and that she was trying to locate extras from the interpreting agency in town, but had no luck at this point. Patrick had a good mind to refuse to interpret the presentations. He, too, was over-worked this semester and felt this course had been stressful enough, even though it was only 50 minutes long. What should he do?

Suggested Best Practice   Working with the interpreter coordinator is certainly appropriate but it is not the only approach to Patrick's dilemma. Talking with the instructor about the anticipated demands of the presentations might lead to some alternatives, even if he gets another interpreter. Copies of each presentation well enough in advance to permit rehearsal would make a difference. Setting up a practice time for any students who agreed to a dry run would also reduce the stress of the fast-paced presentations and alert the students involved to the need for pauses. Requesting several breaks in the presentation schedule, and sequencing the presentations so that faster speakers are alternated with slower speakers would also be helpful. In all of this planning, Patrick should arrange to work with the deaf student, too, in ensuring a smooth sign-to-voice delivery during her presentation.

Departure Questions for Discussion

1. Would this problem be avoided if the instructor had sufficient orientation in working with an interpreter, well before the syllabus was completed?
2. Couldn't students be given more time, so that their presentations could be slower?
3. What's wrong with just refusing to interpret?

Summary

Interpreting in higher education is extremely challenging. The growing number of high school students who enter postsecondary programs are also language learners who continue to develop discourse skills. The current generation of students is the first generation who may have received all formal schooling with educational interpreters. These students and older nontraditional college students are alike in some ways, but also very different in their interpreting and technology preferences. Interpreters who work in postsecondary settings are likely to be comfortable with both the diversity and individuality that characterize these consumers. Interpreters in college settings are encouraged to be aware of their own need for continued learning. Web-based education and mentorship programs were discussed as two possible approaches to continuing education. Challenging cases in higher education closed this chapter.

REFERENCES

Aggarwal, A. (2000). *Web-based learning and teaching technologies: Opportunities and challenges.* Hershey, PA: Idea Group Publishing.

Cerney, B. (1996). Interpreter working conditions: Sharing the vision. *RID Views, 13,* 1, 32.

Clark, T. S. (1995). *Mentorship: A sign of the times: A guide to mentoring in the field of sign language interpretation.* Stillwater, OK: National Clearing House of Rehabilitation Training Materials.

Cokely, D. (1992). *Interpretation: A sociolinguistic model.* Burtonsville, MD: Linstok Press.

Dahl, C., & Wilcox, S. (1990). Preparing the educational interpreter: A survey of sign language interpreter training programs. *American Annals of the Deaf, 135,* 275–279.

Daloz, L. A. (2000). Foreword. In L. J. Zachary, *The mentor's guide: Facilitating effective learning relationships* (xiii–xiv). San Francisco, CA: Jossey-Bass.

Davis, J. E., & Griffin, M. (2002). Preparing interpreters via distance learning technology. *RID Views, 19,* 10–11.

Flexer, C., Wray, D., & Leavitt, R. (1990). *How the student with hearing loss can succeed in college: A handbook for students, families, and professionals.* Washington, DC: Alexander Graham Bell Association for the Deaf.

Gajar, A., Goodman, L., & McAfee, J. (1993). *Secondary schools and beyond: Transition of individuals with mild disabilities.* New York: Macmillan.

Grisham, J. (1997). Using oral interpreters: A college student makes a good decision. *RID Views, 14, 9.*

Hirano-Nakanishi, M. J. (1994). Methodological issues in the study of diversity in higher education. In D. G. Smith, L. E. Wolf, & T. Levitan (Eds.), *Studying diversity in higher education* (pp. 63–85). San Francisco: Jossey-Bass.

Karson, M., Karson, S., & O'Dell, J. (1997). *16PF interpretation in clinical practice: A guide to the fifth edition.* Champaign, IL: Institute for Personality and Ability.

Marschark, M., Lang, H. G., & Albertini, J. A. (2002). *Educating deaf students: From research to practice.* New York:. Oxford University Press.

McKeachie, W. (1991). How teachers teach, how students learn. In *Teaching and technology: The impact of unlimited information access on classroom teaching—Proceedings of a National Forum at Earlham College* (pp. 1–13). Ann Arbor, MI: Pierian Press.

Mintz, D. (1993). Correcting interpretation errors. *RID Views, 10, 1, 10.*

Nippold, M. A. (1998). *Later language development: The school-age and adolescent years, 2nd Ed.* Austin, TX: Pro-Ed.

Norton, P., & Sprague, D. (2001). *Technology for teaching.* Boston: Allyn & Bacon.

Olia, F. (1991). The interaction of mental imagery and cognitive styles in the retention of prose among deaf college students. In D. S. Martin (Ed.), *Advances in cognition, education, and deafness* (pp. 409–413). Washington, DC: Gallaudet University Press.

Palloff, R. M., & Pratt, K. (2001). *Lessons from the cyberspace classroom: The realities of online teaching.* San Fransisco, CA: Jossey-Bass.

Porter, J., Camerlengo, R., DePuye, M., & Sommer, M. (1999). *Campus life and the development of postsecondary deaf and hard of hearing students: Principles and practices.* A report of the National Task Force on Quality of Services in the Postsecondary Education of Deaf and Hard of Hearing Students. Rochester, NY: Northeast Technical Assistance Center, Rochester Institute of Technology.

Rawlings, B. W., & King, S. J. (1986). Postsecondary educational opportunities for deaf students. In A. N. Schildroth & M. A. Karchmer (Eds.), *Deaf children in America* (pp. 231–257). San Diego: College-Hill Press.

Roth, F. P., & Spekman, N. J. (1984). Assessing the pragmatic abilities of children: Part 1. Organization framework and assessment parameters. *Journal of Speech and Hearing Disorders, 49,* 2–11.

Roy, C. B. (2000). *Interpreting as a discourse process.* New York: Oxford University Press.

Sanderson, G., Siple, L., & Lyons, B. (1999). *Interpreting for postsecondary deaf students.* A report of the National Task Force on Quality of Services in the Postsecondary Education of Deaf and Hard of Hearing Students. Rochester, NY: Northeast Technical Assistance Center, Rochester Institute of Technology.

Shroyer, E. H., & Compton, M. V. (1994). Educational interpreting and teacher preparation: An interdisciplinary model. *American Annals of the Deaf, 139,* 472–479.

Smith, D. G., Wolf, L. E., & Levitan, T. (1994). Introduction to studying diversity: Lessons from the field. In D. G. Smith, L. E. Wolf, & T. Levitan (Eds.), *Studying diversity in higher education* (pp. 1–8). San Francisco: Jossey-Bass.

Stewart, D. A., & Kluwin, T. N. (2001). *Teaching deaf and hard of hearing students.* Boston: Allyn & Bacon.

Tannen, D. (1986). *That's not what I meant!* New York: Ballantine Books.

Troiano, C. A. (2000). Training is available for oral transliterators: Twelve years of training educational oral transliterators. *RID Views, 17, 8.*

Zachary, L. J. (2000). *The mentor's guide: Facilitating effective learning relationships.* San Francisco: Jossey-Bass.

7 Educational Interpreting Research

Students in research courses often approach research questions, methods, tools, and analyses with attitudes of detachment. This chapter is written to provide college students, practicing interpreters, and interested researchers a practical and personal experience with current research literature and with future research opportunities.

Question 1: Why is research on educational interpreting important?

In this chapter, *research* is defined as the systematic approach to asking and answering questions about educational interpreting. Research is a process that requires adherence to rules associated with the scientific method. The scientific method, by convention, employs two routes to problem solving: a deductive route, in which we apply general findings to specific cases; and an inductive route, in which we apply findings from specific cases to the general population. Research that involves the behaviors of humans is frequently referred to as behavioral research; all fields that involve humans as social beings are referred to as the social sciences. Research on educational interpreting, then, because it involves the behaviors and relationships of humans, is subject to the same criticisms that research in all behavioral and social sciences must accept. These criticisms rest largely in the complexity of humans. No single individual is completely identical to another individual; furthermore, no single individual is completely consistent from one moment to the next. Humans are different, both from others and within themselves. Consequently, generalizing research findings from specific cases to the general population, and applying general research findings to specific cases, must be done with great caution.

Educational interpreting is both a profession and a discipline. One of the features of any academic discipline, either a traditional discipline or a new discipline, is that it seeks to study and understand itself. One of the characteristics of a profession, either an established profession or a newly emerging profession, is that the professionals—those engaged in the discipline—seek to understand themselves and their discipline. Learning about a discipline as a profession improves the status of the discipline and promotes status for the professionals engaged in the discipline. If educational interpreting is to continue growing as a discipline, it must be researched. If educational interpreters are to continue growing in professional status, we must embrace research about ourselves, our consumers, and our practices.

Donald Moores, in several writings (e.g., 1990), addressed problems inherent in research involving children who are deaf and hard-of-hearing. Education of the deaf historically has been divisive. Issues involving communication methods, educational placements, and the curriculum have been passionately battled by well-intended educators who all too often misapply research findings from general cases to specific students and/or from specific students to the general population of deaf and hard-of-hearing students. Student variables (especially the student's ability, communication skills, and social development) and instructional variables (especially time engaged in learning and the quality of instruction provided) must be carefully described before applications, either specific to general or general to specific, can be made appropriately.

Donna Mertens (1991) also addressed dilemmas facing researchers who investigate educational interpreting. She described the complications involved in collecting data from a teacher–interpreter–student communication triad, in which each party's effective communication is dependent on at least one, but usually both, of the other parties.

> [R]esearchers in deafness and cognition . . . need to formulate questions regarding what the teacher knows, what the student knows, how the student mediates information received from the teacher, and what impact these factors have on performance. Increased attention will also need to be given to the subject matter being studied (1991, pp. 345–346).

The challenge to all professionals involved in educational interpreting research—to those who generate research questions and designs, to those who conduct research, to those who interpret and evaluate research, and to those who apply research findings—can be formidable.

One of the benefits we have today in meeting the challenges that Moores and Mertens described is the access we have to knowledge. Learning what others have learned from their research on educational interpreting no longer involves hours and days and weeks in library stacks. Access to previous research is now as simple as typing the appropriate keywords into the appropriate search engine. The following section represents such a literature review (plus days in the library stacks), offered with this caution: Many reports and articles on educational interpreting have been published in recent years. *RID Views* continues to be a significant depository of these reports, especially with its annual educational interpreting issue. RID published several of these articles in *Educational interpreting: A collection of articles from Views, 1996–2000.* The editors of *Odyssey: New Directions in Deaf Education* (2001) also devoted a publication to educational interpreting,

Interpreting theory and practice: Reaching out to teach deaf children. These numerous articles, some of which I claim as research (e.g., "Educational Interpreters Document Efforts to Improve," Seal, 1999) are not included here, not because they are not important to the profession and discipline, but largely because, in the sacrifice of space, they do not constitute *refereed* research. That is, they have not received blind reviews from editorial staff who could accept them for publication in their journals or books.[1]

Question 2: What research has been done to date on educational interpreting?

A review of the current literature on educational interpreting from 1986 to 2002 revealed several patterns that fit these categories: (1) the current status of and consequential need for educational interpreters; (2) the evaluation of interpreters engaged in sign language interpreting; (3) interpreting in postsecondary education; and (4) a miscellaneous or "other" category for research that did not fit into one of the previously mentioned areas. Some overlap exists between the categories (e.g., an article that focused on evaluating interpreters' use of the cloze process was placed in category 2 but it also involved interpreters in college classrooms, category 3). Table 7.1 provides an annotated bibliography that spans these 16 years.

TABLE 7.1   Research on Educational Interpreting from 1986 to 2002

Author(s)	Year	Brief Description
Category 1: The Status of and Need for Educational Interpreters		
Zawolkow & DeFiore	1986	Reported on the prevalence of educational interpreters, their roles, responsibilities, and needs for training
Rittenhouse, Rahn, & Morreau	1989	Surveyed teachers, deaf college students, and interpreters regarding characteristics and skills of educational interpreters
Dahl & Wilcox	1990	Surveyed program directors regarding educational interpreting services
Mertens	1990	Surveyed, observed, and interviewed deaf adolescents and interpreters regarding implications of interpreting on the learning experience

(continued)

[1]As mentioned in Chapter 6, an online search led to 13,600 hits, most of which are online reports. If, in my efforts to cover only those articles from *refereed* works, I have omitted a favorite print or online article, please know it was not intentional.

TABLE 7.1   (continued)

Author(s)	Year	Brief Description
Category 1: The Status of and Need for Educational Interpreters		
Wilcox, Schroeder, & Martinez	1990	Reported on a model interpreting program in Albuquerque, NM, schools
Luetke-Stahlman	1992	Reported on needs of interpreters in preschool settings
Hayes	1992	Surveyed and interviewed interpreters regarding their roles
Shroyer & Compton	1994	Provided a curriculum for a degree program in Educational Interpreting
Kluwin	1994	Interviewed interpreters on their training, skills, roles, and styles
Taylor & Elliott	1994	Surveyed interpreters, students in ITPs, and teachers who had interpreters in their classrooms on knowledge, skills, and attitudes of educational interpreters
Salend & Longo	1994	Reported on the roles of educational interpreters for classroom teachers and administrators
Afzali-Nomani	1995	Reported on need for trained and certified interpreters for successful inclusion programs
Beaver, Hayes, & Luetke-Stahlman	1995	Surveyed teachers about inservice needs and benefits
Ford & Fredericks	1995	Reported on the need and guidelines for interpreting for a deaf-blind student
Elliott & Powers	1995	Described Alabama's four-university consortium for educational interpreters
Stewart & Kluwin	1996	Reported on practices of interpreters in 15 school districts
Powers	1997	Reported on need for training interpreters in Alabama and Florida
Ramsey	1997	Reported on a longitudinal study of mainstreamed deaf children in primary grades and the roles of their interpreters
Jones, Clark, & Soltz	1997	Profiled 222 educational interpreters in three midwestern states regarding their background and experiences
Antia & Kreimeyer	2001	Reported on a longitudinal study of interpreters in inclusive classrooms with young deaf children

TABLE 7.1   (continued)

Author(s)	Year	Brief Description
Category 1: The Status of and Need for Educational Interpreters		
Yarger	2001	Reported on the qualifications and experiences of 63 educational interpreters in two rural states
Category 2. Evaluation of Interpreters Engaged in Interpreting		
Cokely	1986	Reported on lag time and error patterns
Rudser	1986	Compared changes in interpreters' skills between 1973 and 1985
Smith & Rittenhouse	1990	Reported on students' preferences of RTGD, interpreter only, and combined RTGD and interpreter use
Johnson	1991	Reported on interpreter miscommunications
Winston	1992	Reported on demands of instructional communication on interpreters and students
Siple	1993	Reported on pausing behaviors of interpreters as they interpreted and transliterated
Isham & Lane	1994	Reported on interpreters' cloze procedures
Nover	1995	Reported on comparative analysis of deaf and hearing students' access to English
Shaw & Jamieson	1997	Reported on an 8-year-old's interaction patterns with his interpreter
Siple	1998	Reported on the additions 15 educational interpreters used in their transliteration
Schick, Williams, & Bolster	1999	Reported on evaluation results of 58 interpreters with the EIPA
Sofinski, Yesbeck, Gerhold, & Bach-Hansen	2001	Reported on the transliterations of 15 educational interpreters
Cawthon	2001	Reported differences in teacher language directed to deaf students and their interpreters
Category 3. Interpreting in Postsecondary Educational Settings		
Jones	1986	Reported on deaf graduates of the California State University at Northridge and their use of interpreters
Lawrence	1987	Reported on specialized training for interpreting technical vocabulary
Shaw	1987	Examined register in interpreted and transliterated lectures

(continued)

TABLE 7.1   (continued)

Author(s)	Year	Brief Description
Category 3. Interpreting in Postsecondary Educational Settings		
Petronio	1988	Interviewed deaf-blind students regarding their needs
Cokely	1990	Compared the effectiveness of teacher lecturing with an interpreter and lecturing in simultaneous communication
Locker	1990	Reported on interpreter errors
Khan	1991	Described LaGuardia Commununity College's interpreting program
Livingston	1991	Compared student's interpreting and transliterating preferences for reading comprehension
Mallory & Schein	1992	Surveyed colleges on their use of interpreters
Roy	1993	Reported on the role of the interpreter during a faculty-doctoral student meeting
Siple	1993	Described the interpreter's role in the college classroom
Manning	1994	Reported on teaching a deaf graduate student who used interpreters
Bond	1995	Reported on the needs of deaf students in his hearing classes
Roy	2000	Provided analysis of the discourse patterns of a postsecondary interpreter
Martin & Lytle	2000	Described the importance of the interpreter to successful student teaching of deaf undergraduates
Seal, Wynne, & MacDonald	2002	Described an interpreting training program in undergraduate chemistry research
Napier	2002	Compared Auslan interpreters' styles as either free interpretation or literal transliteration
Marschark, Sapere, Convertino, Seewagen, & Maltzen	In Press	Compared students' comprehension of a lecture that was either interpreted or transliterated; compared deaf students' comprehension to hearing students' comprehension of the same lecture
Category 4. "Other" Research		
Hurwitz	1986	Reported on sign-to-voice interpreting under ASL and PSE conditions
Rudser & Strong	1986	Reported on characteristics that predict high skill level in educational interpreters

TABLE 7.1   (continued)

Author(s)	Year	Brief Description
Category 4. "Other" Research		
Stedt	1989	Reported on Carpal Tunnel Syndrome in educational interpreters
Cohen & Jones	1990	Examined interpreters' roles in interpreting research instruments
Smith, Kress, & Hart	2000	Reported on hand/wrist disorders in postsecondary interpreters
Seal	2000	Reported on the working relationships of 72 educational interpreters with their students' speech-language pathologists
Seal	In Press	Reported on the psychological test results of 28 interpreters

Category 1: The current status of and consequential need for educational interpreters

Reports of demographic data made available through annual surveys of hearing-impaired children and youth, such as those conducted by researchers at the Gallaudet Research Institute and reported in the *American Annals of the Deaf,* and the *U.S. Department of Education's Annual Reports to Congress,* have provided estimates of the increasing numbers of deaf and hard-of-hearing students who are being educated in school programs with educational interpreters. In addition, four national reports have provided state-of-the-union information on educational interpreting needs and services. These include: (1) *Toward Equality: Education of the Deaf* (Commission on Education of the Deaf, 1988); (2) *Educational Interpreting for Deaf Students: Report of the National Task Force on Educational Interpreting* (Stuckless, Avery, & Hurwitz, 1989); (3) *Educational Interpreters for Students who are Deaf and Hard of Hearing* (Linehan, 2000), a report of the National Association of State Directors of Special Education (NASDSE) in cooperation with the U.S. Department of Education's Office of Special Education Programs; and, (4) the report on *Interpreting for Postsecondary Deaf Students* (Sanderson, Siple, & Lyons, 1999) from the National Task Force on Quality of Services in the Postsecondary Education of Deaf and Hard of Hearing Students (chaired by Stuckless). Comparing the two latter reports to the two earlier reports reveals continued needs in both the quantity and quality of educational interpreting services, but also a sense of growth and improvement in these services over the 16-year span.

Because of these demographic and national status reports, several researchers have investigated the characteristics of educational interpreters and interpreter training. Zawolkow and DeFiore (1986) estimated the prevalence of interpreters in elementary and secondary classrooms and reported on their roles and responsibilities. Dahl and Wilcox (1990) analyzed questionnaires sent to 50 program directors regarding training of educational interpreters and areas that needed improvement. Results pointed to inadequate training of educational interpreters, particularly a lack of courses about the education of deaf children, language systems, and classroom interpreting situations. Jones, Clark, and Soltz (1997) reported on 222 educational interpreters across three midwestern states. Their results revealed educational interpreters in K–12 programs to be white and female, between 31 and 40 years old, with 5 years of experience or less, and in need of formal training. Yarger (2001) also investigated the qualifications and experiences of 63 educational interpreters in two rural states. Her results were consistent with these earlier reports—the majority of interpreters needed further training, not only to interpret but also to meet roles outside of interpreting.

Salend and Longo (1994) explained the responsibilities and roles of educational interpreters to classroom teachers and to administrators, with guidelines for administrative evaluations of interpreters. Stewart and Kluwin (1996) reported on educational interpreters from 15 different school districts and revealed discrepancies between interpreters and students' perceptions of what was interpreted. They also reported that interpreters' practices often fell outside the school system's guidelines. Ramsey, in her 1997 report, and Antia and Kreimeyer, in their 2001 report, offered longitudinal evidence of the role of interpreters in primary grades. Their observations and interviews revealed that the interpreters not only met their primary responsibilities in facilitating communication, but the teachers also saw them as integral members of the students' instructional teams.

Shroyer and Compton (1994) reported on the University of North Carolina at Greensboro's Educational Interpreter Training Program as an interdisciplinary model. They described the curriculum as meeting the previously recommended guidelines of the CED/RID Ad Hoc Committee on Educational Interpreting. Wilcox, Schroeder, and Martinez (1990) examined the interpreter services within the Albuquerque, New Mexico public school system. They reported that the school system changed its original standards for hiring interpreters to restrict newly hired interpreters to those who were college educated and RID certified. Wilcox and associates presented the Albuquerque program as a model program. Elliott and Powers (1995) and Powers (1997) also reported a need for improved training for educational interpreters in Alabama and Florida schools. The undergraduate program they developed emerged from a consortium of Alabama universities and focused both on interpreting in rural settings and with multicultural students.

Taylor and Elliott (1994) surveyed 71 professional interpreters, students in interpreting training programs, and teachers who use classroom interpreters according to their perceived needs for educational interpreters. Responses showed a variety of perceptions among the three groups. They disagreed on the skills, knowledge, and attitudes needed by educational interpreters, but agreed on the need for proficiency in English and ASL, and sensitivity to student needs. Rittenhouse, Rahn, and Morreau (1989) reported on the availability of educational interpreters. The 24 teachers, 18 deaf college students, and 27 interpreters disagreed about the roles of the interpreter but agreed on these areas: the importance of the interpreter's knowledge of lighting, elevation, seating, and visual background, and the interpreter's knowledge of the content area being interpreted. Burch[3] (1999) investigated perceptions of competencies, responsibilities, and educational levels for entry-level interpreters in precollege settings. His survey data revealed only one area of strong agreement among the 247 subjects surveyed: Inservice training was considered esential to those who work with interpreters.

Hayes (1992) interviewed and surveyed educational interpreters about their roles and responsibilities. Results indicated that 81% of the interpreters tutored students, 75% assisted students with homework, 75% developed signs for technical vocabulary, 72% served as a link between regular and special education students, and 56% worked with regular education students. Kluwin (1994) interviewed 40 interpreters for deaf students from 13 different programs on their training and experience, assessment of their skills, perception of the role of the interpreter in the classroom, and individual styles of interpreting. He distinguished four types of interpreters by certification and responsibility: professional interpreters, educational interpreters, communication aides, and aides who interpreted. Wide variation was reported across the four types of interpreters in the quality of interpreting services provided to deaf children in public schools.

Luetke-Stahlman (1992) discussed the special skills necessary for interpreting for mainstreamed deaf preschoolers. She identified 11 issues that were important in clarifying the job of the preschool interpreters. Among these issues were recommendations for encouraging communication among the hearing and deaf children. Mertens (1990) reported that her observations of, interviews with, and questionnaires completed by deaf adolescents revealed students to be generally dissatisfied with their interpreters when they took on disciplinary roles. She also reported that teachers were not knowledgeable enough about the roles of interpreters. Ford and Fredericks (1995) reported on the need for interpreter-tutoring services for a deafblind student. Their outline of required knowledge and skills for interpreting for deaf-blind students was offered as a model for other interpreters.

Afzali-Nomani (1995) reported on conditions related to successful full-inclusion programs for deaf and hard-of-hearing children. Her survey of regular educators in Kansas who participated in full-inclusion programs revealed that they viewed the availability of trained and certified interpreters as important to the achievement of their deaf and hard-of-hearing students. Beaver, Hayes, and Luetke-Stahlman (1995) reported on 59 elementary and secondary teachers who worked with educational interpreters. Their survey results revealed that only 33% of the teachers had attended inservices that dealt with educational interpreting. The teachers who attended inservices reported being more comfortable with educational interpreters than those who had not participated in any programs.

---

[3]Dissertations are generally not treated as refereed research. Four dissertation reports are included here in the text review, to applaud doctoral-level research that we hope to see in future refereed journals or books.

Category 2: Evaluation of interpreters engaged in interpreting

This second area of research includes several descriptive research reports. Winston's (1992) ethnographic study of the demands placed on both educational interpreters and deaf students revealed that many instructional situations, particularly those that require students to listen and watch simultaneously, are incompatible for interpreting and transliterating. Isham and Lane (1994) examined four Comprehensive Skills Certificate (CSC) interpreters for their cloze completions during interpreting and transliterating. Results indicated that the interpreters were less accurate in making inferential clozes than in making recall clozes, both in interpreting and transliterating.

Johnson (1991) analyzed 32 hours of videotaped classroom sessions involving sign language interpreters. Numerous miscommunications, which led to student confusion, were exposed. These miscommunications were more serious when the interpreters reported lack of familiarity with the subject and when diagrams were used. Miscommunications also occurred when the deaf students were expected to look at the board and the interpreter at the same time. Cokely's (1986) research involved four interpreters and their miscues. Interpreters with longer lag time made fewer errors.

Rudser (1986) reported on the performance of two sign language interpreters as they interpreted and transliterated two English texts, first in 1973 and again in 1985. Both interpreters showed increases in their use of four ASL features: classifiers, rhetorical questions, noun–adjective word order, and nonmanual negation. Sofinski, Yesbeck, Gerhold, and Bach-Hansen (2001) analyzed 15 educational interpreters' transliteration. Their analyses revealed two approaches used by the interpreters in rendering a target message. Sign-driven approaches included nonmanual markers, topicalization, spatial referencing, and ASL lexical choices. Speech-driven influences included English syntax, oral shadow accompanying fingerspelling, selective initialization, and use of prepositions. Individual variability was also observed across the interpreters' use of these approaches.

Siple (1993b) reported on the pausing behaviors of 20 master sign language interpreters as they interpreted and transliterated monologues. When transliterating, the interpreters were observed to render the source message pauses with visible signals. When interpreting, however, they used different kinds of auditory pauses: gaze shifts, held signs, and filled and empty pauses. In a later project, Siple (1998) reported on 15 educational interpreters' use of addition in their transliteration. She identified five groups of ASL features: (1) use of cohesion markers, (2) clarification, (3) modality adaptations (stress in the auditory message), (4) repetition (for emphasis), and (5) reduplication (for plurality).

Smith and Rittenhouse (1990) reported on four hearing-impaired students from the Arkansas School for the Deaf mainstreamed in an English class with 28 hearing students. The communication support provided the students was divided into three phases. First, all communication was transliterated by an interpreter; then, a stenotypist who used real-time graphic display (RTGD) was added to the interpreter condition. Finally, the interpreter was phased out, leaving the RTGD. At the end of the year, two students preferred the interpreter-only condition; two preferred the interpreter plus the RTGD condition.

Nover's (1995) ethnographic research on the communication patterns of four deaf students in a public high school of over 2,000 hearing students involved discourse analysis of the transliteration provided by one of the interpreters. He reported that whereas hearing students heard 182 spoken English words within a two-minute period, the deaf student saw only 12 fingerspelled English words and 79 ASL signs. Nover concluded that deaf students miss much of the English in the hearing classroom, even when their interpreters provide transliteration. Shaw and Jamieson (1997) reported on an 8-year-old student's interaction patterns in his mainstream classroom. They reported that the student interacted primarily with his interpreter, who also provided more direct instruction than the teacher. Cawthon's (2001) research of teacher language directed to deaf students revealed that hearing teachers in inclusive classrooms, although open to the diverse needs of their deaf students and to the roles of educational interpreters, still directed fewer utterances to their deaf students than to their hearing students.

Another area of research projects within this category of engaged interpreter performance includes research that has focused on appraising educational interpreters. Schick, Williams, and Bolster (1999) reported on their application of the Educational Interpreter Performance Assessment over a three-year period with 58 educational interpreters. No statistical differences were found in interpreting performance according to interpreters' years of experience. Results also revealed that educational interpreters scored significantly higher in the area of vocabulary than they scored in voice-to-sign skills, sign-to-voice skills, and overall performance. Concerns were raised over 29 of the 58 interpreters who repeated the test during the three years and failed to show improvement.

Hill's dissertation research (2000) focused on a deaf student's writing skills and the educational interpreter's role in facilitating writing improvement through English-like interpretation. Both the interpreter and student indicated preferences for ASL interpretation, but English writing improvement was facilitated with transliteration. La Bue's dissertation (1998) also focused on a single interpreter's rendition of a teacher's spoken language in an English class. Analysis of the interpreter's target language revealed several deletions, particularly of pronouns and cohesive elements, and a general exclusion of the deaf student in classroom discussions.

Category 3: Interpreting in postsecondary educational settings

Mallory and Schein (1992) surveyed postsecondary institutions with significant numbers of deaf students. The 63 responding institutions reported a broad range of methods for recruiting, orienting, and supervising sign language interpreters. Managing interpreting systems was discussed from an advantage and disadvantage perspective. Khan (1991) described LaGuardia Community College's (Long Island City,

NY) division of adult and continuing education. This model program increased its technology and faculty orientation to deafness largely through its interpreters. Jones (1986) reported on California State University at Northridge's mainstreamed hearing-impaired students. Five hundred and thirty-eight (538) had completed degrees between 1964 and 1986. The success of the students was attributed to adequate support services, including notetaking and sign language interpreting. Seal, Wynne, and MacDonald (2002) described the use of interpreters-in-training in an undergraduate chemistry research program that included deaf collegiate and high school students. The model program was offered as an approach to improve the shortage of interpreters in laboratory sciences. Kavin's (2001) dissertation research investigated changes in the Midwest Center for Postsecondary Outreach in its student census, preferences for training, and level of support services for deaf and hard-of-hearing students. Technical assistance services were reported to have the most positive change and included captioning, transcription, notetaking, tutoring, and interpreting services.

Siple (1993a) discussed the use of sign language interpreters for deaf college students in terms of the interpreter's role, classroom organization, pacing of speech, testing, and class discussions. She encouraged teachers to use the interpreter's presence and expertise as an opportunity to assess and enhance classroom communication dynamics. Petronio (1988) reported on interviews with 10 deaf-blind college students who explained their needs and expectations from sign language interpreters. The interview and observational data of deaf-blind interpreting situations revealed the types of signing, modifications needed to the signing, and visual information that needs to be conveyed.

Manning (1994) reported on her reactions, expectations, and interactions with interpreters when she, as a professor, experienced having a deaf graduate student in four different classes for the first time. Bond (1995) also reported on the differences required of him as a professor when five deaf students were enrolled in his class. Concerns about the communication gap that occurred, especially when humor was used to illustrate the class material, and concerns about grades well below what the students were capable of achieving, were presented with suggestions to help bridge that gap. Martin and Lytle (2000) reported on a student-teaching program in which deaf students from Gallaudet University participated as interns in local "hearing" schools. Their use of certified sign language interpreters was considered essential to the success of the program.

Roy's (1993, 2000) research involving a videotaped meeting between a professor, a doctoral student, and the interpreter revealed a unique role of the interpreter when the primary speakers talked and signed simultaneously. Rather than serving as a neutral conduit, the interpreter remained active, monitoring the social and linguistic knowledge of the communicative situation, including language competence and appropriate "ways of speaking." The interpreter was described as a discourse manager in the intercultural communication event. Livingston (1991) compared strategies for reading comprehension used by two deaf college students as they discussed assigned readings with their teacher and classmates. One of the two students preferred English-like sign language from his interpreter while the other preferred ASL from the interpreter. The student who preferred English-like signing showed a higher proportion of inaccurate interpretations and paraphrases than the student who preferred ASL. Results indicated that the students' competence in reading was more closely related to their performance than the face-to-face language each reader brought to the text.

Shaw (1987) examined portions of two lectures delivered in ASL and interpretations of each. Nine hearing and five deaf listeners saw and heard the ASL lecture and English interpretation. Analysis of register indicated different registers were observed between the English interpretations of the ASL speaker. Cokely (1990) compared the effectiveness of presenting information to deaf college students with the teacher lecturing in sign language alone, with an interpreter signing and the teacher speaking, and with the teacher signing and speaking simultaneously. Comparisons failed to show that any one method was superior to the other.

Locker (1990) investigated the accuracy of transliterated messages produced by sign language interpreters in college classrooms. Causes of interpreter errors fell into three categories: misperception of the source message, lack of recognition of the source form, and failure to identify a target language (tL) equivalent. Lawrence (1987) reported on an experimental design involving 20 educational interpreters: 10 beginning (with fewer than 300 hours of educational interpreting) and 10 advanced interpreters (with more than 1500 hours of educational interpreting). Five interpreters in each group were chosen for specialized training on terms and concepts related to "cell division" one day before they were asked to interpret a lecture on the same topic in a college biology class. Videotaped performance of the interpreters revealed significantly more accurate transliteration performance for both the beginning and the advanced interpreters who received prior training.

Napier (2002) reported on the analysis of ten Australian Sign Language (Auslan) interpreters who were videotaped as they interpreted a pre-recorded lecture. Their interpretations of three randomly selected sentences were rated on a continuum from an extreme dominant literal (transliteration) style to an extreme dominant free (interpretation) style. Results were varied, with six interpreters demonstrating a dominant free interpretation style and four demonstrating a dominant literal style. Several interpreters also demonstrated code switching between the two approaches. No correlations were found between the interpreters' educational levels and interpreting style. Marschark, Sapere, Convertino, Seewagen, and Maltzen (in press) also compared interpreting and transliterating for their differential effect on student comprehension. In a series of three experiments involving more than 100 college students who reported an interpreting or transliterating preference, tests of student comprehension (number of correct answers to questions from the interpreted or transliterated lecture) revealed no differences between the interpreting or transliterating condition. Comparisons of the deaf students' comprehension with hearing students' comprehension of the same lecture, however, revealed statistically lower scores for the deaf students whose access to the lecture was through an interpreter. Deaf students were also more likely to misjudge their performance on the comprehension test than hearing students.

Category 4: Other research

A variety of other research reports and articles, which span a wide array of topics, has been published in the past 16 years. Cohen and Jones (1990) examined sign language interpreters' participation in translating quantitative instruments used in research projects from written English into ASL. Concerns about translation methodology and the use of a back-translation process pointed to the need for research interpreters to be native ASL users with a comprehensive knowledge of both languages, familiarity with deaf culture, and ability to participate effectively on research teams.

Hurwitz (1986) divided 32 interpreters into two groups of 16, based on their interpreting experience and professional certification. A deaf storyteller presented two different stories, each in two different sign language types (one in ASL and one in Pidgin Sign English). Each interpreter was measured on accuracy and quality of voice interpreting under each of the two different treatment conditions. Results showed that experience with interpreting did not play a significant role in the effectiveness of voice interpreting, in either PSE or ASL conditions. Overall, the interpreters were able to voice PSE stories better than the ASL stories.

Stedt's (1989) paper on carpal tunnel syndrome described the ramifications of the syndrome for educational interpreters. The syndrome's incidences, causes, diagnostic procedures, medical and surgical intervention, and prevention guidelines were presented. Smith, Kress, and Hart (2000) also reported data collected on hand and wrist disorders from postsecondary interpreters. Twenty-six percent (26%) had problems significant enough to limit work. Women were more likely to suffer problems and seek medical assistance than men.

Rudser and Strong's (1986) research focused on the characteristics that predict high skill levels in sign language interpreters. Data collected on 25 interpreters were evaluated with an objective instrument for their interpreting skills and were analyzed on a measurement of personal variables. Multiple regression analysis revealed the importance of certain personality traits, which differed according to whether interpreters came from hearing or deaf families. Seal (2000) reported survey data from 72 educational interpreters on their work with speech-language pathologists. Results indicated that only 42% had working relationships with these professionals who are responsible for the communication evaluation and treatment of deaf and hard-of-hearing students. Guidelines were offered for effective partnerships with interpreters and speech-language pathologists in three areas: evaluating the communication skills of the students, including their ability to work with interpreters; establishing treatment goals and delivering treatment services; and providing inservice workshops to the teaching staff. Seal (in press) also reported on 28 interpreters who participated in a battery of psychological tests, to determine if a psychological profile distinguished interpreters as a group and at different levels. Results showed that scores from only one test, the d2 Test of Attention, had significant predictor value. Most interpreters also scored extremely high on measures of abstract reasoning.

Question 3: What research questions remain to be asked?

In spite of the growing body of literature just described, Kluwin and Stewart reported (2001) that we have little empirical evidence that indicates how well deaf students understand their interpreters. Indeed, the research just presented reveals that the deaf or hard-of-hearing student or consumer is examined far less as a variable of research interest than program and interpreter variables. Another trend in previous and current research is the predominance of attention to higher education. National outreach programs such as PEPNet work to support the growing number of deaf students who are enrolled in higher education programs, and this trend—*growing* enrollments of deaf and hard-of-hearing students in postsecondary programs over the past 10 years—may indeed be just the piece of empirical evidence that is missing. Increased college enrollments means increased acceptance of deaf and hard-of-hearing students from secondary programs. In fact, Kluwin (1993) reported that students in mainstream programs were more likely to be on grade level and to take college-bound courses than their peers in special schools. Mainstreamed students are also more likely to have educational interpreters. Increased eligibility for and increased enrollments in college programs therefore imply (inductive logic working here) that educational interpreting has made a difference in the outcomes of these students. We assume that students who go on to college understood their interpreters in high school.

Concerns about the need for more research on the student consumer are still reasonable, however. Donna Mertens (1991) addressed a concern in data collection. She recommended videotaping the interpreter-student dyad with one camera and the teacher with another camera in order to avoid confounding the collection of data. Videotaping provides a wonderful source for data. The ability to watch a videotape repeatedly ensures reliability within and among viewers. Mertens also recommended detailed narratives of the context in which data are collected. Specifics regarding class, student characteristics, teaching style, interpreter performance, and so on, are frequently sacrificed in the professional literature for lengthier sections on theory that support the research questions and on discussion that support application of the research results. Mertens suggested that researchers attend closely to the details when designing, conducting, evaluating, and reporting their research investigations. She also recommended consistency in transcribing. At least two knowledgeable transcribers or coders or raters of videotaped data should be used. Deaf adults who are knowledgeable users of interpreters and native users of signed languages provide a frequently untapped resource for data coding and transcribing.

Howard Pollio and Marilyn Pollio (1991) have provided us with an additional thought on the student or consumer as a research variable:

How are we to determine that what the teacher (or student) says, the student (or teacher) understands? How do we determine how the world appears from the

> first-person perspective of the student, and how does that perspective agree with the third-person perspective of the instructor or the researcher? (pp. 435–436)

Clearly, several of the articles reviewed over the past 16 years involved questions to the consumer, particularly the college student, and, to a lesser degree, the high school student, about their comprehension of opinions, and perceptions of educational interpreting. Even less attention has been given to the student's role while engaged in learning with an educational interpreter.

Pollio (1984), in his earlier research of the thinking behaviors of deaf college students, used a "thought sampling method" that involved interrupting students at random times to ask them to record what they were just thinking about. He reported that only 61% of deaf undergraduates, when interrupted to ask about their thoughts, were actually engaged mentally in the lecture. This same approach has important applications to educational interpreting research, at least at the secondary- and middle-school levels and, perhaps for some deaf and hard-of-hearing students at the elementary-school level. Students attending to an interpreter could be interrupted to ask about their thoughts, to determine if they are mentally engaged in the teacher's lecture, demonstration, discussion, or assignment, as they learn through their interpreter. One of the recommendations Pollio made, to avoid obtrusive interruptions, is to place a beeper on the student and to beep the student at certain intervals in order for the student to record what he or she is mentally engaged in. He also recommended videotaping the student and cueing recall at a later time while watching the videotape: "What were you thinking at this point?"

The value of this line of research is probably obvious without lengthy discussion. Educational interpreters know well that even though a student's eyes can be fixed on the interpreter, the student's thoughts can be "off" to another time, place, or person. (Is the same possibility true for interpreters?) Determining the "on" behaviors of students who use educational interpreters should answer many research questions about their potential for learning through an interpreter. If we assume, for example, that a student cannot learn without attending, we can determine if students who attend through interpreters are more or less likely than their hearing peers who do not attend through interpreters to be "on." We can also compare a student's "on" behaviors in one class or with one interpreter or with one interpreting approach (e.g., oral versus sign language interpreting) to those in another class or with another interpreter or with another approach. Research that involves repeated measures of a single or small group of students should result in findings that would be beneficial to interpreters, and to teachers in programming for a student with special learning or attending needs. Deaf students who are diagnosed with autistic disorder, learning disabilities, and with attention deficit disorder are also assigned interpreters. The degree to which the interpreter facilitates communication for these students who are at risk for additional communication and learning disorders has not been investigated.

Another area of consumer research that requires thoughtful design and implementation involves hard-of-hearing students, particularly the growing number of students with cochlear implants. Wide variability has been reported in their communication profiles and needs. Many of these students have sufficient auditory skills to take in some or most of their academic and social communication through listening, yet they may also benefit from the oral transliteration, cued speech or sign language transliteration, and interpreting provided by an educational interpreter. Videotaping these student-interpreter pairs should offer answers to questions about the effects of reduced student need, either real or perceived, on interpreter performance. To date, we know very little about the interdependence that exists between student and interpreter, or the degree to which interpreter performance and student support are compromised when that interdependence loses its reciprocity. Students who watch their interpreter only to catch what they missed, or to confirm what they thought they heard, may find their interpreters have reduced their cognitive engagement with the source language and are consequently unable to provide the needed target language. Videotaping and "thought sampling" are both appropriate in investigating this phenomenon, but the sampling must occur with interpreters as well as with students.

Directing questions about the effectiveness of educational interpreting to our interpreter colleagues who practice in educational settings is also important to advancing research in the discipline. In fact, the popular use of surveys, questionnaires, and interview data in the literature review probably says more about the youth of our profession than it says about our research background. We still want very much to know what others *think* when it comes to questions involving educational interpreting. At least two sources of qualitative data should be exploited in the name of research and the consumer. These sources involve collecting data from educational interpreters at workshops, conferences, and other professional gatherings, and collecting data from student consumers in interviews, classes, end-of-year evaluations, and so on.

One of the questions that is of some interest should serve to illustrate how *NOT* to ask research questions. The question involves the consumer's attitude toward *bad* interpreters. On several occasions, with panels of deaf and hard-of-hearing students, I have posed this question: Is it better to have a lousy interpreter or no interpreter at all in your classes? Among deaf adolescents ($N = 8$) the answer has been unanimous: "a bad interpreter is bad, but having no interpreter at all is much worse." Among deaf adults (college students) ($N = 6$), the answer to the same question has not been unanimous, but still very firm: 5 of 6 (83%) of the deaf adults have answered, "I'd rather have a bad interpreter than no interpreter at all." The same question, when posed to educational interpreters, provided similar responses: "Is it better for a school to provide a lousy interpreter or no interpreter at all?"—4 of 5 (80%) of the interpreters I asked in panel situations agreed that a lousy interpreter is better than no interpreter at all. Surprised?

The nature of self-disclosed data, especially when it is offered in a public forum like a panel, is subject to peer influence. If the second person's answer is similar to the first person's answer and the third person answers like the first two, then what is the likelihood that the fourth person will answer with a different response? The cumulative influence of each respondent's answer can skew the reliability of the total respondents' answers. With this influence in mind, then, the answer to this question, "Is it better to have a bad interpreter than no interpreter at all?" must be carefully considered. Quite frankly, I do not think there is an absolute answer to this question. I would anticipate that on any given day when a qualified interpreter is sick and the only available substitute is less than qualified (details would be needed to define "qualified"), then an unqualified interpreter is better than no interpreter at all. But, I can also anticipate that some desperate school systems could use the results of this panel data to justify hiring less qualified, even lousy, interpreters for their students who are deaf or hard of hearing.

The critical point is this: research questions that remain to be asked must be asked, answered, and reported with the highest standard of ethical responsibility. This question, "Is a bad interpreter better than no interpreter at all?" should probably not be asked—for the same reasons we would not ask: "Is a bad doctor better than no doctor at all? Is a bad teacher better than no teacher at all? Is a bad parent better than no parent at all?" These questions do not conform to the rigors of social and behavioral sciences mentioned at the beginning of this chapter.

Many important questions that focus on the consumer or student who learns through an educational interpreter do remain to be asked. The following paragraphs explore some questions and answers from 49 educational interpreters who participated in educational interpreting workshops and volunteered, at the close of the workshops, to record their anonymous thoughts on these *difficult* questions.[4]

> *Research Question 1:* At what age or stage does a student come to realize that an interpreted message is that: interpreted?
>
> a. Cognitively:
> 1. during the preoperational period
> 2. during the concrete operational period
> 3. during the formal operational period
>
> b. Linguistically:
> 1. during the single word/sign stage
> 2. when he or she starts to form sentences
> 3. when he or she becomes aware of different communication styles
>
> c. Chronologically:
> 1. 4 or 5 years old
> 2. 8 to 10 years old
> 3. 12 to 15 years old

Sixty-five percent (65%) of the participating interpreters responded that students come to know that their interpreter is representing the language of others during the concrete operational stage. This cognitive stage corresponds roughly to ages 7 through 11 and matches the responses of the interpreters (64%) who chose "8 to 10 years old" for the chronological part of this question. The same percentage of interpreters (64%), but not necessarily the same interpreters, selected "2" for the answer to the linguistic part of the question. This answer poses a discrepancy in

---

[4]An earlier version of this research was published in *RID Views*; segments of that article, "Educational Interpreters on Child Development" (Seal, 1996), are reprinted here with permission from The Registry of Interpreters for the Deaf, Inc.

the overall pattern of responses. As indicated in Chapter 3, children start to form sentences around age 2 and refine their development of sentences by age 5 or 6, or while they are still in the preoperational cognitive stage.

Interpreting the results of the responses to this developmental question must be done carefully. A look at the distribution of the other responses is appropriate to this interpretation: 12.5% of the interpreters selected the preoperational stage as the answer to the cognitive question, 12.5% chose the formal operational stage, and 10% wrote: "It varies from child to child." With this distribution, we could consider the potential for *all* answers to be accurate. If the interpreters responded from their experiences, and if we assumed a one-to-one correspondence between interpreter and student, then we could also assume that most interpreters (65%) worked with students who discovered that their interpreter was representing the language of others somewhere around age 8, that another 12% to 13% worked with students who made that discovery earlier, and another 12% to 13% worked with students who made that discovery later. Another 10% of the interpreters could fall on either end of this distribution, explaining the "it varies" response that 10% of the interpreters selected. Plotting this type of data distribution yields what researchers recognize as closely fitting a *normal distribution* (see Figure 7.1).

The normal distribution concept, often depicted by a bell-shaped curve, assumes that many human characteristics, like intelligence, are distributed normally throughout the population. This concept also implies that once an average or mean characteristic is established, all deviations from that average will fall within certain standard or expected intervals. As seen in Figure 7.1, we might explain variability within the interpreters' answers according to the normal distribution. That is, if we assume that 8 is the mean age at which deaf and hard-of-hearing students come to realize that their interpreter is interpreting, and if we assume that the standard deviation in this case is 2 years, then we can expect 68% of students who use educational interpreters to reach this milestone of awareness between the ages of 6 and 10. Another 27% would lie 2 standard deviation points from the mean, with half (13.5%) coming to the realization between the ages of 4 and 6, and the other half (13.5%) reaching this milestone between the ages of 10 and 12. The remaining 5% of the population would divide at either end of the curve: 2.5% of children would have the knowledge that their interpreter is representing the language of others before age 4, and 2.5% would not acquire that knowledge until after age 12.

This explanation of the responses to Research Question 1 stretches the rigors of scientific study far beyond scholarly boundaries, but the stretch should serve to explain the variability that can occur with group data and to introduce the concept of individual data. Single-subject research designs promise both practicality and rigor in research that focuses on the student consumer of educational interpreting. Because of its focus on individuals (any one subject or small groups of subjects can be studied), single-subject research enables questions about dependent variables (the student's learning, the student's grades, the student's communication with others, as examples) to be answered before, during, and after the independent variables (the presence of the interpreter, the nature of the interpreting, the

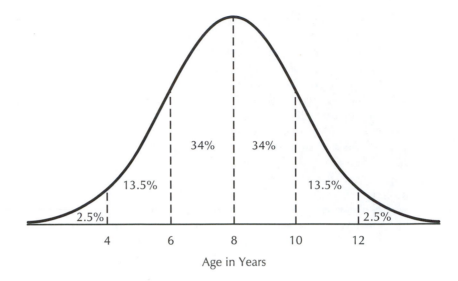

FIGURE 7.1   A normal-distribution approach to questions about the onset of children's awareness that the interpreter is interpreting.

frequency of interpreting, as examples) are manipulated. Questions about the effectiveness or appropriateness of an interpreter for young children lend themselves well to single-subject research.

Imagine that the parents of a 5-year-old deaf child want their child to be enrolled in a full-inclusion kindergarten program with an educational interpreter who provides sign language interpreting. Imagine that the school is prepared to provide this service but questions whether the young student will be able to learn as well with the interpreter as she might in a self-contained class with a special teacher trained in deaf education and fluent in sign language. The school proposes an experimental design—one in which the student is mainstreamed with an interpreter in the kindergarten class for the same reading instruction the teacher provides to the entire class. The dependent variable, the student's performance on measures of site vocabulary, is chosen and will be examined at three-week intervals. The first three-week interval involves the student's participation in the kindergarten reading class without an interpreter (the A condition); sight vocabulary is measured and recorded at the end of this baseline period. The second three-week interval involves the same participation in the same instructional program, but this time, with the addition of the interpreter (the B condition); sight vocabulary is measured and recorded at the end of this treatment period. Then the interpreter is withdrawn for three weeks (returning to the A condition) and the student's sight-reading vocabulary is measured and recorded again. This ABA pattern continues until the student's scores reveal a learning preference. If the student's scores drop considerably during the withdrawal period yet go up again during the reinstatement period, then the effectiveness of the interpreter for the student's learning is clearly documented. If, however, the student's scores show no change with or without the interpreter, the effectiveness of the interpreter is questionable.

Several variations of the single-subject design have been documented that enable multiple baselines to be collected, that control for the problems of repeated measures, that reduce the potentially negative effects of withdrawal, and so on (Hedge, 1987). The values of this design and its variations (e.g., the BAB, ABAB designs), especially for young deaf and hard-of-hearing students, and for those students who present with mixed communication profiles, as discussed in Chapter 4, offer many possibilities for asking and answering research questions that deal with the effectiveness or appropriateness of educational interpreting.

> *Research Question 2:* Is there a relationship between skill level of the interpreter and learning of the student?
> > a. Yes, but not a perfect relationship (a poorly skilled interpreter can hurt a student's learning).
> > b. Yes, but too many other variables (the student's cognitive, communication, and social skills) impact on learning to put all the weight on the interpreter's skills.
> > c. No, a talented student will learn in spite of a poor interpreter.
> > d. No, a student with learning problems will struggle to learn in spite of a skilled interpreter.

Responses to this question did not distinguish a particularly strong attitude toward a single selection. Fifty-three percent (53%) selected *b;* 45% selected *a,* 38% selected *c,* and 38% selected *d*—the sums do not equal 100% because the interpreters could select "all that apply." Eighteen of the 47 interpreters who responded to this question (38%) marked all four answers as being true; another 19% marked *a, b,* and *d* as true, eliminating *c* as a choice.

Much of the descriptive research in behavioral sciences involves the word *relationship.* Research questions frequently address the relationships between variables for several reasons: A wealth of information can come from the answers without having to experiment or control variables. In fact, correlational analysis often serves as the foundation or justification for later experimental designs. Correlational analysis does not suggest a cause–effect relationship, whereas experimental designs can. Correlational research does provide information on the strength of relationships between variables and the direction of the relationships between variables.

If we investigated the relationship between a student's learning and the skill level of the interpreter, we would need to establish the variables of interest. Interpreters who have higher credentials—perhaps more years of experience in educational interpreting settings, or more credits in educational interpreting coursework, or higher performance levels on state or national interpreter tests— could be compared to students' performance levels—perhaps grades in a given subject, attentiveness during a lecture, reading levels as measured on a standard-ized test, achievement test scores, and so on. Imagine, too, that we have a reason-able sample to investigate, and perhaps 40 or 50 students and interpreters who agree to participate.[5] Statistically, a comparison between the entire sample of interpreters' levels and students' scores could be calculated to reveal the direction and strength of the relationship. If the resulting correlation is positive, we would determine that the higher the interpreters' level, then the better the students' scores. If the correlation is negative, we would determine the opposite. Positive and negative in correlation studies refer only to directionality, not to judgments about the research data or results. In addition to direction, we can judge the strength of the correlation. The closer the correlation coefficient is to 1.0 (either +1.00 or -1.00), the stronger the relationship between the student's demonstrated learning and the interpreter's demonstrated skill level. Statistical analysis would also offer the probability of the correlation coefficient being significant; significant findings are considered more generalizable than nonsignificant findings.

What we *cannot* determine from relationship studies is a cause–effect rela-tionship between the variables investigated. We could never conclude that a strong positive relationship between an educational interpreter's skill level and a student's performance level is causal, or that a highly skilled interpreter *causes* high performance in student learning. Too many other variables, as indicated in the popularity of the *a, b,* and *d* choices of Research Question 2, impact learning.

> *Research Question 3:* Does a student benefit more from having a variety of inter-preters or the same interpreter across the years?
> > a. in the primary grades?
> > b. in middle school?
> > c. in the elementary grades?
> > d. in high school?

Responses to this question yielded a pattern of opinions or a trend. Fifty-six percent (56%) of the interpreters reported that they favored the use of the same interpreter during the primary years, 32% favored a variety of interpreters, and 12% were unsure. The percentage favoring a variety of interpreters increased from 56% at the primary level to 61% at the elementary levels, and continued to increase at the middle-school level (90%), and reached its highest level at the sec-ondary stage—93% of the interpreters reported that high school students should have a variety of interpreters; the other 7% were unsure.

Analyzing data to determine patterns or trends is important to research. Pri-marily, analysis of trends enables long-term comparisons of what happened in the past and what is happening in the present in order to predict what is likely to happen

---

[5]Researchers who involve human subjects (students and/or interpreters) in their investigations must go through a review process that ensures protection of the subjects' confidentiality and other rights. Signatures on informed-consent forms are often required as evidence that the subject has knowingly participated.

in the future. A return to the published research from 1986 to 2002 shows a strong interest in describing the state of educational interpreting. The question of "same" or "varied" interpreters over the school years also represents trend analysis. Not only do we see a trend in attitudes favoring a variety of interpreters as students mature, but we can also use this data to establish a point of reference from which the same question can be asked in two years, in five years, in the next decade, and onward. If we find that the trend is stable over the years, then administrators and interpreter trainers can safely predict that a greater pool of "different" interpreters will be needed in secondary programs than in elementary- and middle-school programs, and that a stable pool of "same" interpreters will be needed for primary-aged students.

This predictive knowledge should impact scheduling and hiring of interpreters. If we find a change in the trend's direction, then administrators, interpreter trainers, and educators must prepare for the change. Many interpreter training programs have benefited from federal and state funding that has been made available because of trend analysis. As more and more students who are deaf and hard of hearing have been educated in local schools, more and more interpreters have been needed. Federal and state support, particularly grant funding, is a product of trend analysis.

Analyzing longitudinal data for trends leads to the topic of replication. *Replication* is highly valued in behavioral and social sciences research. Replication studies involve asking the same research questions that were investigated earlier with the same research design and the same analysis procedures. Direct replication involves exact replication, involving subjects who are just like those used earlier; systematic replication involves varying some aspect of the research, such as using elementary students instead of high school students. Individuals who are interested in research on educational interpreting should be encouraged to pursue replication studies, as well as original research. A replicated study that reveals results similar to those of an earlier study can add to the reliability and generalizability of the earlier study's results. A replicated study that reveals different results can add to our knowledge of change in trends.

Research Question 4: What attributes (personal or professional) do you think are most critical for interpreters?
   a. at the primary level?
   b. at the elementary level?
   c. at the middle school level?
   d. at the high school level?

This final survey question deviates from focusing on the student consumer, but the student is at the heart of most answers provided by the interpreters. Responses to the question were analyzed for frequency of occurrence and similarity across the categories. Only those attributes listed at least twice by different interpreters are included here (see Table 7.2).

Discussion of this question and its answers is directed to interpreters on a personal level. If we accept that one of our responsibilities as professionals is to

TABLE 7.2 Attributes Critical to Educational Interpreters

At All Levels	Frequency of Response
Flexibility	6
Patience	6
Knowledge of/skill in languages	3
Knowledge of language development	3
Knowledge of deafness	2
Knowledge of psychological development	2
Understanding the interpreter's role	2
Ability to work cooperatively with staff	2
Sense of humor	2

At the Primary Level	Frequency of Response	At the Elementary Level	Frequency of Response
Flexibility	10	Flexibility	9
Patience	8	Patience	7
Caring/kindness/compassion	4	Sense of humor	4
Well-developed skills	3	Background in education	3
Background in early childhood	3	Background in development	2
Knowledge of language development	3	Comfortable with children	2
Background in psychology	2	Highly skilled	2
Ability to sign at child's level	2	Knows when to pull away	2
Proficiency in the language	2		

At the Middle School Level	Frequency of Response	At the High School Level	Frequency of Response
Patience	4	Knowledge of the subjects	6
Flexibility	3	Extensive vocabulary	3
Knows when to pull away	3	Self-disciplined (will study)	3
Good interaction skills	2	Professional demeanor	2
Quick thinking	2		
Good vocabulary	2		

apply research findings, then each of us can meet that responsibility by asking ourselves if we possess this list of attributes or competencies. We may create our own list of attributes independently and compare it to those listed here. This kind of research, because it involves self-inspection or self-supervision (as discussed in Chapter 2), results in interpersonal findings that should lead to our own experimentation and trend analysis over the years.

A final question of related research interest to many interpreters, interpreter educators, and employers involves psychological characteristics of interpreters. In a recent investigation of cognitive, fine-motor, personality, and attention skills, I analyzed test scores of 28 interpreters (in press).[6] Fourteen of these 28 worked full-time in K–12 programs; the other 14 were community interpreters, although 10 of them also interpreted part-time in postsecondary programs. The 28 interpreters were further divided into three groups: Group 1 interpreters ($N = 8$) held level II screenings from the Virginia Quality Assurance Screening test; group 2 ($N = 9$) held level III VQAS scores; and group 3 ($N = 11$) held RID certification.

The interpreters participated in a battery of six tests. Results of two tests are reported here. The Wonderlic Personnel Test (Wonderlic, 1998) is a test of general cognitive ability—the ability to learn, understand instructions, and solve problems. Fifteen interpreters scored at or above the 90th percentile and nine of those scored above the 95th percentile. Only two interpreters scored below the 50th percentile. Group 3 interpreters scored higher than group 2, who scored higher than group 1, but their differences were not statistically significant.

The 28 interpreters also completed the Sixteen Personality Factor Questionnaire (16PF) (Cattell, Cattell, & Cattell, 1994), a test that measures 16 personality traits across four domains: cognitive, affective, preferential, and behavioral. The participating interpreters had many extreme traits or attributes that fell outside the average range. They averaged 6.8 extreme traits (range from 3 to 12).

Extremely high scores in *abstract reasoning* stood out as the most remarkable cognitive trait on the 16PF. Eighteen interpreters (four in Group 1, five in Group 2, and nine in Group 3) scored extremely high on questions that tapped abstract reasoning. An even split was found between the educational and community interpreters, with nine in each group. Other extreme attributes tended to have relatively symmetrical distributions. For example, five interpreters scored extremely high on *warmth*, five scored extremely low, and all others scored in the average range. Four scored extremely high on *self-control,* and four scored extremely low. Two scored high in *privateness,* and three scored low. Three scored extremely high in *self-reliance,* and three scored low. Four scored high on *sensitivity,* while three scored low. Four scored extremely high on *social boldness,* and six scored extremely low. Six scored high on *apprehension,* while eight scored low. Five interpreters scored extremely high on *extraversion* and four scored extremely low.

---

[6]This research was sponsored by the Virginia Department of Education. Preliminary results were presented at the 2002 National Educational Interpreting Conference.

At least three findings are suggested from these data. First, the interpreters who participated collectively tested well above average on cognitive measures. If we plotted their percentile rankings on Figure 7.1, 26 of the 28 interpreters would be above the 50th percentile, or midline point, and 15 would be above the 90th percentile point. Intelligence is a factor in the second finding, too; 18 of the 28 scored extremely high in abstract reasoning, and no one scored low. Third, the personality traits of these 28 interpreters tended to be extreme, but their extremes were fairly widespread or evenly distributed. Variability in personal traits tends to dismiss the notion of a singular personality type. Instead, these interpreters appeared very diverse or heterogenous in their distinguishing affective, behavioral, and preferential traits. This heterogeneity seems particularly fitting, especially after reflecting on the broad variability of student consumers described throughout the chapters of this book.

Caution must be advised in generalizing these cognitive and personality results for many reasons. One involves the small number of participants. Another involves the volunteer participation. The fact that most of these interpreters performed at or above the 90th percentile on tests of cognition suggests that interpreters are exceptionally bright. Their volunteer participation, though, colors the potential that another group who doubted their superior cognitive performances may not have come forward to participate in the tests. At the same time, these results may have important implications for our training programs, for interpreting assignments in schools, and for future research on our consumer, teaming, and mentoring relationships.

Summary

Educational interpreting as a new discipline offers us many exciting opportunities for research. We should approach the previously published research presented here, as well as new research, with a spirit of learning and a desire to apply what we learn to our own practices. We should also approach our practices with an attitude of questioning that spawns new and replicated research. And, finally, where personal growth is the desired outcome of research, we should hold our questions and those of our colleagues who pursue research to the highest ethical and scientific standards.

REFERENCES

Afzali-Nomani, E. (1995). Educational conditions related to successful full inclusion programs involving deaf/hard of hearing children. *American Annals of the Deaf, 140,* 396–401.

Antia, S. D., & Kreimeyer, K. H. (2001). The role of interpreters in inclusive classrooms. *American Annals of the Deaf, 146,* 355–365.

Beaver, D. L., Hayes, P. L., & Luetke-Stahlman, B. (1995). In-service trends: General education teachers working with educational interpreters. *American Annals of the Deaf, 140,* 38–46.

Bond, M. M. (1995, May). Have you ever seen a voice talking? . . . Well, I have! Paper presented at the annual international conference of the National Institute for Staff and Organization Development on Teaching Excellence and Conference of Administrators, Austin, TX.

Burch, D. D. (1999). Essential competencies, responsibilities, and education of sign language interpreters in pre-college educational settings. (Doctoral dissertation, Southern University and Agricultural and Mechanical College, 1999). *Dissertation Abstracts International, 62,* 10A.

Cattell, R. B., Cattell, A. K. S., & Cattell, H. E. P. (1994). *The Sixteen Personality Factor Questionnaire (16PF), Fifth Edition.* Champaign, IL: Institute for Personality and Ability Testing.

Cawthon, S. W. (2001). Teaching strategies in inclusive classrooms with deaf students. *Journal of Deaf Studies and Deaf Education, 6,* 212–225.

Cohen, H., & Jones, E. G. (1990). Interpreting for cross-cultural research: Changing written English to American Sign Language. *Journal of the American Deafness and Rehabilitation Association, 24,* 41–48.

Cokely, D. (1986). The effects of lag time on interpreter errors. *Sign Language Studies, 53,* 341–375.

———. (1990). The effectiveness of three means of communication in the college classroom. *Sign Language Studies, 69,* 415–442.

Commission on Education of the Deaf. (1998). *Toward equality: Education of the deaf, a report to the President and the Congress of the United States.* Washington, DC: U.S. Government Printing Office.

Dahl, C., & Wilcox, S. (1990). Preparing the educational interpreter: A survey of sign language interpreter training programs. *American Annals of the Deaf, 135,* 275–279.

Elliott, R. N., & Powers, A. R. (1995). Preparing interpreters to serve in educational settings. *A.C.E.H.I. Journal, 21,* 132–140.

Ford, J., & Fredericks, B. (1995). Using interpreter-tutors in school programs for students who are deaf-blind. *Journal of Visual Impairment and Blindness, 89,* 229–234.

Gallaudet University Laurent Clerc National Deaf Education Center. (2001). Interpreting theory and practice: Reaching out to teach deaf children. *Odyssey, 2,* 2.

Hayes, L. (1992). Educational interpreters for deaf students: Their responsibilities, problems, and concerns. *Journal of Interpretation, 5,* 5–24.

Hedge, M. N. (1987). *Clinical research in communicative disorders: Principles and strategies.* Boston: College-Hill Press.

Hill, P. A. (2000). Studies of the impact of sign modality. (Doctoral dissertation, University of Alberta, 2000). *Dissertation Abstracts International, 62,* 05A.

Hurwitz, A. T. (1986). Two factors related to effective voice interpreting. *American Annals of the Deaf, 131,* 248–252.

Isham, W., & Lane, H. (1994). A common conceptual code in bilinguals: Evidence from simultaneous interpretation. *Sign Language Studies, 85,* 291–317.

Johnson, K. (1991). Miscommunication in interpreted classroom interaction. *Sign Language Studies, 70,* 1–34.

Jones, B. E., Clark, G. M., & Soltz, D. F. (1997). Characteristics and practices of sign language interpreters in inclusive education programs. *Exceptional Children, 63,* 257–268.

Jones, R. L. (1986). Can Deaf students succeed in a public university? *A.C.E.H.I. Journal, 12,* 43–49.

Kavin, D. S. (2001). Two-year postsecondary educational institutions in the midwest serving persons who are deaf/hard of hearing: Technical assistance needs and programmatic changes related to services provided by the Midwest Center for Postsecondary Outreach (1997–2000) (Doctoral dissertation, Northern Illinois University, 2001). *Dissertation Abstracts International, 62,* 08A.

Khan, F. J. (1991). Transitional services for hearing impaired young adults using continuing education division of a community college. *Journal of the American Deafness and Rehabilitation Association, 25,* 16–27.

Kluwin, T. N. (1993). Cumulative effects of mainstreaming on the achievement of deaf adolescents. *Exceptional Children, 60,* 73–81.

Kluwin, T. N. (1994). Interpreting services for youngsters who are deaf in local public school programs. *Journal of the American Deafness and Rehabilitation Association, 28,* 21–29.

Kluwin, T. N., & Stewart, D. A. (2001). Interpreting in schools: A look at research. *Odyssey, 2,* 15–17.

La Bue, M. A. (1998). Interpreted education: A study of deaf students' access to the content and form of literacy instruction in a mainstreamed high school English class. (Doctoral dissertation, Harvard University, 1998). *Dissertation Abstracts International, 59,* 04A.

Lawrence, R. W. (1987). Specialized preparation in educational interpreting. *Jouranl of Interpretation, 4,* 87–90.

Linehan, P. (2000). *Educational interpreters for students who are deaf and hard of hearing. Project Forum at NASDE.* U.S. Office of Special Education Programs.

Livingston, S. (1991). Comprehension strategies of two deaf readers. *Sign Language Studies, 71,* 115–130.

Locker, R. (1990). Lexical equivalence in transliterating for deaf students in the university classroom: Two perspectives. *Issues in Applied Linguistics, 1,* 167–195.

Luetke-Stahlman, B. (1992). Sign interpretation in preschool. *Perspectives in Education and Deafness, 10,* 12–15.

Mallory B. L., & Schein, J. D. (1992). Mediated communication for deaf postsecondary students in the United States. *Journal of the American Deafness and Rehabilitation Association, 25,* 28–31.

Manning, K. (1994). Expectations and surprises in learning to teach a member of the Deaf Culture. *Journal on Excellence in College Teaching, 5,* 77–88.

Marschark, M., Sapere, P., Convertino, C., Seewagen, R., & Maltzen, H. (In Press). Comprehension of sign language interpreting: Deciphering a complex task situation. *Sign Language Studies.*

Martin, D. S., & Lytle, R. R. (2000). Deaf teacher candidates in hearing classrooms: A unique teacher preparation program. *American Annals of the Deaf, 145,* 15–21.

Mertens, D. M. (1990). Teachers working with interpreters: The deaf student's educational experience. *American Annals of the Deaf, 136,* 48–52.

———. (1991). Implications from the cognitive paradigm for teacher effectiveness research in deaf education. In D. S. Martin (Ed.), *Advances in cognition, education, and deafness* (pp. 342–347). Washington, DC: Gallaudet University Press.

Moores, D. F. (1990). Research in educational aspects of deafness. In D. F. Moores & K. P. Meadow-Orlans (Eds.), *Educational and developmental aspects of deafness* (pp. 11–24). Washington, DC: Gallaudet University Press.

Napier, J. (2002). University interpreting: Linguistic issues for consideration. *Journal of Deaf Studies and Deaf Education, 7,* 281–301.

Nover, S. M. (1995). Full inclusion for deaf students: An ethnographic perspective. In B. Snider (Ed.), *Inclusion? Defining quality education for Deaf and Hard of Hearing students* (pp. 33–50). Washington, DC: Gallaudet University Press.

Petronio, K. (1988). Interpreting for deaf-blind students: Factors to consider. *American Annals of the Deaf, 133,* 226–229.

Pollio, H. R. (1984). *What students think about and do during college lectures: Teaching–learning issues.* Knoxville, TN: Learning Research Center Reports.

Pollio, H. R., & Pollio, M. R. (1991). Some observations from a different point of view. In D. S. Martin (Ed.), *Advances in cognition, education, and deafness* (pp. 429–442). Washington, DC: Gallaudet University Press.

Powers, A. R. (1997). The preparation of educational interpreters for rural education settings. *Rural Special Education Quarterly, 16,* 24–32.

Ramsey, C. L. (1997). *Deaf children in public schools: Placement, context, and consequences.* Washington, DC: Gallaudet University Press.

Registry of Interpreters for the Deaf, Inc. (2000). *Educational interpreting: A collection of articles from Views: 1996–2000.* Silver Spring, MD: RID Publications.

Rittenhouse, R., Rahn, C., & Morreau, L. (1989). Educational interpreter services for hearing-impaired students: Provider and consumer disagreements. *Journal of the American Deafness and Rehabilitation Association, 22,* 57–63.

Roy, C. B. (1993). A sociolinguistic analysis of the interpreter's role in simultaneous talk in interpreted interaction. *Multilingua, 12,* 341–363.

———. (2000). *Interpreting as a discourse process.* New York: Oxford University Press.

Rudser, S. F. (1986). Linguistic analysis of changes in interpreting: 1973–1985. *Sign Language Studies, 53,* 332–340.

Rudser, S. F., & Strong, M. (1986). An examination of some personal characteristics and abilities of sign language interpreters. *Sign Language Studies, 53,* 315–331.

Salend, S. J., & Longo, M. (1994). The roles of the educational interpreter in mainstreaming. *Teaching Exceptional Children, 26,* 22–28.

Sanderson, G., Siple, L., & Lyons, B. (1999). *Interpreting for postsecondary deaf students.* A report of the national task force on quality of services in the postsecondary education of deaf and hard of hearing students. Rochester, NY: Northeast Technical Assistance Center, Rochester Institute of Technology.

Schick, B., Williams, K., & Bolster, L. (1999). Skill levels of educational interpreters working in public schools. *Journal of Deaf Studies and Deaf Education, 4,* 144–155.

Seal, B. C. (1996). Educational interpreters on child development. *RID Views, 13,* 14.

———. (1999). Educational interpreters document efforts to improve. *RID Views, 16,* 30–33.

———. (2000). Working with educational interpreters. *Language, Speech, and Hearing Services in Schools, 31,* 15–25.

———. (in press). Psychological testing of sign language interpreters. *Journal of Deaf Studies and Deaf Education.*

Seal, B. C., Wynne, D., & MacDonald, G. (2002). Deaf students, teachers, and interpreters in the chemistry lab. *Journal of Chemical Education, 79,* 239–243.

Shaw, R. (1987). Determining register in sign-to-English interpreting. *Sign Language Studies, 57,* 295–322.

Shaw, J., & Jamieson, J. (1997). Patterns of classroom discourse in an integrated, interpreted elementary school setting. *American Annals of the Deaf, 142,* 40–47.

Shroyer, E. H., & Compton, M. V. (1994). Educational interpreting and teacher preparation: An interdisciplinary model. *American Annals of the Deaf, 139,* 472–479.

Siple, L. A. (1993a). Working with the sign language interpreter in your classroom. *College Teaching, 41,* 139–142.

———. (1993b). The use of pausing by sign language interpreters. *Sign Language Studies, 79,* 147–179.

Siple, L. A. (1998). The use of addition in sign language transliteration. In A. Weisel (Ed.), *Issues unresolved: New perspectives on language and deaf education* (pp. 65–75). Washington, DC: Gallaudet University Press.

Smith, S. B., & Rittenhouse, R. K. (1990). Real-time graphic display: Technology for mainstreaming. *Perspectives in Education and Deafness, 9,* 2–5.

Smith, S. M., Kress, T. A., & Hart, W. M. (2000). Hand/wrist disorders among sign language communicators. *American Annals of the Deaf, 145,* 22–25.

Sofinski, B. A., Yesbeck, N. A., Gerhold, S. C., & Bach-Hansen, M. C. (2001). Features of voice-to-sign transliteration by educational interpreters. *Journal of Interpretation: Millennial Edition,* 47–68.

Stedt, J. D. (1989). Carpal tunnel syndrome: The risk to educational interpreters. *American Annals of the Deaf, 134,* 223–226.

Stewart, D. A., & Kluwin, T. N. (1996). The gap between guidelines, practice, and knowledge in interpreting services for deaf students. *Journal of Deaf Studies and Deaf Education, 1,* 29–39.

Stuckless, E. R., Avery, J. C., & Hurwitz, T. A. (Eds.) (1989). *Educational interpreting for deaf students: A report on the national task force on educational interpreting.* Rochester, NY: NTID/RIT.

Taylor, C., & Elliott, R. N. (1994). Identifying areas of competence needed by educational inter-preters. *Sign Language Studies, 83,* 179–190.

Wilcox, P., Schroeder, F., & Martinez, T. (1990). A commitment to professionalism: Educational interpreting standards within a large public school system. *Sign Language Studies, 68,* 277–286.

Winston, E. (1992). Mainstream interpreting: An analysis of the task. In L. Swabey (Ed.), *The challenge of the 90s: New standards in interpreter education* (pp. 51–67). Proceedings of the Eighth National Convention of the Conference of Interpreter Trainers. Pomona, CA.

Wonderlic, E. F. (1937–1998). *The Wonderlic Personnel Test.* Northfield, IL: Wonderlic and Associates.

Yarger, C. C. (2001). Educational interpreting: Understanding the rural experience. *American Annals of the Deaf, 146,* 16–30.

Zawolkow, E., & DeFiore, S. (1986). Educational interpreting for elementary- and secondary-level hearing-impaired students. *American Annals of the Deaf, 131,* 26–28.

APPENDIX

RID Standard Practice Paper

Standard Practice Papers are available in brochure format through the National Office. RID encourages use of these brochures for public distribution and advocacy.

Interpreting In Educational Settings (K–12)

Following the passage of a number of laws concerning the education of deaf children, educational interpreting has become more common in elementary and secondary schools. This is a growing profession and can be one way of making school programs and services more accessible to children who are deaf. As a member of the educational team, the interpreter should be an educated and qualified professional.

What is the role of the educational interpreter?

The fundamental role of an interpreter, regardless of specialty or place of employment, is to facilitate communication between persons who are deaf and hard of hearing and others. Educational interpreters facilitate communication between deaf students and others, including teachers, service providers, and peers within the educational environment. Many educational environments have a communication policy which should be clearly defined to the interpreter applicant. The educational team may be composed of school personnel and parents and may be more structured in some school districts than others. The educational interpreter is a member of the educational team and should be afforded every opportunity to attend meetings where educational guidelines are discussed concerning students who are provided services by that interpreter.

What responsibilities are appropriate for an educational interpreter?

Interpreting is the primary responsibility of the interpreter. The interpreter may perform this responsibility in a variety of settings, in and outside of the classroom including:

- instructional activities
- field trips
- club meetings
- assemblies
- counseling sessions
- athletic competitions

Interpreting is the educational interpreter's primary role, and must take priority over any other demands. In some schools, interpreters may also interpret for deaf parents, deaf teachers, and other deaf employees.

- Interpreters may have additional responsibilities when not interpreting.[1] In determining appropriate responsibilities, it is important to utilize specialized competencies and skills of the interpreter and assign only those responsibilities for which the interpreter is qualified.

Responsibilities that maximize the interpreter's effectiveness during non-interpreting periods of time might include:

- planning and preparing for the interpreting task
- presenting in-service training about educational interpreting
- working with teachers to develop ways of increasing interaction between deaf students and their peers
- if qualified, tutoring the student who is deaf or hard of hearing
- if qualified, teaching sign language to other school staff and to pupils who are not deaf

Responsibilities that tend to reduce the interpreter's effectiveness may include:

- copying and filing
- playground supervision
- bus attendant duty
- lunchroom duty
- monitoring study hall

The educational interpreter's responsibilities and the relative proportion of time between interpreting and non-interpreting responsibilities are likely to vary from one work setting to another and may be influenced by a number of factors which may include:

- number of students who are deaf or hard of hearing in the school or district and distribution across grade levels and school buildings
- possibility of physical injury due to stress or overuse[2]
- nature of the employment; full-time, part-time, or hourly
- interpreter's background, knowledge, skill, and competencies
- qualifications and availability of the interpreting staff

[1]see Multiple Roles
[2]see Cumulative Motion Injury

How can confusion about the interpreter's responsibilities be avoided?

The role and responsibility of the interpreter is distinct from that of the teacher and that of other professionals in the educational setting. This distinction must be kept clear. For example, for the interpreter to provide classroom instruction and discipline directly to a student would be inappropriate because that is the teacher's responsibility.

A clear and detailed job description, prepared in advance of hiring and shared with the interpreter applicant and with others who need to understand the interpreter's duties, will help avoid confusion and misunderstanding.

Who should supervise the educational interpreter?

A member of the educational administration staff who has an understanding of interpreting should supervise the interpreter. In most cases, hiring an agency outside the educational institution or using a teacher in whose class the educational interpreter works would not be appropriate. The interpreter's supervisor may have interpreting skills, which is valuable, but the supervisor should at least know what interpreting is, how the interpreter functions best as a member of the educational team, and when interpreting is or is not the most appropriate service. If the supervisor is not qualified to evaluate interpreting skills or performance, an outside consultant knowledgeable in interpreter assessment and skill development should be hired.

What qualifications should the educational interpreter have?

Interpreting is a highly specialized professional field; simply knowing sign language does not qualify a person as an interpreter. Professional sign language interpreters develop their specialization through extensive training and practice over a long period of time. In addition, skills in oral transliteration may be needed. Throughout their careers, interpreters improve their skills, knowledge, and professionalism through continued training and through participation in RID. The use of a comprehensive written professional development plan will guide the educational interpreter to meet professional goals, including that of certification.

In interpreting, as in other professions, appropriate credentials are an important indicator of competence. RID awards certification to interpreters who successfully pass national tests. The tests assess not only language knowledge and communication skills, but also knowledge and judgment on issues of ethics, culture and professionalism which form the essential foundation for quality interpreting. The assessments do not test for additional specialist skills necessary in educational settings. Many interpreters working in educational settings either already have or are working toward certification. An increasing number of states are requiring educational interpreters to have interpreting credentials.

Educational interpreting is a specialty requiring additional knowledge and skills. In the classroom, the instructional content varies significantly, and the skills and knowledge necessary to qualify an interpreter vary accordingly. In the primary grades, the interpreter needs a broad basic knowledge of the subject areas such as mathematics, social studies, and language arts, and should have an understanding of child development. At the secondary level, the interpreter needs sufficient knowledge and understanding of the content areas to be able to interpret highly technical concepts and terminology accurately and meaningfully.

How is reasonable compensation determined for the educational interpreter?

Pay levels and employee benefits for educational interpreters should be competitive with that of other professional school employees. They should be based on interpreting skills, education, experience, certification, performance, and job responsibilities. Creation of positions with appropriate pay and benefits is a key to attracting and keeping qualified professional interpreters.

How does the RID Code of Ethics apply to educational interpreters?

The RID Code of Ethics is the statement of ethical principles for all interpreters, including those who work in educational settings. Within the boundaries of the educational team, the Code of Ethics deals fairly with the major issue of confidentiality.

Where can I learn more about educational interpreting?

The National Task Force on Educational Interpreting published a report entitled "Educational Interpreting for Deaf Students" which can be obtained from Rochester Institute of Technology, National Technical Institute for the Deaf.

The Association believes that educational interpreting is one way of making school programs and services more accessible to children who are deaf. The educational interpreter should be an RID certified, highly trained and qualified professional who can function as a member of the educational team.

RID has a series of Standard Practice Papers available upon request. Footnotes frequently reference these materials.

Code of Ethics of The Registry of Interpreters for the Deaf, Inc.

Introduction

The Registry of Interpreters for the Deaf, Inc. [RID, Inc.] refers to individuals who may perform one or more of the following services:

- Interpret spoken English to American Sign Language and American Sign Language to spoken English;
- Transliterate spoken English to manually coded English/pidgin signed English, manually coded English/pidgin signed English to spoken English, and spoken English to paraphrased nonaudible spoken English;
- Gesticulate/mime to and from spoken English.

The Registry of Interpreters for the Deaf, Inc., has set forth the following principles of ethical behavior to protect and guide interpreters and transliterators and hearing and deaf consumers. Underlying these principles is the desire to ensure for all the right to communicate.

This Code of Ethics applies to all members of The Registry of Interpreters for the Deaf, Inc., and to all certified nonmembers:

1. Interpreters/transliterators shall keep all assignment-related information strictly confidential.
2. Interpreters/transliterators shall render the message faithfully, always conveying the content and spirit of the speaker using language most readily understood by the person(s) whom they serve.
3. Interpreters/transliterators shall not counsel, advise, or interject personal opinions.
4. Interpreters/transliterators shall accept assignments using discretion with regard to skill, setting, and the consumers involved.
5. Interpreters/transliterators shall request compensation for services in a professional and judicious manner.
6. Interpreters/transliterators shall function in a manner appropriate to the situation.
7. Interpreters/transliterators shall strive to further knowledge and skills through participation in workshops, professional meetings, interaction with professional colleagues, and reading of current literature in the field.
8. Interpreters/ transliterators, by virtue of membership or certification by the RID, Inc., shall strive to maintain high professional standards in compliance with the Code of Ethics.

Reprinted from Membership Directory 1995 with permission from The Registry of Interpreters for the Deaf, Inc.

The RID Certification Maintenance Program

The Certification Maintenance Program is the vehicle through which the continued skill development of certified interpreters is monitored. Certification maintenance provides an avenue through which practitioners maintain their skill level and stay abreast of the developments in the field, and assures consumers that a certified interpreter means quality interpreting services. Many professions utilize continuing education as a way to maintain standards of their certified practitioners. Nurses, CPAs, and lawyers are just a few examples of professions that require continuing education to maintain certification. The RID Certification Maintenance Program began operation on July 1, 1994 with almost 2,500 participants. The system relies on RID Approved Sponsors to provide appropriate educational activities for the participants. These activities can be either group activities (such as workshops, lectures, or conferences) or independent study activities (such as mentoring or self-study). Sponsors must go through an application process whereby the Professional Development Committee (PDC) reviews their qualifications to provide appropriate activities. Those applicants [who] meet the standards developed by the PDC are approved as sponsors. Sponsors are monitored on a regular basis to ensure their activities maintain high quality.

RID uses a common method of administering a continuing education program by requiring participants to earn a specific number of continuing education units, or CEUs, in a specific time frame. The CEU is a nationally recognized unit of measurement for activities that meet established criteria for increasing knowledge and competency. One CEU is defined as 10 contact hours of participation in an organized continuing education experience under responsible sponsorship, capable direction, and qualified instruction. As part of RID's Certification Maintenance Program, certified interpreters are required to earn nine CEUs in a three-year cycle.

Participants are encouraged to acquire CEUs in a variety of content areas so that their particular educational needs can be met. Creativity is allowed and even encouraged when designing a plan for completion of the CEU requirement. It is recognized that a wide variety of experiences benefit one's interpreting skills, and this fact is incorporated into RID's Certification Maintenance Program.

Reprinted from the Membership Directory 1995 with permission from The Registry of Interpreters for the Deaf, Inc.

Cued Speech Transliterator Assessments

**Earl Fleetwood, M.A., and
Melanie Metzger, Ph.D.**

Guidelines have been derived and set forth to regulate and give direction to the profession of Cued Speech transliteration as well as to furnish a foundation on which job expectations are formulated and quality services are cultivated. This foundation serves as a national standard, defining the bounds of judgment and practice that distinguish Cued Speech transliteration from other professions. If the evaluation, licensing, and certification of Cued Speech transliterators is to be of value, the knowledge and skills of practitioners must be scrutinized in deference to this standard. Currently, two evaluation tools are recognized as serving this purpose: The Cued Speech Transliterator State Level Assessment (CSTSLA) and the Cued Speech Transliterator National Certification Examination (CSTNCE).

Cued Speech Transliterator State Level Assessment

The CSTSLA Written Assessment is a 50-question, multiple-choice medium through which an individual's knowledge of information fundamental to the role and responsibilities of a Cued Speech transliterator can be measured and documented. Included are questions pertaining to the Cued Speech Transliterator Code of Conduct, the Code of Ethics of the Registry of Interpreters for the Deaf, various populations of deaf people, Cued Speech research, and interpreting/transliterating terminology.

The CSTSLA Performance Assessment is designed to serve as a medium through which the quality of an individual's Cued Speech transliterating skills can be measured and documented. Five (5) expressive tasks are presented: two-part dialogue/performance, first-grade story w/AES, freelance paraphrasing, and foreign language in educational setting. Two (2) receptive tasks are presented for voicing. The voicing tasks utilize one individual whose cueing intelligibility is good and one whose cueing intelligibility is moderate. Each receptive and expressive task is approximately two minutes. Written and spoken directions are given before each task. Total performance assessment time is approximately 20 minutes. A warm-up videotape parallels the tasks presented in the Performance Assessment and provides practice for voicing the deaf individuals who appear on the actual assessment.

Scoring of the CSTSLA Performance Assessment is performed by a panel of three (3) trained raters. Each panel contains at least one (1) deaf and one (1)

hearing rater. Raters compare the performance standard for Cued Speech transliteration with the actual performance modeled by the individual being assessed.
Various aspects of individual performance are rated on a scale of 0 to 10, with
10 being a perfect score. Scores are computed separately for expressive and receptive tasks.

The CSTSLA package consists of one (1) written assessment, one (1) warm-
up performance videotape, and one (1) performance videotape. A second version
of the performance assessment videotape can be purchased with the aforementioned package. The CSTSLA package may be purchased by state agencies who are
responsible for the evaluation of interpreters and transliterators in keeping with
state mandates. The state agency determines levels of compliance with the mandates and awards transliterator performances accordingly.

Cued Speech Transliterator National Certification Examination

The Cued Speech Transliterator National Certification Examination (CSTNCE) is a
six-part test of job-related knowledge and skill and is administered through Training, Evaluation, & Certification Unit (TECUnit). The CSTNCE is described as
follows:

The Basic Cued Speech Proficiency Rating   [BCSPR] provides a framework for assessing and categorizing expressive cueing proficiency and formulating
diagnostic feedback. As part of the CSTNCE, the BCSPR is recorded on videotape
for subsequent analysis, scoring, and determination of recommendations.

The Syllables-Per-Minute Assessment   provides a framework for analyzing and assessing expressive cueing fluency during the process of transliteration.
The certification candidate's ability to maintain modeled cueing proficiency (as
determined by the BCSPR profile) is analyzed for transliterating tasks ranging
from two (2) to five (5) syllables per second. This subsection of the CSTNCE is
based on the average conversational speaking rate of three (3) syllables per second
(as determined by Dr. Daniel Ling). The certification candidate is videotaped.

The Cued Speech Reading Test   provides a framework for determining
whether or not an individual can utilize Cued Speech receptively toward the comprehension of spoken messages (without the aid of sound). The individual views a
videotape and records responses on an answer form.

The CSTNCE Written Assessment   is a 150-question multiple-choice test
designed to measure the certification candidate's knowledge of the role and function of a Cued Speech transliterator as specified by the Cued Speech Transliterator
Code of Conduct (1989 Fleetwood & Metzger), the Code of Ethics as established
by The Registry of Interpreters for the Deaf, Inc. (1989 RID, Inc.) as well as other
information related or significant to the various duties of a professional Cued

Speech transliterator. Included are questions pertaining to: deafness in general, language development, audiology, speech (development/production), linguistics, inservicing, Cued Speech research, cue reading, Cued Speech oral coding, cue notation, organizations related to deaf/hard-of-hearing people in particular, interpreting terminology, interpreting ethics, various tactics for facilitating communication, and issues related to sign language and the Deaf community.

The CSTNCE Performance Assessment is designed to allow each certification candidate an opportunity to demonstrate the ability to implement knowledge, conduct, and skills relevant to Cued Speech transliteration. Factors considered include: eye contact, cueing delivery, voicing of deaf/hard-of-hearing consumers, expression, appearance, indication of sound source, and adherence to the Code of Conduct and Code of Ethics. Other evaluated factors include the candidate's ability to paraphrase/summarize and convey dialectical details, dramatic material, and Auditory Environmental Stimuli (AES). The certification candidate is videotaped.

The CSTNCE Commentary requires that the candidate view a videotape of Cued Speech transliterators working in various situations/circumstances and comment on functional considerations related to the role, responsibilities, and/or duties expected of and modeled by these transliterators in deference to the Cued Speech Transliterator Code of Conduct.

Scoring of the CSTNCE Performance Assessment is performed by a panel of three (3) trained raters, at least one (1) of whom is hearing and one (1) of whom is deaf/hard-of-hearing. A videotape of a CSTNCE applicant's performance is utilized as the source of CSTNCE performance information. Raters compare the performance standard for Cued Speech transliteration with the actual performance modeled by the individual being assessed. Raters are directed, via a rating booklet to record the applicant's abilities for 13 specific criteria for each of 11 tasks. Various aspects of individual performance are rated on a scale of 0 to 10, with 10 being a perfect score. Scores are computed separately for expressive and receptive tasks.

The remaining sections of the CSTNCE are rated according to specific subtest scoring criteria, producing both a score and diagnostic feedback for the CSTNCE applicant. TECUnit awards national certification at one of three levels in deference to the degree to which an individual is able to meet knowledge and performance standards. (In keeping with other professions, as the availability of training opportunities and materials expands, certification categories that reflect more limited knowledge and skills will be eliminated.)

Significance

The CSTSLA and the CSTNCE are currently the only measurement tools recognized as testing for the knowledge and performance standards that define the role and function of a Cued Speech transliterator. While the CSTSLA is not as comprehensive as the CSTNCE, it does test for the same standards of knowledge and performance. This is significant in that the nature and scope of transliterator training is provided a backdrop of consistently defined goals. Such consistency allows Cued Speech transliterators to better understand the focus of their efforts and thereby provide deaf/hard-of-hearing consumers the quality services they deserve.

Various states are in the process of formulating or revising regulations that relate to interpreters and transliterators for deaf/hard-of-hearing people. If you would like assistance in ensuring that such regulations include recognition of the CSTSLA and/or CSTNCE, please contact TECUnit at 1616 Parham Road, Silver Spring, MID 20903, (301) 439–5766–V/TTY.

Levels of Certification and Credentials

Each of the six (6) sections of the Cued Speech Transliterator National Certification Examination (1988 Fleetwood & Metzger, Williams-Scott, rev. 1991) is scored and weighted with regard for its impact on effective job performance. This series of weighted scores is used to determine each candidate's level of certification, as appropriate. Currently, there are three levels of certification:

TSC: 2 - Functional	Performs with *adequate* skills and/or knowledge of function. However, breadth of skills and/or knowledge might limit realization of deaf/hard-of-hearing consumer potential. Certification expires in two (2) years.
TSC: 3 - Competent	Performs with *intermediate* skills and knowledge of function. Certification expires in three (3) years.
TSC: 4 - Expert	Performs with *comprehensive* skills and knowledge of function. Certification expires in four (4) years.

Individuals who receive national certification as Cued Speech transliterators are, thereby, awarded a nationally recognized credential. This credential distinguishes them from other working Cued Speech transliterators in that it is not simply a job title or its abbreviation. The credential of a nationally certified Cued Speech transliterator should read like one of the following:

TSC: 2 - Functional
TSC: 3 - Competent
TSC: 4 - Expert

For example, a nationally certified Cued Speech transliterator who has received a level 3 certificate will write his or her name as:

John/Jane Doe, TSC: 3

Note: TSC stands for "Transliteration Skills Certificate"

This indicates the credential he or she has received as a practitioner of Cued Speech Transliteration and will be included among other nationally recognized credentials which may apply, such as CPA and CI/CT. (Eventually, different levels of certification will not be available, at which time no number will be included in the credential.)

For more information regarding the levels of certification and the skills they represent contact TECUnit—1616 Parham Road, Silver Spring, MD 20903, (301) 439-5766–V/TTY; Fax: (301) 593–6571.

The TECUnit Cued Speech Transliterator Code of Conduct

A Cued Speech Transliterator shall:

Facilitate communication between deaf/hard-of-hearing Cued Speech cunsumers and hearing consumers

Cued Speech transliterators serve to remove expressive and receptive communication difficulties/ambiguities between deaf/hard-of-hearing consumers and hearing consumers. Facilitation of communication (spoken), however, should not exclude concurrent consideration for and conveyance of auditory environmental stimuli.

Provide sound-based environmental information to deaf/hard-of-hearing consumers of Cued Speech

Cued Speech transliterators should include appropriate representation of auditory environmental stimuli as it occurs, without the influence of personal judgment as to its value to the deaf/hard-of-hearing consumer. This conveyance of auditory environmental stimuli should serve to facilitate a common mainstream experience. Inclusion of auditory environmental stimuli, however, should not exclude concurrent consideration for and facilitation of spoken communication.

Provide appropriate training to deaf/hard-of-hearing consumers to allow for proper transliterator utilization

Cued Speech transliterators serve in an ongoing training capacity with regard to client-transliterator utilization. The development of transliterator usage skills should always be facilitated with tact, reasonable judgment, and prudent regard for the rights of the deaf/hard-of-hearing client.

Provide hearing consumers with appropriate demonstration/explanation of the transliterator role

It is reasonable to assume that hearing consumers are unfamiliar with or do not understand the aspects of a transliterating situation which are intended to preserve the equal access rights of the deaf/hard-of-hearing consumer. Consequently,

Cued Speech transliterators must secure the confidence and support of said consumers through role demonstration and/or explanation in order to appropriately implement methods used to preserve these equal access rights.

Demonstrate and implement ongoing reverence for the preservation and promotion of complete and equal access

Cued Speech transliterators should always employ the skills and conduct necessary to preserve the equal access rights of the deaf/hard-of-hearing consumer. This includes appropriate remediation of the lack of logistical and/or ethical consideration on the part of others. Equal access rights include unconventional as well as conventional factors available to the mainstream population.

Promote the progression of events as if circumstances do not necessitate transliterator presence

Cued Speech transliterators strive to maintain an atmosphere, environment, and consequent experience unaffected, even incidentally, by their necessary presence and function. Most individuals rarely come in contact with a working transliterator in a mainstream situation. Consequently, the common mainstream experience is not influenced by the presence of a transliterator. Therefore, to allow the deaf/hard-of-hearing consumer equal access to this common experience, transliterators must avoid influencing the atmosphere, environment, and resulting experience of the mainstream.

Adhere to the ethical standards of transliterating for deaf/hard-of-hearing consumers

Deaf/hard-of-hearing consumers must be able to trust through Cued Speech transliterator utilization they are consequently afforded the same conventional and unconventional rights, privileges, and opportunities as individuals who need not utilize such services. Ethical standards* have been adopted and must be practiced by transliterators to secure the trust of consumers and offer them fair and equal access.

*The Code of Ethics of The Registry of Interpreters for the Deaf, Inc., 1989 RID, Inc.

Support the profession of Cued Speech transliteration by striving to improve related skills and knowledge and the application thereof

The deaf/hard-of-hearing consumer is entitled to receive the most effective service available in the field of Cued speech transliteration. Therefore, it is the professional responsibility and ethical obligation of Cued Speech transliterators to adhere to and implement the currently accepted philosophies and techniques in the field.

Oral Transliterating Defined

(www.clarkeschool.org.)

An Oral Trnasliterator repeats to a student who is deaf or hard-of-hearing everything that is said in class discussions, lectures, meetings or assemblies. The Transliterator sits in the front of the room facing the student and repeats in an unaudible whisper everything that is said. In this way, the student is able to receive all of the information from different speakers in different parts of the room by just watching one person.

The Transliterator's job is a challenging one, involving listening and "talking" at the same time. The more structured the speaker's remarks, the easier the Transliterator's job. The less structured the communication process is, the more difficult the Transliterator's job.

Although the Transliterator is involved in the educational process, she is not the student's teacher. If the student is confused and needs help, or wants to ask a question, the student asks the teacher. The Transliterator's sole responsiblity is to pass along to the student anything that is said. The student's success, or lack of it, may not reflect the quality of the Transliterator's work.

After years of experience observing the communication process in regular schools, the staff of The Mainstream Center [at Clarke] believes there should be someone who is knowledgeable about oral transliterating in every school that has a student with hearing loss. This does not mean that we are recommending full time oral transliterating for every student, although this might be needed in some cases. It is merely the recognition that this service is needed on at least an occasional basis. We believe that a trained member of a school staff (e.g., teacher aide, tutor, or library aide) would be ideally suited to provide this service on an occasional basis.

Evaluating Educational Interpreters Using Classroom Performance

Brenda Schick and Kevin Williams

Educational Interpreting in the Schools

In the two decades since the passage of P. L. 94-142, public school programs have increasingly assumed the role of educating Deaf and Hard-of-Hearing children in a regular classroom setting. These students are frequently mainstreamed, with an educational interpreter whose role is to provide a visual representation of the classroom discourse. As of 1984, more than 60% of deaf children have been educated in public school day classes (Moores, 1992). For many of these students, a mainstreamed placement is possible only with the use of an interpreter.

While the need for interpreters in public school settings has increased, the discipline of educational interpreting is still relatively new. Interpreting has traditionally been a service for deaf adults, and most of the standards in training, practice, and evaluation were established with them in mind (Stuckless, Avery, & Hurwitz, 1989). However, adult consumers are very different from children in educational settings, and training programs are only beginning to address the special needs of children as consumers. Many professionals are well aware of this problem (see Gustason, 1985; Moores, Kluwin, & Mertens, 1985; Stedt, 1992) but for the most part, training practices have not accommodated the special preparation needed for educational interpreting (Hurwitz, in press).

There are a few exceptions, such as the training program at the National Technical Institute for the Deaf, which offers a degree in educational interpreting, and the University of Tennessee, which is developing a curriculum for educational interpreters. But in states with rural populations, the situation is far from adequate. For example, Schick and Williams surveyed 30 educational interpreters in the state of Colorado and found that only four had any formal training and none had any specialized training in educational interpreting. Most of the interpreters had developed their skills in isolation, through occasional workshops and friends. For these interpreters, the professional responsible for supervision was unable to judge skill levels in sign communication. While there are individuals who are attempting to develop evaluation systems for educational interpreters, there is no system that evaluates the criteria we felt were critical for educational interpreters, as will be explained in the following section.

Difficulties in Evaluating Educational Interpreters

There are difficulties using traditional evaluation methods to assess educational interpreters (see Table A.1). First, many evaluation or rating systems evaluate the use of American Sign Language (ASL) which is rarely used in its pure form in schools. Other evaluation tools, such as that created by Gustason for SEE II, focus on a pure form of manually coded English (MCE). These finely focused evaluation tools often do not take into account the variety of sign systems that occur in an educational setting and the modifications of pure languages or systems that an individual program may make. For example, a school system may adopt Signed English but decide to not use any of the inflectional markers. Woodward and Allen (1988) found that while nearly 60% of teachers reported that they used some form of MCE, when asked questions about how they signed certain sentences, only 12% of the teachers followed the system they said they used. Observations in school systems support the notion that modifications of pure MCE systems are very common. Current evaluation tools are not flexible enough to consider modifications without penalizing the interpreter. This also means that the interpreter can be evaluated on how closely they follow the goals set forth in the IEP which may specify modifications to be made for an individual child.

Second, most current assessments do not assess what is actually required in the classroom. Rather they focus on the interpreter's ability to sign in ASL. Most educational programs use some form of MCE, such as SEE II or Signed English (Woodward & Allen, 1988). While it is highly desirable for an interpreter to know ASL as well as some form of MCE, it is not valid to assume that MCE skills would be equal to those in ASL. That is, an interpreter's skills in communicating in MCE may not be obvious by evaluating their ASL skills. The fact that current tools evaluate pure ASL or pure MCE presents potential legal problems. For example, if the interpreter is required to interpret in MCE in school, the interpreter has a right to be evaluated on performance using that sign system. Evaluating the interpreter's skills in another sign language or sign system is not a valid reflection of what the interpreter is required to do in the actual classroom.

There are numerous issues surrounding the use of ASL or MCE systems in school systems. The EIPA/CPA is not intended as a political statement. It is an attempt to evaluate interpreters while they are signing what is required by the educational program. However, even when someone is signing MCE, there are principles of good sign communication that should be borrowed from ASL and incorporated into their signs.

Third, current evaluation methods assess adult-to-adult communication, and do not consider whether the interpreter is able to make adjustments that are appropriate for children. Deaf adults sign differently to children just as hearing adults speak differently to children. There is a need for a tool that recognizes the differences in communication register required by classroom interpreters, particularly for younger children. Educational interpreters also must understand children's signing, a difficult task given that children sign differently than adults. Even formally trained interpreters have little to no training in reading child signers. The child's full inclusion in the classroom is as dependent on being understood by hear-

Table A.1   Problems with Existing Methods of Interpreter Evaluation

1. Evaluate pure forms of ASL or sign systems

2. Do not reflect actual job requirements

3. Do not evaluate signing to children

4. Do not evaluate ability to understand children's signing

5. Do not evaluate a broad range of skills

6. Provide minimal feedback about skills

ing peers and teachers, as on understanding the spoken communication in the classroom.

Fourth, some of the tools that have been designed specifically to evaluate MCE focus on vocabulary skills. That is, an interpreter who has a large sign vocabulary can obtain a relatively high rating even if their signing is not good visual communication. Interpreting is more than having a dictionary of signs to match with spoken words, and an evaluation tool should reflect this.

Finally, most tools result in a single numeric description of the interpreter. These types of instruments provide little feedback to the interpreter concerning strengths and weaknesses. Schools also need more complete feedback in order to place interpreters appropriately, to ensure that children are receiving the educational program specified in their IEP, and to provide inservice training. Without specific feedback, interpreters and schools are left with little information to guide training and skill development.

The Educational Interpreter Performance Assessment: EIPA

The purpose of this paper is to describe a tool, the Educational Interpreter Performance Assessment, or EIPA, that is designed to evaluate the skills of educational interpreters in a classroom setting. The EIPA is not limited to any one sign language/system nor is it limited to any one grade level. The EIPA uses a specially trained evaluation team and videotaped samples from the interpreter's classroom environment and with a deaf child in the class. The following section will present the EIPA process in more detail. First, the broad assessment goals of the EIPA (see Table A.2) will be discussed, followed by an overview of the EIPA process.

Reflect Actual Classroom Performance

In order to evaluate the educational interpreter, a sample of their interpreting in the actual classroom and a sample involving an interview with a child or youth

TABLE A.2 Assessment Goals of the EIPA

1. Reflect actual classroom performance

2. Reflect program philosophy

3. Reflect a philosophy of interpreting

4. Evaluate more than one sign language or systems

5. Evaluate signing for young children, not adults

6. Evaluate interpreter's skills across all grade levels

7. Evaluate a broad range of skills, not just vocabulary

8. Evaluate both voice-to-sign and sign-to-voice

9. Provide a skill portfolio for the interpreter

10. Provide feedback to the interpreter and school program

from their classroom are collected. Prior to the sampling, detailed information from the school program is obtained to determine what should be signed (e.g., ASL, Signed English, PSE) and what modifications to the "pure" system can be made by the interpreter. Given this, the interpreter is evaluated on exactly what they are asked to do in the classroom and not some idealized system or language, as described by individuals outside the school program.

Reflect Program Philosophy

School districts often make programmatic decisions concerning the use of a specific sign system or language, either throughout the program or with an individual child. The EIPA is designed to evaluate whether an interpreter's performance is consistent with the goals set on a child's IEP or with the program as a whole. By requiring the supervisor or administrator to specify which sign system or language should be used and what modifications are acceptable, a dialogue is created among the professionals responsible for the educational program for an individual child. Many times the supervisor, administrator, or the multidisciplinary team may not be aware of exactly what the educational interpreter is using in the classroom. The EIPA provides a structured means of collaboration and agreement. This also means that the interpreter knows exactly what they will be expected to use in the classroom.

Reflect a Philosophy of Interpreting

The ability to interpret requires much more than knowing the signs for a large number of English words. The EIPA is designed to evaluate whether an interpreter is actively involved in analyzing the incoming message from a "top-down" perspective. The interpreter should be aware of the speaker's goals and integrate the speaker's use of prosody into their signed or spoken interpretations. Many educational interpreters focus solely on the lexical or word/sign level, often missing the "big picture" presented during the communication. This type of interpreting appears as an unrelated stream of signs or words, and thus is not representative of the actual communication that is occurring.

Evaluate More Than One Sign Language or System

The EIPA is designed to evaluate more than one sign language or system. It was designed to be sufficiently flexible so that school personnel could specify, using a series of questions modeled after Woodward and Allen (1988), what types of modifications are acceptable while interpreting. This information is used by the evaluation team to assess whether changes the interpreter has made in the standard MCE system are consistent with what the school wants. Flexibility is also accomplished by changing the team of evaluators who assess a given interpreter. Evaluation teams are selected to best match the target sign language or system, as explained in more detail later in this paper.

Evaluate Signing for Young Children, Not Adults

A classroom interpreter's performance should be evaluated with the consideration of the age and grade level of the child. What constitutes "good interpreting" differs depending whether the child is in preschool, elementary school, and junior high and high school. Because the EIPA collects a sample of actual classroom performance, evaluators can assess how well the interpreter is able to sign in a register appropriate for the particular age group of children or adolescents. The vocabulary and language used throughout a child's educational program differs as the child changes grades. An interpreter who knows the vocabulary needed to interpret for high school may not know the appropriate vocabulary for an elementary child.

In addition to signing appropriately for young children, the EIPA evaluates how well the educational interpeter can understand the child they work with. This is accomplished by an interview procedure where the deaf child is asked questions by a hearing adult. The child's responses are interpreted for the hearing individual. The receptive sample is composed of this sign-to-voice translation.

Evaluate a Broad Range of Skills, Not Just Vocabulary

The EIPA evaluates a broad range of skills, not just vocabulary knowledge. One of our original motivations to develop this tool was our belief that good signing, which includes all MCE signing, requires a person to borrow heavily from visual language principles found in ASL. This is consistent with the principles laid out for every English sign system. Good English signing involves the use of facial expression, body movement, and the use of space, as does good ASL signing. Although some evaluation tools have considered these features, the weighting given to incorporating ASL features was generally light in comparison with the weighting given vocabulary knowledge. This means that an interpreter who did not use ASL features, but had a large English sign vocabulary, could score relatively high even when their signing was visually unacceptable. We wanted a tool that would reflect what Deaf individuals felt were good sign principles, regardless of the sign system or sign language used. This is accomplished by the inclusion of skills specifically evaluated and by the weighting of skills in the rating form.

Evaluate Both Voice-to-Sign and Sign-to-Voice

The EIPA evaluates both voice-to-sign, or how well a person signs, as well as sign-to-voice, or how well a person understands sign. Many interpreters function reasonably well when they have to sign but have limited comprehension of sign. This means that only half of the classroom needs are met, and the child is at high risk for not have his or her message communicated fully or accurately.

Provide a Skill Portfolio for the Interpreter

Historically, most evaluation tools provide a single summative rating number that attempts to reflect the interpreter's skills in all settings. The EIPA takes a very different approach in that interpreters, over time, collect a portfolio of EIPA evaluations that reflect their performance. An interpreter with a high level of skills will be able to demonstrate high levels of performance regardless of the age or grade level of a child. This notion parallels how other professionals are evaluated in that they do not receive a single numeric rating on job performance, but instead are evaluated on their overall skills over time. For an interpreter who has demonstrated proficiency in a variety of settings, a supervisor has a wide variety of placemetn options. In contrast, an interpreter who has been successful in a narrow range of assignments will have limited placement flexibility. Skill portfolios also allow a school system to adjust pay scales based on performance.

Provide Feedback to the Interpreter and School Program

The EIPA provides feedback to the interpreter and the school program that can help in skill improvement and the placement of interpreters. It is not very informative for interpreters to find out a single number without information regarding their strengths and weaknesses. The evaluation should be a learning process for the interpreter to determine targets for improving their skills. This is especially true since many interpreters have often not discussed principles that contribute to clear signing. It is our experience that interpreters appreciate this type of information because they can actively work on areas of weakness, rather than simply fearing their next evaluation.

In addition, program supervisors and adminsitrators will have information detailing the interpreter's skills that will aid in placing interpreters with specific children. For example, an interpreter who has weak skills in fingerspelling may not be best placed in a high school biology class, which requires fingerspelling of numerous technical terms.

The EIPA Process

The EIPA is most appropriately termed a process because the actual rating or evaluation is only one step in the entire procedure. Figure A.1 shows a flow chart outlining the overall process. In this section we will describe each component of the evaluation.

Collect Program and Classroom Information

First, information is collected about the program, such as what sign system or sign language is used and whether the interpreter can or should modify signs or language for an individual child. This information is collected by means of a checklist that is completed by the supervisor and, hopefully, the classroom interpreter. The questions that elicit that information purposefully ask how grammatical structures and vocabulary should be signed, how idioms should be conveyed, and to what extent inflectional morphemes should be signed. Because many interpreters and professionals are not always aware of how much they deviate from a pure system or language, this information cannot be obtained by simply asking a school program what they use in the classroom (Woodward & Allen, 1988).

Collect the Videotaped Samples

Two samples of interpreting are collected. First, the interpreter is videotaped while interpreting a lesson in the classroom to obtain the expressive sample. Second, the receptive sample is collected during a specially designed interview procedure with a deaf child from the class. For this example, a hearing adult asks the child a series of questions, which elicit extended conversation (provided with the EIPA). The interpreter provides a voice translation of the child which is also videotaped.

The quality of the samples of interpreting is very important. For the expressive portion, the goal is to collect a sample of performance in a situation that is reasonably challenging. In previous evaluations of educational interpreters, we found that some interpreters will choose to videotape themselves during classes that are not representative of the child's day, such as during an art class. We want to see a sample of performance during the child's most challenging classes. It should be collected in a course that contains content material that is not review, preferably a reading, science, or social studies class. The material that will be interpreted should be cognitively challenging, meaning that it should be information

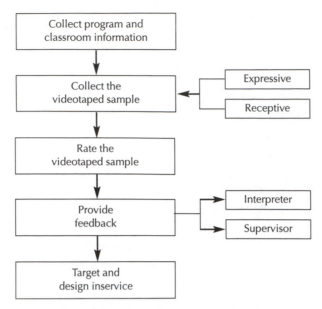

FIGURE A.1   A Flowchart Showing the EIPA Evaluation Process

that may be difficult for the child. We feel that if the interpreter can function well in this type of environment, then it is likely that all other environments will be similar.

In order to assume this, the teacher and supervisor must approve the class that will be videotaped. In doing this, the evaluation team can be certain that the sample they rate represents what the interpreter should be able to do.

Rate the Videotaped Sample

After the sample is collected, evaluators trained in the EIPA process view the videotape and rate the sample. The basic philosophy that the IEPA follows is that individuals who are fluent in a language can evaluate language skill when they are specially trained to do so. Evaluators do not need special academic degrees, rather their own skills and abilities needed to discuss what is involved in skillful interpreting are more important. These evaluators are from the region and are selected for training by an area coordinator who knows both Deaf and hearing individuals in the community.

Once a group of evaluators is trained, teams are constructed on an "as needed" basis. Any given team should be comprised of three trained evaluators, with at least one team member proficient in the specific sign system being evaluated and one team member proficient in ASL. Because Deaf individuals are the best judges of fluent signing, regardless of whether the target is MCE or ASL, they should be an integral part of each evaluation team.

Each team should have a "captain" who acts as a group leader, and a tie-breaker, if one is needed. The captain is the evaluator whose signing skills best match the target sign language/system identified in the program information checklist. Once each evaluator rates the sample, the scores are averaged across all evaluations. This becomes the score the interpreter receives. The team captain also summarizes the evaluation team's feedback for the interpreter.

Provide Feedback

The evaluation team provides the school adminstrator and the interpreter with the completed rating forms. Along with the overall evaluation score, interpreters and supervisors receive evaluation scores for specific areas of performance as detailed on the EIPA evaluation form. Feedback comments are also included on the evaluator's rating forms. The interpreter also receives a copy of the videotape so he or she can review their performance evaluation by watching the tape in addition to reading the evaluation. These items become part of the interpreter's professional portfolio.

Target and Design Inservice

Using the feedback provided, interpreters and program administrators can set goals for skill improvement and design the types of inservice training that will help the interpreter achieve those goals.

Conclusion

The EIPA is an evaluation process that is particularly useful for interpreters working in an educational setting. Because it assesses actual performance, the EIPA is a valid means of evaluating skills, given that school systems vary so widely in the sign language and systems they use, and the degree to which they may have special modifications and signs specific to their own program. In addition, the EIPA is sensitive to the variation of interpreting that occurs across grade levels and with different children. One strength of the EIPA is that it allows a school to address the specific needs of an individual child, which is consistent with the concept of an IEP. The EIPA is intended to be a consumer product in that states and regions train teams of evaluators. It involves Deaf individuals to ensure that the interpreter's product is good visual communication, regardless of whether the goal is MCE, CASE, or ASL. The use of regional teams ensures that interpreters use the signs most common to that particular area. Finally, the EIPA provides feedback in sufficient detail so that interpreters and school programs can target areas for skill growth, and programs can place an interpreter in assignments that best fit the interpreter's constellation of skills.

REFERENCES

Gustason, G. (1985). Interpreters entering public school employment. *American Annals of the Deaf, 130,* 265–266.

Hurwitz, T. A. (In press). Interpreters in the educational setting. In B. Schick & M. P. Moeller (Eds.), *Issues in language and deafness: Sign language in education.* Omaha, NE: Boys Town Press.

Moores, D. (1992). A historical perspective on school placement. In T. N. Kluwin, D. F. Moores, & M. G. Gaustad (Eds.), *Toward effective public school programs for deaf students: Context, process, and outcomes* (pp. 7–29). New York: Teachers College Press.

Moorse, D., Kluwin, T., & Mertens, D. (1985). High school programs for deaf students in metropolitan areas (Monograph No. 3). Washington, DC: Gallaudet College, Gallaudet Research Institute.

Stedt, J. D. (1992). Issues of educational interpreting. In T. N. Kluwin, D. F. Moores, & M. G. Gaustad (Eds.), *Toward effective public school programs for deaf students: Context, process, and outcomes* (pp. 83–99). New York: Teachers College Press.

Stuckless, E. R., Avery, J. C., & Hurwitz, T. A. (Eds.). (1989). *Educational interpreting for deaf students: Report of the National Task Force on Educational Interpreting.* Rochester, NY: National Technical Institute for the Deaf.

Woodward, J., & Allen, T. (1988). Classroom use of artificial sign systems by teachers. *Sign Language Studies, 61,* 405–418.

Reprinted from *RID Views, 11,* 15, 21, 23–24 (1994) with permission from The Registry of Interpreters for the Deaf, Inc.

NIOSH Evaluates Musculoskeletal Disorders

Marie Haring Sweeney, Martin Peterson, and Virginia O'Neill

In May, 1992, the Ohio Chapter of the Registry of Interpreters for the Deaf (OCRID) requested the National Institute for Occupational Safety and Health (NIOSH) to evaluate the problem of musculoskeletal disorders among interpreters for the deaf. In response, NIOSH conducted an investigation among active members who attended a conference held by the national Registry of Interpreters for the Deaf (RID) for Region III in Cleveland, Ohio, in September, 1992. The study was conducted using sign language interpreters who attended the Ohio conference and who volunteered to participate in the study.

The evaluation included a self-administered questionnaire which obtained data on musculoskeletal symptoms of the upper extremity (neck, shoulders, elbows, fingers, hands, and wrists) and low back. If the symptoms occurred in the past year, more information was obtained regarding the symptoms' onset, duration, frequency, and severity. The questionnaire also included information on age and preexisting conditions related to nonoccupational musculoskeletal disorders and traumatic or acute injuries to the area of interest.

Occupational history was also obtained and included amount of time spent per week working as a sign language interpreter, preferred method of signing, and usual location of interpreting jobs. All participants completing the questionnaire were offered a physical examination of their upper extremities. The standard examination consisted of inspection, palpation, passive movements, resisted movements, and a variety of maneuvers to define upper-extremity musculoskeletal conditions. The examining physician was blind to the participants' symptom histories.

Based on the questionnaire and physical examination, two case definitions were created: "symptom" cases based on questionnaire data, and "symptom exam" cases based on physical exam findings. Associations between workplace factors and the two case definitions were assessed by multiple logistic models generated for each area of interest: neck, shoulders, elbows, fingers, hands, and wrists. A total of 106 individuals were included in the analysis of the symptom questionnaire data, and 105 in the analysis of the examination data.

More than 92% of the participants reported symptoms in at least one part of the body during the year prior to the study. Of those reporting discomfort at a particular site, up to 64% also reported that symptoms occurred in the week prior to the study. For each body site, at least 32% of the respondents reporting discomfort during the past year described it as moderate to severe. Over 20% of participants met the symptom case definition for the shoulder, elbow, and fingers, and more than 30% met the symptom case definition for the neck and hand. Only 8% met the case definition for the back. In the logistic regression models, statistically significant elevated age-adjusted odds ratios were found for neck and finger symptoms in sign language interpreters who worked for 10 or more years relative to those working less than one year, and for shoulder pain in sign language interpreters who worked, on average, more than 20 hours per week.

Approximately 23% of the study participants were found to have tenderness or pain in the hand/wrist area on palpation or manipulation during the physical examination. For the elbow area, 6.7% of participants had such problems. The case definition was met my 13% of the participants; 9% met the case definition for the hand/wrist area; 3% met the case definition for carpal tunnel symdrome. Prevalence rates of neck, elbow, finger, or shoulder disorders were each less than 2%.

Reprinted (with minor edits) from *RID Views, 12,* 10 (1995) with permission from The Registry of Interpreters for the Deaf, Inc.

If I Had It to Do Over Again . . .

P. Lynn Hayes

Educational interpreting is the fastest growing area in the field of interpreting. A full-time job working with children and youth, summers off, a steady income, and the possibility of fringe benefits are just a few of the reasons why over 50% of the graduates of Interpreter Preparation Programs (IPPs) are working in educational settings.

Although an increasing number of IPPs focus specifically on educational interpreting, the fact still remains that a large majority of interpreters working in educational settings have not had an opportunity to attend such progams. If educational interpreters had it to do over again, what courses would they take? Thirty-two educational interpreters were surveyed regarding the classes they felt would be the most beneficial to interpreters currently working in educational setting. A variety of responses were given to this question, the seven most frequent are discussed here.

1. *Public speaking.* Because educational interpeting is such a new and unique field, interpreters are constantly explaining their role and responsibilties to everyone from the administration to the janitorial staff. Educational interpreters frequently serve as liaisons for persons (e.g., administrators, faculty, staff, students) throughout the school. They are often the only persons in the school district with some understanding of deafness, making them likely candidates for civic groups and educational organizations seeking a speaker. Good communication skills are essential; therefore, a class in public speaking would be beneficial.

2. *Human growth and development.* How do children and youth grow and mature? What aspects of a child's development are different at age 9 versus age 14? Understanding where a child is developmentally (i.e., cognitively, physically, linguistically) gives the interpreter a better sense of how best to do his or her job in an educational setting.

3. *Educational interpreting.* Interpreters want courses that focus specifically on educational interpreting. In most of the curricula used by IPPs the focus is on freelance interpreting; there is little about the various roles and responsibilities of the educational interpreter, working in a classroom, adapting to the educational environment, or problem-solving techniques necessary to survive in an educational setting.

4. *MORE sign language/systems.* It is no surprise that educational interpreters want to see more sign language/systems classes offered both in the community and in IPPs. It is understandable that the curricula of IPPs cannot be altered to the point that all is being taught are sign classes when it is apparent that students need to take a variety of classes (e.g., interpreting, deaf studies); however, we should be concerned about the skills our interpreters are graduating with and if they are appropriate for educational interpreting. Are we preparing future interpreters to work in settings where the preferred mode of communication is American Sign Language, Signed English, Pidgin Signed English (i.e., a contact language), or Signing Exact English (SEE II)? It would be literally impossible to complete a two-year program and be fluent in each of these modes of communication. A teacher who graduates from a teacher training program does not graduate with all the necessary skills just as an interpreter does not. Educational interpreters must look to their community or local IPPs for additional sign classes in an effort to upgrade their skills.

5. *Deaf culture.* A majority of educational interpreters have not had a course in Deaf culture or Deaf studies. They are unfamiliar with the rich culture of the Deaf community. How can we expect an interpreter to effectively work with a person whose culture they are unfamiliar with? Fortunately, many programs do have Deaf studies classes or something of that nature that would include information about culture, language, and community. Interpreters who are already working in educational settings should be encouraged to take such a class in the future.

6. *Deaf education and regular education.* Why should an educational interpeter take classes in education? They are not in the classroom to teach but to facilitate communication. No matter how many times we say an educational interpreter's jopb is to INTERPRET, the fact remains that a majority of educational interpreters have various roles and responsibilities in the classrom such as tutoring students or working with the teacher on class projects. Interpreters are often hired as "paraprofessionals" or "aides." The educational community often sees the interpreter as another adult in the classroom who serves both hearing and deaf children and is expected to assist the teacher in whatever way necessary to promote a successful classroom. A general knowledge of education, current legislation of education, or even the array of acronyms (e.g., LD, BD, IEP, IFSP, EMR), constantly used and rarely defined, provide the interpreter with basic information for working in an educational setting. In addition, interpreters also need more information about how to work with students who are deaf or hard-of-hearing and may have additional disabilities (e.g., fine- and gross-motor abnormalities, vision impairment, mental retardation).

7. *Practica at each educational level.* Interpreters surveyed were adamant about the need for a variety of practica experiences. The types of educational interpreting experiences are endless, ranging from working in an infant/toddler program to interpreting for a doctoral student; therefore, exposure to a variety of educational placements is valuable.

* * *

There is no way we can prepare educational interpreters for every experience they will encounter. However, we can take into consideration the areas of concern expressed by educational interpreters and encourage them to upgrade their skills by attending classes or participating in community events. All these efforts will make the interpreter a more valuable member of the eduational team.

Reprinted (with minor edits) from *RID Views, 12,* 3, 25 (1995) with permission from The Registry of Interpreters of the Deaf, Inc.

INDEX